Prenatal Alcohol Use and Fetal Alcohol Spectrum Disorders: Diagnosis, Assessment and New Directions in Research and Multimodal Treatment

Editor

Susan A. Adubato

and

Deborah E. Cohen

Prenatal Alcohol Use and Fetal Alcohol Spectrum Disorders: Diagnosis, Assessment and New Directions in Research and Multimodal Treatment

Editors: Susan A. Adubato and Deborah E. Cohen

eISBN: 978-1-60805-031-4

ISBN: 978-1-60805-690-3

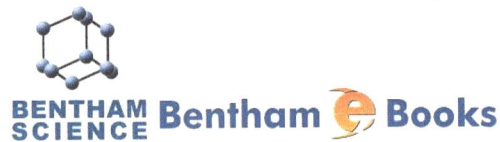

BENTHAM SCIENCE **Bentham** **e Books**

LET US PUT OUR MINDS TOGETHER AND SEE WHAT LIFE WE CAN MAKE FOR OUR CHILDREN
Sitting Bull

This e book is dedicated to all of our families, who continue to show us what we need to learn

CONTENTS

FOREWORD

This book is being published at just the right time in the history of efforts to address Fetal Alcohol Spectrum Disorders. It is not only timely but supported by the thinking of some of the most talented scientists in the field. Many, I have had the pleasure of working with and I know well their selfless dedication to this field of work.

It was 1995 when I joined the National Institute on Alcohol Abuse and Alcoholism, National Institutes of Health, as the Associate Director for Collaborative Research. My career in government began 28 years prior with the conduct of studies on the effects of thalidomide and the potential for other prescription drugs to cause unanticipated fetal damage. Unsuspecting pregnant mothers consumed thalidomide hoping to escape the discomfort of nausea and brought to term children damaged for life. I took an immediate interest in the effects of alcohol consumption on pregnancy outcomes and child development. Once again, I thought the answer would be simple. Since no one willingly and knowingly wants to harm or in any way damage their developing child, the prevention of Fetal Alcohol Syndrome (FAS) had to be a straight forward task. Simply make it known and the incidence and prevalence would be reduced; the problem eliminated. The state of the research on the cause and consequences of prenatal exposure to alcohol was clear. Case studies and population studies confirmed the findings of Jones and Smith that prenatal alcohol exposure can cause a pattern of deficits that are permanent. Many research questions remained unanswered because of the low prevalence of affected children in the United States of the same age, in the same general location, and with their birth families. A major problem at the time was in the fact that only those children with the documented distinctive facial features of FAS were being counted. With the face as the only recognized biomarker for the disorder, it was puzzling to be shown a child with normal appearance and told that he or she was affected by FAS.

The breakthrough occurred in 1997, when Dr. Denis Viljoen, a pediatrician, alerted the Institute to the high prevalence of affected children in the wine growing areas of South Africa. A site visit by research scientists from many disciplines was organized by me and Dr. Kenneth Warren, currently Acting Director of the Institute, and led by Dr. TK Li, then a distinguished Professor at Indiana University and subsequently Director of the Institute until his retirement in 2008. The resulting research and studies advanced the state of knowledge and understanding of the disorder and pointed to the need for further collaborations with the governments and research scientists in other countries. And so it went and has continued until now. Many countries have joined in the research, recognized that the problem exists in their populations, and taken steps toward prevention. There now is documentation of prenatal alcohol effects in different populations with the realization that there is truly a spectrum of effects. The most devastating is not the facial features, but the behavioral patterns and cognitive deficits that are problematic and costly for families and governments.

What is now accepted widely as Fetal Alcohol Spectrum Disorders (FASD) can be prevented. Just stop drinking during pregnancy. I have travelled to many countries and seen many pamphlets, displays and tee shirts that were developed as a prevention effort. The winner in my opinion was in South Africa. The tee shirt read, "Mommy please don't hurt my brain". It had a picture of a pregnant woman drinking alcohol with an x through the alcohol- straight forward and clearly stated. Did it work? We have yet to determine but for those who do not read pamphlets and books, it is worth a try.

I cannot overlook the contributions of the agencies that joined with NIAAA in an Interagency Coordinating Committee on Fetal Alcohol Spectrum Disorders. Representatives from Federal agencies in the Department of Health and Human Services, the Department of Justice and the Department of Education have worked tirelessly since 1997 to address FASD within the mission of their organizations. As the former Chair for this Committee, I am grateful and I am certain that the families of affected children are encouraged by the progress that has been made under the leadership of these agencies: websites were developed, state FAS coordinators met annually, grants for interventions and prevention approaches increased, a Center for Excellence for FASD was created in one agency, interventions for affected children were tested in another, numerous effective workshops and symposia were held, and teachers and physicians and social workers were alerted. This work continues.

The realization that any significant progress in research (basic and translational), in prevention, and in intervention development for FASD requires multi-disciplinary and trans-disciplinary partnerships and collaborations nationally and internationally was a breakthrough. There are few persons on the planet who won't recall where they were on September 11, 2001when the World Trade Center in the United States was destroyed by explosives. An international group of FASD research scientists will always remember that they were meeting in Valencia, Spain to determine the feasibility of advancing the state of research on FASD through closer working relationships between basic research scientists and those that studied affected children. They identified the research questions that were plaguing each group and left with a determination that significant progress would be made from more intensive interactions. NIAAA published requests for applications that encouraged the open exchange of information, nurtured partnerships and encouraged the formation of teams of scientists representing multiple disciplines. And this continues.

I cannot paint the picture of progress and continuing efforts without a mention of the national and international non-profit organizations that stood by the scientists and government agencies that fought and educated in the arenas and settings in which they could be effective. I especially applaud the work of the National Organization on Fetal Alcohol Syndrome. This work continues.

Again, I think this book brings it all together. It is comprehensive and well informed and it is my hope that it will be used as a teaching tool as well as renewed motivation and re-dedication to make progress for affected children and their families.

Faye J. Calhoun
Retired Former Deputy Director
National Institute on Alcohol Abuse
Alcoholism, National Institutes of Health
Bethesda, Maryland

PREFACE

Welcome to the first E-book on prenatal alcohol exposure and Fetal Alcohol Spectrum Disorders (FASD). When we first set out to do this E book, our intent was to compile a text that presented a past, present, and future directions perspective, but our authors had their own ideas. This book has turned out to be a look, not only at present research but, more importantly, innovations of research and clinical interventions. In addition, while the thematic basis for this E-book is the consequences of consuming alcohol during pregnancy, each chapter offers a different perspective resulting from prenatal exposures. As such, each chapter can "stand alone". This E book provides a phenomenal opportunity in that it allows readers to "link" directly to relevant websites, and to view real time videos within the text.

Although the use of the term "FASD" was not officially accepted for general use until 2004, many clinicians in the field used it previously. Please note that many of the authors for this E book use FASD generically for their discussions regarding any prenatal alcohol exposure, even when discussing issues prior to 2004. In addition, the term "intellectual disability" has replaced the term "mental retardation".

Our first chapter begins with an oft-times debatable topic- diagnosis. Susan Astley provides a provocative chapter on such a heated topic. Presenting the various models in use today, Dr. Astley provides the reader with the choices for diagnosing an FASD and the strengths and weaknesses of each model.

The second chapter, by Jennifer Thomas and Ed Riley, presents the fascinating and relatively new research on choline and other interventions. Drawn from basic science research, the interventions discussed seem to hold some promises for improving the effects of prenatal exposure to alcohol in the coming years.

The chapter by Natalie Novick Brown, Kieran O'Malley and Anne Streissguth addresses the challenges of diagnosing, assessing and treating psychiatric problems that are associated with prenatal alcohol exposure and co-occurring issues.

Chapters 4-6 provide a life span look at the difficulties encountered by families dealing with prenatal alcohol exposure, and some of the innovative work being done for and with our families. Heather Carmichael Olson and Rachel Montaque, begin this journey with a chapter that addresses the importance of early interventions and other related issues for young children. Claire Coles, Elles Taddeo and Molly Millians discuss very interesting and innovative interventions that are assisting school aged children to reach their potential. And finally, Mary DeJoseph completes the life span approach in her discussion of the continuing needs of adolescents and adults that are exacerbated by the paucity of scientific research for, and what some of the clinicians in the field have been suggesting, are effective intervention.

Kay Kelly provides very practical approaches for navigating the sometimes difficult and confusing social and legal systems in Chapter 7.

The next chapter by Kathy Mitchell and Mary DeJoseph allows the reader to understand what it means to struggle with addiction, recovery and an FASD on a daily basis through interviews with and individual vignettes written by family members whose lives have been touched by FASD. Very little of this chapter was edited, so readers will get a firsthand account from the individuals themselves.

For the final chapter, the co-editors, Debbie Cohen and Susan Adubato present the "state of the states": descriptions of federal programs as well as initiatives that have been undertaken in three States and Common wealth are presented. This chapter illustrates differing ways state programs have evolved to address the need for screening for prenatal alcohol consumption, FASD assessment, diagnosis and treatment, and service system enhancement. The chapter concludes with information about the role of and need for joining forces with voluntary agencies to address FASD.

The last word for the E book is a personal journey for one family and offers hope for families that their family member affected by prenatal exposure to alcohol can develop, mature, find love and success and be happy.

Please remember: The opinions expressed in this e book are those of the individual authors, and do not necessarily reflect the views of the editors.

All proceeds for this E book will go to further training through NOFASNJ.

We would like to thank Cara Castiglio, who works for the Southern New Jersey Prenatal Cooperative for our cover art. We also are most appreciative to Ellen Dunn, NJ Office For the Prevention of Developmental Disabilities, for her careful review of this manuscript.

The editors also would like to thank Bentham Publishers for taking a chance on this E-book, and an extra "thank you" to Bushra Siddiqui, whose patience and direction made the journey much easier.

While we both work in the field of FASD, one of the greatest benefits for us in compiling this E-book is that our knowledge of the consequences of prenatal exposure to alcohol and the possibilities of interventions and treatment grew. It is our hope that you will benefit from this E-book in similar ways and that it stimulates your interest to continue to learn more about FASD. To this end, as this book is to be produced, one new publication has been released on basic research in FASD: [Alcohol, 2011:45(1):1-104] and two recently published are: Looking at legal and justice issues for individuals with FASD [Journal of Psychiatry & Law, 2010;38(4);Winter], and Alcohol Research and [2011,34(1);summer]. Both discuss various topics and new innovations in FASD, including new developments in imaging.

Susan A. Adubato
University of Medicine and Dentistry of New Jersey
New Jersey Medical School
USA

&

Deborah E. Cohen
Office for the Prevention of Developmental Disabilities, New Jersey
USA

CONTRIBUTORS

Susan Adubato

Associate Director for Clinical Services, Division for Developmental and Behavioral Pediatrics, University of Medicine and Dentistry of New Jersey- New Jersey Medical School; Director, New Jersey/Northeast FASD Education and Research Center; Director, Northern New Jersey FAS Diagnostic Center; Assistant Professor, Departments of Pediatrics and Psychiatry, UMDNJ-NJMS, Newark, New Jersey, USA

Susan J. Astley

Professor of Epidemiology/Pediatrics; Director, WA State FAS Diagnostic & Prevention Network, University of Washington, Seattle, Washington, USA

Faye Calhoun

Retired, Former Deputy Director, National Institute on Alcohol Abuse and Alcoholism at NIH; Special Assistant to the Vice Chancellor for Graduate Education and Research, North Carolina Central University, Durham, North Carolina, USA

Deborah E. Cohen

Former Director, New Jersey Office for the Prevention of Developmental Disabilities, Trenton, New Jersey, USA

Claire D. Coles

Director, Fetal Alcohol and Drug Exposure Clinic, Marcus Autism Center, Children's Health Care of Atlanta, and Professor, Departments of Psychiatry and Behavioral Sciences and Pediatrics, Emory University School of Medicine, Atlanta, Georgia, USA

Natalie Novick Brown

Program Director, FASD Experts; Clinical Faculty, Department of Psychiatry and Behavioral Medicine, University of Washington, Seattle, Washington, USA

Mary DeJoseph

Consultant, New Jersey/NE FASD Education and Research Center, UMDNJ-NJMS, Newark, NJ, USA

Kathryn Kelly

Project Director, FASD Legal Resource Center, Fetal Alcohol and Drug Unit, Department of Psychiatry and Behavioral Sciences, School of Medicine, University of Washington, Seattle, Washington, USA

Molly N. Millians

Special Educator Evaluator, Fetal Alcohol and Drug Exposure Clinic, Marcus Autism Center, Children's Health Care of Atlanta, Atlanta, Georgia, USA

Rachel A. Montague

Graduate Student, Department of Clinical Psychology, Seattle Pacific University, Seattle, Washington, USA

Kathleen Tavenner Mitchell

Vice President, International Spokesperson, National Organization for Fetal Alcohol Syndrome, Washington, DC, USA

Heather Carmichael Olson

Department of Psychiatry and Behavioral Sciences, University of Washington School of Medicine, Seattle Childrens' Hospital Child Psychiatry Outpatient Clinic, Fetal Alcohol Syndrome Diagnostic and Prevention Network, Families Moving Forward Research Program, Seattle, Washington, USA

Kieran D. O'Malley

Child and Adolescent Psychiatrist, Lucena Clinic, Child Adolescent Mental Health Services (CAMHS), Dublin, Ireland

Edward P. Riley

Director, Center for Behavioral teratology, Professor, Department of Psychology, San Diego State University, San Diego, California, USA

Ann P. Streissguth

Professor Emerita, Department of Psychiatry and Behavioral Sciences, Founding Director, Fetal Alcohol & Drug Unit, University of Washington School of Medicine, Seattle, Washington, USA

Elles Taddeo

FAS Research Education Specialist, Emory University School of Medicine, Department of Psychiatry and Behavioral Sciences, Atlanta, Georgia, USA

Jennifer D. Thomas

Professor, Department of Psychology, Center for Behavioral Teratology, San Diego State University, San Diego, California, USA

Prenatal Alcohol Use and FASD: Diagnosis, Assessment and New Directions in Research and Multimodal Treatment, 2011, 3-29

CHAPTER 1

Diagnosing Fetal Alcohol Spectrum Disorders (FASD)

Susan J. Astley*

Departments of Epidemiology and Pediatrics, University of Washington, Seattle, Washington, USA

While we try to teach our children about life, our children teach us what life is all about

Angela Schwindt

Abstract: Fetal Alcohol Syndrome (FAS) is a permanent birth defect syndrome caused by maternal consumption of alcohol during pregnancy. Almost four decades have passed since the term FAS was first coined. The condition is now recognized as a spectrum of disorders: Fetal Alcohol Spectrum Disorders (FASD). Substantial progress has been made in developing specific criteria for delineating diagnoses under the umbrella of FASD. In the 14 years since the publication of the seminal report on FAS by the Institute of Medicine in 1996, clear consensus has been reached on two fundamental issues: 1) an FASD diagnostic evaluation is best conducted by a team of professionals from multiple disciplines (medicine, psychology, speech-language, occupational therapy) and 2) the team should use rigorously case-defined and validated FASD diagnostic guidelines. This chapter will provide a brief overview of the discovery of FASD, diagnostic challenges, how diagnostic guidelines and clinical models have evolved over time to address these challenges, and how new technology may influence the future of FASD diagnosis.

INTRODUCTION

What is FASD?

Fetal Alcohol Syndrome (FAS) is a permanent birth defect syndrome caused by maternal consumption of alcohol during pregnancy. The definition of FAS has changed little since the 1970's when the condition was first described and refined [1-5]. The condition has been broadly characterized by prenatal and/or postnatal growth deficiency, a unique cluster of minor facial anomalies, and central nervous system (CNS) abnormalities. FAS is the leading known preventable cause of intellectual disabilities in the Western World [6]. The prevalence of FAS is estimated to be 1 to 3 per 1,000 live births [1] in the general population, but has been documented to be as high as 10 to 15 per 1,000 in some higher-risk populations such as children residing in foster care [7,8].

The physical, cognitive, and behavioral deficits observed among individuals with prenatal alcohol exposure are not dichotomous, that is either normal or clearly abnormal. Rather, the outcomes, and the prenatal alcohol exposure, all range along separate continua from normal to clearly abnormal and distinctive [9-12]. This full range of outcomes observed among individuals with prenatal alcohol exposure has come to be called Fetal Alcohol Spectrum Disorders (FASD). Diagnoses like FAS, Partial FAS (PFAS), and Alcohol-Related Neurodevelopmental Disorder (ARND) fall under the umbrella of FASD.

The Diagnostic Challenge

FASD can present a daunting, but not insurmountable challenge for diagnosis. Individuals with prenatal alcohol exposure present with a wide range of outcomes, most of which are not specific to prenatal alcohol exposure and often manifest differently across the lifespan. Professionals from multiple disciplines (medicine, psychology, speech-language pathology, occupational therapy, etc.) are needed to assess and interpret accurately the broad array of outcomes that define the diagnoses. The pattern and severity of outcomes are dependent on the timing, frequency, and quantity of alcohol exposure (which is rarely known with any level of accuracy), and is frequently confounded by other adverse prenatal and postnatal exposures and events.

---

*Address correspondence to Susan J. Astley: FAS DPN, Center on Human Development & Disability, Box 357920, University of Washington, Seattle WA 98195-7920, USA; E-mail: astley@u.washington.edu

Susan A. Adubato and Deborah E. Cohen (Eds)

In the absence of objective, accurate, and reproducible methods for measuring and recording the severity of exposures and outcomes in individual patients, diagnoses have varied widely from clinic to clinic [1,13-16]. From a clinical perspective, diagnostic misclassification leads to inappropriate patient care, increased risk for secondary disabilities [17], and missed opportunities for primary prevention [18]. From a public health perspective, diagnostic misclassification leads to inaccurate estimates of incidence and prevalence [1,14,16,19]. Inaccurate estimates thwart efforts to allocate sufficient social, educational, and health care services to this high-risk population, and preclude accurate assessment of primary prevention intervention efforts. From a clinical research perspective, diagnostic misclassification reduces the power to identify clinically meaningful contrasts between FAS and control groups and between FASD clinical subgroups like FAS and ARND [9,14,20]. Non-standardized diagnostic methods also thwart valid efforts to compare outcomes between research studies [9,10, 21].

DISCOVERY OF FETAL ALCOHOL SYNDROME

Reference to the harmful effects of maternal drinking on infant outcome date back to biblical times (Behold, thou shalt conceive, and bear a son; and now drink no wine or strong drink…Judges 13:7) [22], with several remarkably comprehensive descriptions by physician groups in the 1700s and 1800s [23-25]. But several hundred years would go by before another entry would be made to the medical literature. In 1968 Lemoine and colleagues from France published an article describing 147 patients [26]. In 1970, unaware of the Lemoine publication, Ulleland and colleagues from Seattle, Washington published similar observations describing a small group of alcohol-exposed infants admitted to several high-risk maternal-child health clinics at the University of Washington [27, 28]. Dr. Ulleland's findings were accepted for presentation at the American Pediatric Society-Society for Pediatric Research meeting, held in Atlantic City New Jersey in 1970 [27]. Through a presentation to the University of Washington pediatric faculty, David Smith, M.D., a dysmorphologist, became interested in Dr. Ulleland's research. This would eventually lead to a collaborative publication in 1973 describing the pattern of outcome associated with prenatal alcohol exposure [29] and the publication that coined the term FAS [2].

Initial FAS Diagnostic Guidelines (1973-89)

Progress in refining the FAS diagnosis can be traced by reviewing Clarren and Smith [4], who summarized the available clinical reports from 1973 to 1976, and the reports from the fetal alcohol workshops of the Research Society of Alcoholism in 1980 and 1989 [3,5].

IOM FAS Diagnostic Guidelines (1996)

In recognition of the seriousness of FAS for the individual and society, the U.S. Congress mandated (in Section 705 of Public Law 102-321, the ADAMHA Reorganization Act) the Institute of Medicine (IOM) of the National Academy of Sciences to conduct a study of FAS and related birth defects. A seminal report was published in 1996 covering the full spectrum of issues from prevalence, diagnosis, prevention, to treatment [1]. A chapter entitled "Diagnosis and Clinical Evaluation of FAS" was included. The committee was charged with evaluating existing diagnostic criteria and formulating the best possible diagnostic guidelines reflective of current knowledge. The IOM diagnostic guidelines for FASD are presented in their entirety across Tables **1-4**, as they represent an important baseline from which current guidelines evolved. The IOM committee recognized the following issues as central to delineating FASD:

1. Should a documented history of exposure to alcohol be required for a diagnosis of FAS?

2. Which physical features should be used to define the disorder?

3. Can behavioral or cognitive features be used to define the disorder?

4. Is there a role for ancillary measures (e.g., magnetic resonance imaging [MRI] in making the diagnosis?

5. Can criteria be designed to be used across the lifespan?

6. What is the relationship of so-called fetal alcohol effects to fetal alcohol syndrome?

These issues will be discussed later in this chapter as they relate to both the IOM guidelines and current guidelines.

While the IOM guidelines reflected an important advancement in FASD diagnosis: 1) the IOM committee felt "a medical diagnosis of FAS remained the purview of dysmorphologists and clinical geneticists" (page 79), and 2) the guidelines remained intentionally broad and conceptual (e.g., gestalt) rather than specific and operational (e.g., case-defined) [1].

FASD diagnosis has now advanced beyond the 1996 IOM FASD diagnostic guidelines. While areas of debate still exist, the field has reached consensus on two fundamental issues: 1) an FASD diagnostic evaluation is best conducted by an interdisciplinary team of professionals, and 2) the team should use rigorously case-defined and validated FASD diagnostic guidelines.

Interdisciplinary Diagnostic Approach

The University of Washington FAS Diagnostic & Prevention Network (FAS DPN) first introduced an interdisciplinary approach to FASD diagnosis through a CDC-sponsored FAS prevention project conducted in 1992-97 [18,30-32]. Because of the complexity and broad array of outcomes observed in individuals with prenatal alcohol exposure, an interdisciplinary team is essential for an accurate and comprehensive diagnosis and treatment plan. An interdisciplinary FASD diagnostic team typically includes a medical doctor, psychologist, speech language pathologist, occupational therapist, social worker, and family advocate. Other members of the interdisciplinary team may include, but are not limited to, psychiatrists, neuropsychologists, geneticists, public health nurses, and mental health specialists.

Interdisciplinary models will necessarily vary to accommodate site-specific factors like funding, location (rural versus urban), access to services, target population, etc. The model used by the University of Washington FAS DPN diagnostic clinic targets both a general population and a high-risk foster care population. Individuals from the general population (birth to adult) are referred to the clinic by a broad array of community professionals (medical, educational, social-service, justice). In addition, all children who screen positive for the full FAS facial phenotype from the FAS DPN-Foster Care Passport Program FAS screening program [7,8] are also referred to the clinic.

The patient population served by the FAS DPN has expressed strong preference for an evaluation that can be completed in a single visit. Thus, two patients are evaluated per day, one in the morning and one in the afternoon. The interdisciplinary team includes a pediatrician, two psychologists, a speech-language pathologist, an occupational therapist, a social worker, and a family advocate. Prior to an evaluation, previous medical, school, and social records are collected by the clinic coordinator and reviewed by the lead psychologist. On the day of the evaluation, the lead psychologist presents the case to the team. The child is then assessed by the second psychologist, speech language pathologist, and occupational therapist while the caregivers are interviewed by the pediatrician and lead psychologist. Upon completion of the interview, the pediatrician conducts a physical exam of the patient. The team reconvenes to derive the FASD 4-Digit Code and compose an intervention plan. The team shares the diagnostic results and intervention plan with the family at the end of the 4-hour appointment. A single comprehensive report documenting the diagnostic outcome, all data used to derive the diagnostic outcome, and intervention recommendations are submitted to the patient's medical record.

A more detailed description of the interdisciplinary diagnostic approach used by the University of Washington FAS DPN is presented in Clarren *et al.*, [32]. A short video of an interdisciplinary diagnostic team conducting an FASD diagnostic evaluation can be viewed by clicking on **http://depts.washington.edu/fasdpn/htmls/diagteamvideo.htm** (Fig. **1**).

Figure 1: This video segment portrays an interdisciplinary team conducting an FASD diagnostic evaluation using the FASD 4-Digit Code. The video is a live recording of an actual FASD diagnostic evaluation. The patient is an adolescent adopted from Russia. The interdisciplinary team includes a pediatrician, two psychologists, a speech-language pathologist, an occupational therapist, a social worker, a family advocate, and a public health professional. The child will receive a 4-Digit Code of 4442 (FAS / Alcohol Exposure Unknown). The team conducted a 2-hour interview with the adoptive parents and a 2-hour evaluation of the child. The team has already derived the first two digits of the 4-Digit Code (the Growth and Face Ranks). This segment portrays the team's derivation of the last two digits of the 4-Digit Code (the CNS and Alcohol Ranks). The team will also document all other prenatal and postnatal risk factors that may have contributed to the child's outcomes. This video segment is one of several presented in the FASD 4-Digit Diagnostic Code Online Course offered at the FAS DPN at the University of Washington [33]. Copyright: Susan Astley, University of Washington, Seattle, WA.

Current FAS/D Guidelines (1997-2005)

Four FAS/D diagnostic guidelines have been published since the IOM Guidelines in 1996 [1]: the FASD 4-Digit Code in March 1997 [34,35]; the CDC FAS guidelines in July 2004 [36]; the Hoyme FASD guidelines in January 2005 [19], and the Canadian FASD guidelines in March 2005 [37]. The 4-Digit Code was subsequently updated in January, 1999 [34] and November 2004 [38]. All four guidelines are in current use. This is not to imply the 1996 IOM guidelines are not in use. But each of the four new guidelines purports to have been created to replace or augment the 1996 IOM guidelines.

Why are there four separate guidelines? Their existence reflects the ongoing debate on how best to approach FASD diagnosis. All present with strengths and limitations. Each was developed under different circumstances that influenced their outcome. The 4-Digit Code was investigator initiated in a statewide clinical/research arena using a clinical sample of 1,014 individuals of all races and ages (birth to 51 years of age) [14]. Empirical methods were used both to develop [20,39] and validate the performance of the 4-Digit Code [7-9,14,20,39]. The CDC [36] and Canadian [37] guidelines were federally mandated and commanded a more consensus-driven process. These guidelines were not empirically validated prior to publication. The Hoyme [19] guidelines were also investigator initiated in a clinical/research arena, using a clinical sample of 164 Native American and South African children to augment an existing set of guidelines: the IOM Guidelines.

Each guideline is introduced below. Since the circumstances that surrounded the development of each guideline influenced its outcome, it seemed most appropriate to let each guideline introduce itself (the published abstract or executive summary of each is presented below, with permission).

To facilitate comparisons across the five guidelines, the FAS criteria used by the 4-Digit Code [38], CDC [36], Canadian [37], Hoyme [19], and IOM [1] guidelines are presented in Table **1**. The same format is used to present the criteria for PFAS, ARND, and ARBD (Tables **2-4** respectively).

It is important to note that for the purposes of this chapter, the 4-Digit Code has been translated, as best as possible, into a text, rather than numeric, format across Tables **1-4**. This was done to facilitate comparison to the other guidelines that publish their diagnostic criteria in text format. Diagnostic teams should not use the textual translations of the 4-Digit Code presented in Tables **1-4** to derive a 4-Digit Code. Diagnostic teams should use the numeric format presented in the 2004 Diagnostic Guide [38].

Table 1: FAS diagnostic criteria: Comparison across the five most current FAS/D diagnostic guidelines

	4-Digit Code (2004)[38]	CDC (2004) [36]	Canadian (2005) [37]	Hoyme (2005)[19]	IOM (1996)[1]
Growth	Prenatal and/or postnatal height or weight $\leq 10^{th}$ percentile	Prenatal and/or postnatal height or weight $\leq 10^{th}$ percentile	At least 1 of the following: • Prenatal and/or postnatal height or weight $\leq 10^{th}$ percentile • Weight-to-height ratio ($\leq 10^{th}$ percentile)	Prenatal and/or postnatal height or weight $\leq 10^{th}$ percentile	At least 1 of the following: • Low birth weight • Low weight for height • Decelerating weight
	(Growth Ranks 2-4)	(Growth Ranks 2-4)	(Growth Ranks 2-4)	(Growth Ranks 2-4)	(Growth Ranks 1-4)
Face	All 3 of the following at any age: • PFL $\leq 3^{rd}$ percentile • Smooth philtrum Rank 4 or 5 • Thin upper lip Rank 4 or 5	All 3 of the following: • PFL $\leq 10^{th}$ percentile • Smooth philtrum Rank 4 or 5 • Thin upper lip Rank 4 or 5	All 3 of the following at any age: • PFL $\leq 3^{rd}$ percentile • Smooth philtrum Rank 4 or 5 • Thin upper lip Rank 4 or 5	2 or more of the following: • PFL $\leq 10^{th}$ percentile • Smooth philtrum Rank 4 or 5 • Thin upper lip Rank 4 or 5	Characteristic pattern that includes features such as short PFL, flat upper lip, flattened philtrum, and flat midface.
	(Face Rank 4)	(Face Ranks 3-4)	(Face Rank 4)	(Face Ranks 2-4)	(Face Ranks 1-4)

CNS	At least 1 of the following:
	• Structural/Neurological: (e.g., OFC $\leq 3^{rd}$ percentile, abnormal structure, seizure disorder, hard signs)
	• Severe Dysfunction: (3 or more domains[a] of function with impairment 2 or more SDs below the mean)
		At least 1 of the following:
		• Structural/Neurological: (e.g., OFC $\leq 10^{th}$ percentile, abnormal structure, seizure disorder, hard/soft signs)
		• Dysfunction[b]:
		  ○ 3 or more domains of function with impairment 1 or more SDs below the mean
		  ○ Global deficit (2 or more SDs below the mean)
			At least 3 of the following Structure/Neurological/ Functional domains with impairment[c]:
			• Hard/soft signs, structure, cognition, communication, academic achievement, memory, executive functioning, abstract reasoning, ADD, adaptive behavior, social skills, or communication
				At least 1 of the following:
				• Structural
				  ○ OFC $\leq 10^{th}$ percentile
				  ○ Abnormal structure
					At least 1 of the following:
					• Structural/Neurological:
					  ○ Decreased cranial size at birth
					  ○ Abnormal structure (e.g., microcephaly, partial/complete agenesis of the corpus callosum, cerebellar hypoplasia)
					  ○ Neurological hard/soft signs

	(CNS Rank 3 and/or 4)	(CNS Ranks 2-4)	(CNS Ranks 3 and/or 4)	(CNS Rank 1 or 4)	(CNS Rank 4?)
Alcohol	Confirmed or Unknown	Confirmed or Unknown	Confirmed or Unknown	Confirmed-excessive or Unknown	Confirmed-excessive or Unknown
	(Alcohol Ranks 2,3 or 4)	(Alcohol Ranks 2,3 or 4)	(Alcohol Ranks 2,3 or 4)	(Alcohol Ranks 2 or 4)	(Alcohol Ranks 2 or 4)

a. 4-Digit Code: Domains may include, but are not limited to: executive function, memory, cognition, social/adaptive skills, academic achievement, language, motor, attention, or activity level.

b. CDC: Performance substantially below that expected for an individual's age, schooling, or circumstances, as evidenced by: 1. Global cognitive or intellectual deficits representing multiple domains of deficit (or significant developmental delay in younger children) with performance below the 3rd percentile (2 standard deviations below the mean for standardized testing) or 2. Functional deficits below the 16th percentile (1 standard deviation below the mean for standardized testing) in at least three of the following domains: a) cognitive or developmental deficits or discrepancies b) executive functioning deficits c) motor functioning delays d) problems with attention or hyperactivity e) social skills f) other, such as sensory problems, pragmatic language problems, memory deficits, etc.

c. Canadian: Impairment indicates scores ≥ 2 SDs below the mean, discrepancies of 1.5-2 SDs among subtests, or ≥ 1 SD discrepancy between subdomains.

The equivalent 4-Digit Ranks for Growth, Face, CNS and Alcohol are inserted in red font to facilitate comparison across the guidelines.

Table 2: Partial FAS diagnostic criteria. Comparison across the five most current FAS/D diagnostic guidelines

	4-Digit Code (1997-2004)[38]	CDC[a] (2004) [36]	Canadian (2005)[37]	Hoyme (2005)[19]	IOM (1996)[1]
Growth	Prenatal or postnatal height or weight $\leq 10^{th}$ percentile (Growth Ranks 1-4)	--	No growth deficiency (Growth Rank 1)	Prenatal and/or postnatal height or weight $\leq 10^{th}$ percentile (Growth Ranks 2-4)	At least 1 of the following: • Low birth weight • Low weight for height • Decelerating weight (Growth Ranks 1-4)
Face	All 3 of the following at any age: • PFL $\leq 3^{rd}$ percentile • Smooth philtrum Rank 4 or 5 • Thin upper lip Rank 4 or 5 (Face Ranks 3 or 4)*	--	2 of the following at any age: • PFL $\leq 3^{rd}$ percentile • Smooth philtrum Rank 4 or 5 • Thin upper lip Rank 4 or 5 (Face Ranks 2 or 3)	2 or more of the following: • PFL $\leq 10^{th}$ percentile • Smooth philtrum Rank 4 or 5 • Thin upper lip Rank 4 or 5 (Face Ranks 2-4)	Some components of the pattern of FAS characteristic facial anomalies. (Face Ranks 1-4)

CNS	At least 1 of the following:
	• Structural/Neurological: (e.g., OFC $\leq 3^{rd}$ percentile, abnormal structure, seizure disorder, hard signs)
	• Severe Dysfunction: (3 or more domains[b] of function with impairment 2 or more SDs below the mean)
	
	(CNS Rank 3 and/or 4)
			At least 3 of the following Structure/Neurological/Functional domains with significant impairment[c]:
			• Hard/soft signs, structure, cognition, communication, academic achievement, memory, executive functioning, abstract reasoning, ADD, adaptive behavior, social skills, or communication
			
			(CNS Rank 3 and/or 4)
				At least 1 of the following:
				• Structural
				  o OFC $\leq 10^{th}$ percentile
				  o Abnormal structure
				• Dysfunction
				  o Complex pattern[d] of behavior / cognitive abnormalities
				(CNS Ranks 1-4)
					At least 1 of the following:
					• Structural/Neurological:
					  o Decreased cranial size at birth
					  o Abnormal structure
					  o Hard/soft signs
					• Dysfunction
					  o Complex pattern[e] of behavior / cognitive abnormalities
					(CNS Ranks 2-4)

Additional Criteria	PFAS requires the CNS and Alcohol criteria to be met and allows either the Growth or the Face criteria to be relaxed just slightly. • *If the growth deficiency criteria above are met, one facial feature may be relaxed as follows: (PFL ≤ 1 SD, or Philtrum Rank 3, or Lip Rank 3) or • If the FAS face criteria are met, growth can be relaxed to normal.		None	PFAS requires the Face and Alcohol criteria to be met and only one of the following additional criteria : • Growth • CNS Structural • CNS dysfunction	PFAS requires the Face and Alcohol criteria to be met and only one of the following additional criteria : • Growth • CNS Structural / Neurological • CNS dysfunction
Alcohol	Confirmed (Alcohol Ranks 3 or 4)	--	Confirmed (Alcohol Ranks 3 or 4)	Confirmed-excessive or Unknown (Alcohol Ranks 2 or 4)	Confirmed-excessive (Alcohol Rank 4)

a.   The CDC Guidelines only address FAS.

b.   4-Digit Code: Domains may include, but are not limited to: executive function, memory, cognition, social/adaptive skills, academic achievement, language, motor, attention, or activity level.

c.   Canadian: Impairment indicates scores ≥ 2 SDs below the mean, discrepancies of 1.5-2 SDs among subtests, or ≥ 1 SD discrepancy between subdomains.

d.   Hoyme: Marked impairment in the performance of complex tasks (complex problem solving, planning, judgment, abstraction, metacognition, and arithmetic tasks); higher-level receptive and expressive language deficits; and disordered behavior (difficulties in personal manner, emotional lability, motor dysfunction, poor academic performance, and deficient social interaction).

e.   IOM: Complex pattern of behavior or cognitive abnormalities that are inconsistent with developmental level and cannot be explained by familial background or environment alone: e.g., learning difficulties; deficits in school performance; poor impulse control; problems in social perception; deficits in higher level receptive and expressive language; poor capacity for abstraction or metacognition; specific deficits in mathematical skills; or problems in memory, attention or judgment.

The equivalent 4-Digit Ranks for Growth, Face, CNS and Alcohol are inserted in red font to facilitate comparison across the guidelines.

Table 3: ARND (or its equivalent: Static Encephalopathy/Alcohol Exposed or Neurobehavioral Disorder/Alcohol Exposed) diagnostic criteria. Comparison across the five most current FAS/D diagnostic guidelines

	4-Digit Code (1997-2004)[38]	CDC[a] (2004)[36]	Canadian (2005)[37]	Hoyme (2005)[19]	IOM (1996)[1]
Growth	Normal to deficient (Growth Ranks 1-4)	--	No growth deficiency (Growth Rank 1)	No growth deficiency (Growth Rank 1)	No growth deficiency (Growth Rank 1)
Face	No more than 1 of the following: • PFL ≤ 3rd percentile • Philtrum Rank 4 or 5 • Lip Rank 4 or 5 (Face Ranks 1-2)	--	No FAS facial phenotype (Face Rank 1)	No FAS facial phenotype (Face Rank 1)	Presumably no components of the pattern of FAS characteristic facial anomalies. (Face Rank 1)
CNS	Criteria for "Static Encephalopathy" At least 1 of the following: • Structural/Neurological: (e.g., OFC ≤ 3rd percentile, abnormal structure, seizure disorder, hard signs) • Severe Dysfunction: (3 or more domains[b] of function with impairment 2 or more SDs below the mean) (CNS Rank 3 and/or 4) Criteria for "Neurobehavioral Disorder"[c] • No Structural/Neurological abnormalities. • Moderate Dysfunction: (1-2 domains[b] of function with impairment ≥ 1.5 SDs below the mean) (CNS Rank 2)	--	At least 3 of the following Structure/Neurological/ Functional domains with significant impairment[c]: • Hard/soft signs, structure, cognition, communication, academic achievement, memory, executive functioning, abstract reasoning, ADD, adaptive behavior, social skills, or communication (CNS Ranks 3-4)	At least 1 of the following: • Structural o OFC ≤ 10th percentile o Abnormal structure • Dysfunction o Complex pattern[d] of behavior / cognitive abnormalities (CNS Ranks 1-4)	At least 1 of the following: • Structural/Neurological: o Decreased cranial size at birth o Abnormal structure o Hard/soft signs • Dysfunction o Complex pattern[e] of behavior / cognitive abnormalities (CNS Ranks 2-4)
Additional Criteria	The term ARND is not used. The following terms are used in lieu of ARND: Static Encephalopathy (Severe dysfunction) Neurobehavioral Disorder (Moderate dysfunction)	--	--	--	--
Alcohol	Confirmed (Alcohol Ranks 3 or 4)	--	Confirmed (Alcohol Ranks 3 or 4)	Confirmed-excessive (Alcohol Rank 4)	Confirmed-excessive (Alcohol Rank 4)

a. The CDC Guidelines only address FAS.

b. 4-Digit Code: Domains may include, but are not limited to: executive function, memory, cognition, social/adaptive skills, academic achievement, language, motor, attention, or activity level. MRI research confirms Neurobehavioral Disorder/Alcohol Exposed is a distinct, clinically meaningful subclassification under the umbrella of FASD [9].

c. Canadian: Impairment indicates scores > 2 SDs below the mean, discrepancies of 1.5-2 SDs among subtests, or > 1 SD discrepancy between subdomains.

d. Hoyme: Marked impairment in the performance of complex tasks (complex problem solving, planning, judgment, abstraction, metacognition, and arithmetic tasks); higher-level receptive and expressive language deficits; and disordered behavior (difficulties in personal manner, emotional lability, motor dysfunction, poor academic performance, and deficient social interaction).

e. IOM: Complex pattern of behavior or cognitive abnormalities that are inconsistent with developmental level and cannot be explained by familial background or environment alone: e.g., learning difficulties; deficits in school performance; poor impulse control; problems in social perception; deficits in higher level receptive and expressive language; poor capacity for abstraction or metacognition; specific deficits in mathematical skills; or problems in memory, attention or judgment.

The equivalent 4-Digit Ranks for Growth, Face, CNS and Alcohol are inserted in red font to facilitate comparison across the guidelines.

Table 4: ARBD diagnostic criteria. Comparison across the five most current FAS/D diagnostic guidelines

	4-Digit Code[a] (1997-2004) [38]	CDC[b] (2004) [36]	Canadian[a] (2005) [37]	Hoyme (2005) [19]	IOM (1996) [1]
Growth	--	--	--	Not specified (Growth Rank ?)	Not specified (Growth Rank ?)
Face	--	--	--	2 or more of the following: • PFL $\leq 10^{th}$ percentile • Philtrum Rank 4 or 5 • Lip Rank 4 or 5 (Face Ranks 2-4)	Not specified (Face Rank ?)
CNS	--	--	--	Not specified (CNS Rank ?)	Not specified (CNS Rank ?)
Congenital Defects	--	--	--	1 or more of the following: • Cardiac: Atrial septal defects, Ventricular septal defects, Aberrant great vessels, Tetralogy of Fallot. • Skeletal: Hypoplastic nails, Shortened fifth digits, Radioulnar synostosis, Flexion contractures, Camptodactyly, Clinodactyly, Pectus excavatum and carinatum, Klippel-Feil syndrome, Hemivertebrae, Scoliosis. • Renal: Aplastic/dysplastic/hypoplastic kidneys, Horseshoe kidneys, Ureteral duplications, Hydronephrosis. • Ocular: Strabismus, Retinal vascular anomalies, Refractive problems secondary to small globes. • Auditory: Conductive hearing loss, Neurosensory hearing loss. • Other: Virtually every malformation has been described in some patient with FAS. The etiologic specificity of most of these anomalies to alcohol teratogenesis remains uncertain.	Congenital structural defects in 1 of the following categories, including malformations and dysplasias (if the patient displays minor anomalies only, 2 must be present): • Cardiac: Atrial septal defects, Ventricular septal defects, Aberrant great vessels, conotruncal heart defects. • Skeletal: Radioulnar synostosis, Vertebral segmentation defects, Large joint contractures, Scoliosis. • Renal: Aplastic/dysplastic/hypoplastic kidneys, "Horseshoe" kidney/ureteral duplications. • Eyes: Strabismus, Ptosis, Retinal vascular anomalies, Optic nerve hypoplasia. • Ears: Conductive hearing loss, Neurosensory hearing loss. • Minor Anomalies: Hypoplastic nails, Short fifth digits, Clinodactyly of fifth fingers, Pectus carinatum / excavatum, Camptodactyly, "Hockey stick" palmar creases, Refractive errors, "Railroad track" ears.
Alcohol	--	--	--	Confirmed-excessive (Alcohol Rank 4)	Confirmed-excessive (Alcohol Rank 4)

a.   The 4-Digit Code and Canadian Guidelines do not recognize ARBD as a FASD diagnostic classification.

b.   The CDC Guidelines only address FAS.

The equivalent 4-Digit Ranks for Growth, Face, CNS and Alcohol are inserted in red font to facilitate comparison across the guidelines.

FASD 4-Digit Code (1997, 1999, Nov 2004) [34,35,38]

Rationale for the FASD 4-Digit Code

One year after the release of the 1996 IOM guidelines [1], the FASD 4-Digit Diagnostic Code was created [14,34,35,38] to address the following limitations in the extant gestalt approach to FASD diagnosis.

1.   There have been no standardized operational definitions for FAS or for any of the other diagnoses that fall under the umbrella of FASD. Rather, there have been diagnostic guidelines that physicians have been encouraged to follow, but the guidelines have not been sufficiently specific to assure diagnostic accuracy or precision.

For example, according to the diagnostic guidelines published by Sokol and Clarren [5], which were a minor modification of the 1980 definition of FAS by the Fetal Alcohol Study Group of the Research Society for

Alcoholism [3], which, in turn, were derived from the work of Clarren and Smith [4]: "The diagnosis of FAS can only be made when the patient has signs of abnormality in each of the three categories: 1) Prenatal and/or postnatal growth retardation (weight and/or length below the 10th percentile when corrected for gestational age), 2) central nervous system involvement (including neurological abnormality, developmental delay, behavioral dysfunction or deficit, intellectual impairment, and/or structural abnormalities, such as microcephaly [head circumference below the 3rd percentile or brain malformations found on imaging studies or autopsy] and 3) a characteristic face, currently qualitatively described as including short palpebral fissures, an elongated midface, a long and flattened philtrum, thin upper lip, and flattened maxilla".

The 1996 guidelines for the diagnosis of FAS proposed by the IOM [1] took a similar approach. The diagnosis of FAS can be made when the patient presents with: "1) Evidence of growth retardation, as in at least one of the following: a) low birth weight for gestational age; b) decelerating weight over time not due to nutrition; or c) disproportional low weight to height; 2) Evidence of a characteristic pattern of facial anomalies that includes features such as short palpebral fissures and abnormalities in the premaxillary zone (e.g., flat upper lip, flattened philtrum, and flat midface); and 3) Evidence of CNS neurodevelopmental abnormalities, as in at least one of the following: a) decreased cranial size at birth; b) structural brain abnormalities (e.g., microcephaly, partial or complete agenesis of the corpus callosum, cerebellar hypoplasia);c) neurological hard or soft signs (as age appropriate), such as impaired fine motor skills, neurosensory hearing loss, poor tandem gait, poor eye-hand coordination".

Although these descriptions do provide guidance, they are not sufficiently specific to assure diagnostic accuracy and precision. They reflect a gestalt approach to diagnosis. The guidelines for CNS abnormalities do not address how many areas of deficit must be present, how severe the deficits must be, or what level of documentation must exist to substantiate the presence of the deficit. The guidelines for the facial phenotype are equally nonspecific. How many facial features must be present, how severe must the features be, and what scale of measurement should be used to judge the severity? One need only read the clinical literature or review medical records, birth certificates, birth defect registries or ICD-9 codes to see how variably these criteria are interpreted, applied and reported [1,40-43].

2.   *There has been a lack of objective, quantitative scales to measure and report the magnitude of expression of key diagnostic features.*

For example, although a thin upper lip and smooth philtrum are key diagnostic features [1,2,4,39,44], quantitative measurement scales were never used to measure thinness or smoothness, and guidelines had never been established for how thin or smooth the features must be. Objective quantitative scales not only improve accuracy and precision, but also establish a common numeric language for communicating outcomes in medical records and in the medical literature.

3.   *The term fetal alcohol effects (FAE) was broadly used and poorly defined.*

The term 'suspected fetal alcohol effects' was first introduced into the medical literature in 1978 and was defined as 'less complete partial expressions' of FAS in individuals with prenatal alcohol exposure [4]. Based on this definition, an individual whose mother drank a few glasses of wine intermittently throughout pregnancy and presented with attention deficit hyperactivity disorder would meet the criteria for FAE. So would an individual whose mother drank a fifth of vodka daily throughout pregnancy and presented with microcephaly, severe mental retardation, growth deficiency and no facial anomalies. The broad use of this term and the reluctance to abandon it points to the clear need to develop diagnostic terms for individuals with prenatal alcohol exposure who present with physical anomalies and/or cognitive/behavioral disabilities, but do not meet the criteria for FAS. New diagnostic terms that more finely differentiate the variable exposures and outcomes of individual patients, without implying alcohol as the sole causal agent, were needed.

4.   *Clinical terms like FAE [4,5], alcohol-related birth defects (ARBD) [1] and alcohol-related neurodevelopmental disorder (ARND) [1] imply a causal link between alcohol exposure and outcome in a given individual that cannot be medically confirmed. Leading dysmorphologists in the field of FAS diagnosis have formally requested that the term FAE no longer be used for this reason [13].*

With the likely exception of the full facial phenotype, no other physical anomalies or cognitive/behavioral disabilities observed in an individual with prenatal alcohol exposure are necessarily specific to (caused only by) their prenatal alcohol exposure [1]. Features such as microcephaly, neurological abnormalities, attention deficit, intellectual disability, and growth deficiency frequently occur in individuals with prenatal alcohol exposure, and frequently occur in individuals with no prenatal alcohol exposure. The diagnostic terms ARBD and ARND introduce the same limitation as does FAE, namely, implying alcohol exposure caused the birth defect or neurobehavioral disorder in an individual patient.

5. *Too often diagnoses depicting FASD are reported in the medical records and scientific literature with no documentation of the method used to derive the diagnosis and little or no documentation of the data used to render/support the diagnosis.*

Failure to report this information can limit the patient's ability to qualify for and receive appropriate intervention services from subsequent health care, social service, and educational providers. For example, simply reporting that an individual has FAS does little to convey the individual's strengths and disabilities. Some individuals with FAS have low IQs, some have IQs in the normal range, some have attention deficits, some do not, some have problems with memory, while others have language deficits. From a public health perspective, failure to report these data also prevents surveillance efforts from accurately tracking the prevalence of FASD diagnoses in the population. The supportive data are needed to validate the diagnoses. Accurate surveillance is vital for setting public health policy and assessing the effectiveness of primary prevention efforts. The 4-Digit Code requires that data be collected not just to support the diagnosis, but to derive the diagnosis. The 4-Digit Code provides a comprehensive FASD Diagnostic Form for recording all supportive data and provides a numeric classification scheme that is readily incorporated into clinical, research, and surveillance databases.

6. *FAS is a medical diagnosis and thus has historically been diagnosed by a medical doctor (e.g., dysmorphologist, geneticist). There is now clear consensus that an interdisciplinary team approach is superior [32,35-37].*

Each of the above limitations was largely overcome with the development of the FASD 4-Digit Diagnostic Code in 1997 [35]. Briefly, the 4 digits of the FASD 4-Digit Code reflect the magnitude of expression of the 4 key diagnostic features of FASD, in the following order: (1) growth deficiency, (2) FAS facial phenotype, (3) CNS structural/functional abnormalities, and (4) prenatal alcohol exposure (Figs. **2** and **3**). The magnitude of expression of each feature is ranked independently on a 4-point Likert scale, with 1 reflecting complete absence of the FASD feature and 4 reflecting a strong "classic" presence of the FASD feature. Each Likert rank is specifically case defined. For example if a patient received the following Ranks: Growth = 3, Face = 4, CNS = 4, Alcohol = 4; the resulting 4-Digit Code would be 3444. Code 3444 is one of twelve 4-Digit Codes that meet the criteria for FAS/Alcohol Exposed (Fig. **2**). An interactive, electronic FASD 4-Digit Code Short Form [45] is provided (Fig. **4**) to demonstrate the simple, numeric approach used by the 4-Digit Code to define and derive a diagnosis. There are 256 possible 4-digit diagnostic codes, ranging from 1111 (reflecting complete absence of growth deficiency, FAS facial features, CNS abnormalities, and alcohol exposure) to 4444 (reflecting the most severe presentation of FAS: severe growth deficiency, the full FAS facial phenotype, significant CNS abnormalities, and high exposure to alcohol). Each 4-Digit diagnostic code falls into 1 of 22 unique clinical diagnostic categories (labeled A through V). Seven of the 22 diagnostic categories (4-Digit Categories A–C and E–H) fall broadly under the umbrella of FASD (A. FAS/Alcohol Exposed B. FAS/Alcohol Exposure Unknown, C. Partial FAS/Alcohol Exposed, E-F. Static Encephalopathy/Alcohol Exposed, and G-H. Neurobehavioral Disorder/Alcohol Exposed) (Fig. **2**).

The FASD 4-Digit Diagnostic Code was developed from the clinical records of 1,014 patients of all races and ages evaluated by the FAS DPN interdisciplinary team at the University of Washington. The purpose was not to redefine, but rather, more specifically case-define the key diagnostic components of FAS as presented across several previously published FAS diagnostic guidelines [1,3-5]. The performance of the 4-Digit Code was validated prior to its release [14]. Its performance was compared to the standard gestalt method of diagnosis on the first 454 patients who had received a gestalt diagnosis of FAS, PFAS or possible fetal alcohol effect (PFAE) prior to the development of the 4-Digit Code.

FASD 4-Digit Diagnostic Code				
	3	**4**	**4**	**4**
4	Severe	Severe	Definite	High risk
3	Moderate	Moderate	Probable	Some Risk
2	Mild	Mild	Possible	Unknown
1	None	None	Unlikely	No Risk
	Growth Deficiency	**FAS Facial Features**	**CNS Damage**	**Prenatal Alcohol**

(RANK labels rows 4–1)

Digit Diagnostic Codes within each FASD Diagnostic Category

A. FAS / Alcohol Exposed

2433	3433	4433
2434	3434	4434
2443	3443	4443
2444	3444	4444

B. FAS / Alcohol Exposure Unknown

2432	3432	4432
2442	3442	4442

C. Partial FAS /Alcohol Exposed

1333	1433	2333	3333	4333
1334	1434	2334	3334	4334
1343	1443	2343	3343	4343
1344	1444	2344	3344	4344

E. Sentinel Physical Finding(s) / Static Encephalopathy / Alcohol Exposed

3133	3233	4133	4233
3134	3234	4134	4234
3143	3243	4143	4243
3144	3244	4144	4244

F. Static Encephalopathy / Alcohol Exposed

1133	1233	2133	2233
1134	1234	2134	2234
1143	1243	2143	2243
1144	1244	2144	2244

G. Sentinel Physical Finding(s) / Neurobehavioral Disorder / Alcohol Exposed

1323	2323	3123	3323	4123	4323
1324	2324	3124	3324	4124	4324
1423	2423	3223	3423	4223	4423
1424	2424	3224	3424	4224	4424

H. Neurobehavioral Disorder / Alcohol Exposed

1123	1223	2123	2223
1124	1224	2124	2224

I. Sentinel Physical Finding(s) / Alcohol Exposed

1313	2313	3113	3313	4113	4313
1314	2314	3114	3314	4114	4314
1413	2413	3213	3413	4213	4413
1414	2414	3214	3414	4214	4414

J. No Physical Findings or CNS Abnormalities Detected / Alcohol Exposed

1113	1213	2113	2213
1114	1214	2114	2214

Figure 2: The 4-Digit Code is derived by ranking the severity of growth deficiency, FAS facial features, CNS abnormality, and alcohol exposure on 4-point Likert scales. Each rank is specifically case-defined [38]. The 4-Digit Code 3444 is one of twelve 4-Digit Codes that meet the diagnostic criteria for FAS / Alcohol Exposed.

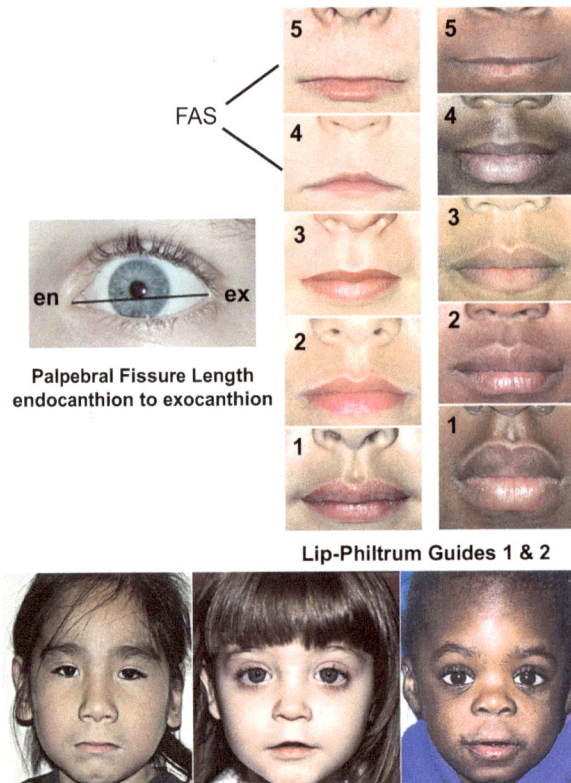

Figure 3: FASD 4-Digit Code FAS facial phenotype. The Rank 4 FAS facial phenotype determined with the 4-Digit Diagnostic Code requires the presence of all 3 of the following anomalies: (1) palpebral fissure length 2 or more standard deviations below the norm; (2) smooth philtrum (Rank 4 or 5 on the Lip-Philtrum Guide), and (3) thin upper lip (Rank 4 or 5 on the Lip-Philtrum Guide). Examples of the Rank 4 FAS facial phenotype for Native American, Caucasian, and African American children are shown. Copyright: Susan Astley, University of Washington, Seattle, WA.

The FASD 4-Digit Diagnostic Code:

1. Greatly increased diagnostic precision and accuracy through the development of objective, quantitative measurement scales (e.g., Lip-Philtrum Guides), facial analysis software, and specific case definitions.

2. Diagnosed the full spectrum of outcomes across the lifespan.

3. Offered an intuitively logical numeric approach to reporting outcomes and exposure that reflects the true diversity and continuum of disability observed in individuals with prenatal alcohol exposure.

4. Established a method for case-defining the highly variable, nonspecific CNS dysfunction that typifies FASD, by quantifying the breadth and magnitude of dysfunction (number of domains of function 2 or more SDs below the mean) without unduly constraining which domains must be impaired.

5. Established diagnostic subclassifications that captured the full spectrum of FASD without inferring alcohol is the sole causal agent.

6. Documents all other prenatal and postnatal adverse exposures and events that can also impact outcome.

7. Provides a quantitative measurement and reporting system (the 4-Digit Code) that can be used independent of the diagnostic nomenclature.

8. Has received extensive assessment/validation of its performance.

9. Was designed for use by an interdisciplinary FASD diagnostic team.

10. Is readily taught to a wide array of health care and social service providers (e.g., FASD 4-Digit Code Online Course[46]), thus greatly expanding the availability of diagnostic services.

Astley SJ. Diagnostic Guide for FASD:

Hold mouse over this green field to view pop-up instructions.

FASD 4-Digit Diagnostic Code - Short Form (2004)- Fillable

Reset Form

Astley SJ. Diagnostic Guide for FASD: The 4-Digit Code, 3rd edition, 2004 Download free pdf of Guide at www.fasdpn.org/pdfs/guide 2004.pdf for full instructions.

Patient Name	John	Doe		Birth date	Jan 1, 2000
Gender	male			Clinic Date	Jan 1, 2008
Race	Caucasian			Age (yrs)	8.00
Clinic Name	FAS DPN			Medical #	xxx

NAME OF DIAGNOSIS

Partial Fetal Alcohol Syndrome

(alcohol exposed)

Link to FASD Diagnostic Guide

FASD 4-DIGIT DIAGNOSTIC CODE

	1	4	3		4	

				Growth	Face	CNS		Alcohol		
Significant	Severe	Definite	4		X			X	4	High risk
Moderate	Moderate	Probable	3			X			3	Some risk
Mild	Mild	Possible	2						2	Unknown
None	None	Unlikely	1	X					1	No risk
Growth Deficiency	FAS Facial Features	CNS Damage		Growth	Face	CNS		Alcohol		Prenatal Alcohol

DATA BELOW WAS USED TO DERIVE / SUPPORT 4-DIGIT CODE

GROWTH

Date	Height measure	Height percentile	Weight measure	Weight percentile
01/01/2000	50.0 cm	50	3,530 g	50
01/01/2004	103.0 cm	57	17 kg	65
01/01/2006	115.0 cm	47	24 kg	84

GROWTH TABLES (Circle ABC Scores to Derive Rank)

Percentile Range	ABC-Scores for: Height	Weight
≤ 3rd	C	C
> 3rd and ≤ 10th	B	B
> 10th	A	A

4-Digit Diagnostic Rank	Growth Deficiency Category	Height-Weight ABC-Score Combinations
4	Severe	CC
3	Moderate	CB, BC, CA, AC
2	Mild	BA, BB, AB
1	None	AA

FACE

Guide 1 Used

	Date	01/01/2008
Right PFL: mm / Z-score	23	-3.5
Left PFL: mm / Z-score	23	-3.5
mean PFL: mm / Z-score	23	-3.5
Philtrum Rank	5: smooth	
Lip Rank	4: fairly thin	
Lip Circularity	98.2	

FACE TABLES (Circle ABC-Scores to Derive Rank)

5-Point Rank for Philtrum or Lip	Z-scores for Palpebral Fissure Length (PFL)	ABC-Scores for: Palpebral Fissure	Philtrum	Upper Lip
4 or 5	≤ - 2 SD	C	C	C
3	> - 2 SD and ≤ -1 SD	B	B	B
1 or 2	> - 1 SD	A	A	A

4-Digit Diagnostic Rank	Level of Expression of FAS Facial Features	Palpebral Fissure - Philtrum - Lip ABC-Score Combinations
4	Severe	CCC
3	Moderate	CCB CBC BCC
2	Mild	CCA. CAC. CBB. CBA. CAB. CAA BCB. BCA. BBC. BAC. ACC. ACB. ACA. ABC. AAC
1	None	BBB. BBA. BAB. BAA ABB. ABA. AAB. AAA

CNS

Rank 4 Check 1 or more	microcephaly	abnormal structural brain image	serizure disorder	/	No evidence
	Other (specify): None				

Rank 2 or 3		Domain / Test / Subtest Name	Score (units)	Date
Evidence of Dysfunciton	1	Cognition / WISC IV / FSIQ	70 (standard score)	01/01/2008
	2	Memory / WRAML / General Memory Index	2 (percentile)	01/01/2008
	3	ADHD diagnosis, effectively medicated with Ritalin	ADHD Diagnosis	05/01/2007

PRENATAL ALCOHAL

Confirmed	Trimester(s): 1.2.3	Ave. drinking days/week: 3 days/wk	Ave. drinks / per occasion: 5
Other (Specify):	Birth mother attended the FASD dignostic evaluation and reported to the best of her recollection		

Other Prenatal and Postnatal Exposures / Events

Risk Rank: (None = 1, Unknown = 2, Some = 3, High = 4)	Prenatal Rank:	3	Postnatal Rank:	3

Figure 4: FASD 4-Digit Diagnostic Code Short Form. In lieu of the more comprehensive 7-page FASD Diagnostic Form, some clinics may prefer to use the **1-page FASD 4-Digit Short Form**. The Short Form allows a clinician to record the minimum amount of data required to derive/support the 4-Digit Code. Diagnostic teams who do not have the time/capacity to complete the more comprehensive form will find this electronic, interactive, Short Form helpful.

The 4-Digit Code has served as the cornerstone of a fully integrated and highly successful screening, diagnostic, intervention, prevention, and surveillance program in Washington State for the past 17 years [7,8,18,1,47-49]. A comprehensive profile of all patients receiving an interdisciplinary FASD diagnostic evaluation using the 4-Digit Code at the Washington State FAS Diagnostic and Prevention network (WA FAS DPN) clinic in the first 12 years of operation is presented in the Astley paper [50]. Hundreds of FASD diagnostic teams have been trained worldwide to use this interdisciplinary FASD diagnostic system [46].

CDC FAS Guidelines, July 2004 [36]

In 2004 the CDC published the following Executive Summary to introduce the CDC FAS guidelines (p. vii-ix, with permission) [36]:

"As part of the fiscal year 2002 appropriations funding legislation, the U.S. Congress mandated that the Centers for Disease Control and Prevention (CDC), acting through the National Center on Birth Defects and Developmental Disabilities (NCBDDD) Fetal Alcohol Syndrome (FAS) Prevention Team and in coordination with the National Task Force on Fetal Alcohol Syndrome and Fetal Alcohol Effect (NTFFAS/FAE), other federally funded FAS programs, and appropriate nongovernmental organizations, would:

Develop guidelines for the diagnosis of FAS and other negative birth outcomes resulting from prenatal exposure to alcohol,

Incorporate these guidelines into curricula for medical and allied health students and practitioners, and seek to have them fully recognized by professional organizations and accrediting boards, and

Disseminate curricula to and provide training for medical and allied health students and practitioners regarding these guidelines.

Through the coordinated efforts of CDC, the NTFFAS/FAE, and a scientific working group (SWG) of experts in FAS research, diagnosis, and treatment, the diagnostic criteria were developed over a 2-year period.

A primary goal of these guidelines is to provide standard diagnostic criteria for FAS so that consistency in the diagnosis can be established for clinicians, scientists, and service providers. The guidelines are based on state-of-the-art scientific research, clinical expertise, and family input regarding the physical and neuropsychological features of FAS. The SWG sought to harmonize these guidelines with other diagnostic systems currently in use in this country and others (e.g., Canada). The SWG strove to provide a balance between conservative and overly inclusive diagnostic systems. Differential diagnosis from other genetic, teratological, and behavioral disorders was emphasized.

These guidelines are not intended to be an endpoint in the discussion of diagnosing FAS. There is a great need to acquire science-based information that will facilitate diagnostic criteria for additional related disorders, such as Alcohol Related Neurodevelopmental Disorder (ARND). These guidelines conclude with a call for further research and continuous refinement of the diagnostic criteria for FAS and related conditions so that affected individuals and their families can receive important services that enable them to achieve healthy lives and reach their full potential."

Hoyme FASD Guidelines, January 2005 [19]

In 2005, Hoyme *et al.*, [19] published the following abstract (p. 39, with permission) to introduce their FASD guidelines:

"The adverse effects of alcohol on the developing human represent a spectrum of structural anomalies and behavioral and neurocognitive disabilities, most accurately termed fetal alcohol spectrum disorders (FASD). The first descriptions in the modern medical literature of a distinctly recognizable pattern of malformations associated with maternal alcohol abuse were reported in 1968 and 1973. Since that time, substantial progress has been made in developing specific criteria for defining and diagnosing this condition. Two sets of diagnostic criteria are now used most widely for evaluation of children with potential diagnoses in the FASD continuum, ie, the 1996 IOM [1] criteria and the Washington criteria. Although both approaches have improved the clinical delineation of FASD,

both suffer from significant drawbacks in their practical application in pediatric practice. Objective. The purpose of this report is to present specific clarifications of the 1996 IOM criteria [1] for the diagnosis of FASD, to facilitate their practical application in clinical pediatric practice. A large cohort of children who were prenatally exposed to alcohol were identified, through active case-ascertainment methods, in 6 Native American communities in the United States and 1 community in the Western Cape Province of South Africa. The children and their families underwent standardized multidisciplinary evaluations, including a dysmorphology examination, developmental and neuropsychologic testing, and a structured maternal interview, which gathered data about prenatal drinking practices and other demographic and family information. Data for these subjects were analyzed, and revisions and clarifications of the existing IOM FASD diagnostic categories were formulated on the basis of the results. The revised IOM method defined accurately and completely the spectrum of disabilities among the children in our study. On the basis of this experience, we propose specific diagnostic criteria for fetal alcohol syndrome and partial fetal alcohol syndrome. We also define alcohol-related birth defects and alcohol-related neurodevelopmental disorder from a practical standpoint. The 1996 IOM criteria [1] remain the most appropriate diagnostic approach for children prenatally exposed to alcohol. The proposed revisions presented here make these criteria applicable in clinical pediatric practice."

Canadian FASD Guidelines, March 2005 [37]

In 2005 Chudley *et al* [37] published the following abstract (p. s1) to introduce the Canadian FASD guidelines:

"A subcommittee of the Public Health Agency of Canada's National Advisory Committee on Fetal Alcohol Spectrum Disorder reviewed, analyzed and integrated current approaches to diagnosis to reach agreement on a standard in Canada. The purpose of this paper is to review and clarify the use of current diagnostic systems and make recommendations on their application for diagnosis of FASD-related disabilities in people of all ages. The guidelines are based on widespread consultation of expert practitioners and partners in the field. The guidelines have been organized into 7 categories: screening and referral; the physical examination and differential diagnosis; the neurobehavioural assessment; and treatment and follow-up; maternal alcohol history in pregnancy; diagnostic criteria for fetal alcohol syndrome (FAS), partial FAS and alcohol-related neurodevelopmental disorder; and harmonization of Institute of Medicine and 4-Digit Diagnostic Code approaches. The diagnosis requires a comprehensive history and physical and neurobehavioural assessments; a multidisciplinary approach is necessary. These are the first Canadian guidelines for the diagnosis of FAS and its related disabilities, developed by broad-based consultation among experts in diagnosis."

Comparison of Current Guidelines

An interdisciplinary approach to FASD diagnosis using more rigorously case-defined guidelines, as originally proposed by the WA FAS DPN [14,32,35] was adopted in principal in all subsequent guidelines. Key contrasts do exist, however (Tables **1-4**). Of the guidelines currently in use, the FASD 4-Digit Code[38] and Canadian FASD guidelines [37] are most similar. Both systems cover the full spectrum of diagnostic outcomes, use FAS facial criteria with confirmed high specificity to prenatal alcohol exposure, and adhere to strict criteria that use the standard medical/statistical definition of "abnormal" (2 or more SDs below the mean or its equivalent $\leq 2.5^{th}$ percentile) [51]. In contrast to the 4-Digit Code and Canadian guidelines, the CDC guidelines [36] address only FAS; have more relaxed facial criteria (with unknown specificity); and have more relaxed CNS criteria (using diagnostic cutoff values for "abnormal" of 1 SD below the mean or $\leq 10^{th}$ percentile). The Hoyme guidelines [19], while addressing the full spectrum of outcomes, diverge considerably from the 4-Digit Code, CDC, and Canadian guidelines, but are closely aligned with the IOM guidelines [1] from which they were derived. For the diagnosis of FAS, the Hoyme guidelines further relax the facial criteria requiring only 2 of the 3 diagnostic features be present while allowing the palpebral fissure length (PFL) to move further into the normal range ($\leq 10^{th}$ percentile). This results in facial criteria that are no longer specific to prenatal alcohol exposure [16]. The Hoyme guidelines for FAS also restrict the CNS criteria to structural abnormalities only; and relax the criterion for small head circumference from the medical definition of microcephaly ($\leq 2.5^{th}$ percentile) [52] to $\leq 10^{th}$ percentile. All 4 sets of guidelines require prenatal alcohol exposure to be documented, but allow a diagnosis of FAS to be rendered if prenatal alcohol exposure is unknown. The Hoyme guidelines, like the IOM guidelines, go further by requiring that the confirmed exposure be "excessive" (e.g., characterized by substantial regular intake or heavy episodic drinking). Features unique to each guideline are: 1) The 4-Digit Code does not use the term ARND and is the only guideline that measures all four features of FAS (growth, face, CNS, and alcohol exposure) on continuous scales; 2) The Canadian guidelines require severe CNS dysfunction be present for a diagnosis of FAS; and 3) The Hoyme guidelines use only physical features to define FAS.

Diagnostic Nomenclature

A number of terms have been established over the years to label the diagnostic subclassifications under the umbrella of FASD. These include FAS, PFAS ARND, Static Encephalopathy/Alcohol Exposed (SE/AE), Neurodevelopmental Disorder/Alcohol Exposed (ND/AE), Alcohol Related Birth Defects (ARBD), and Fetal Alcohol Effects (FAE). Table **5** presents each term, the clinical features that delineate each term, and which guidelines use the terms.

Table 5: FASD diagnostic terms, the clinical features that define each term, and which FAS/D guidelines use each term

FASD Diagnostic Terms	Clinical Features Present					Guidelines That Use the Term				
	Growth Deficiency	FAS Facial Phenotype	CNS Abnormality	Prenatal Alcohol Exposure	Other Congenital Defects	4-Digit[38]	CDC[a][36]	Canadian[37]	Hoyme[19]	IOM[1]
FAS	Yes	Yes	Yes	Yes or Unknown		■	■	■	■	■
PFAS	Yes or No	Yes (Full or Partial)	Yes or No[b]	Yes or Unknown[c]		■	-	■	■	■
ARND			Yes	Yes			-	■	■	■
SE/AE			Yes, Severe	Yes		■	-			
ND/AE			Yes, Moderate	Yes		■	-			
ARBD	Yes and No[d]			Yes	Yes		-		■	■
FAE[e]			Yes	Yes			-			

a.   (-) CDC guidelines currently address only FAS.
b.   The Hoyme and IOM guidelines allow PFAS to be diagnosed in the absence of CNS abnormality.
c.   Only the Hoyme guidelines allow an unknown alcohol exposure for PFAS.
d.   The Hoyme guidelines require the FAS facial phenotype be present for ARBD. The IOM guidelines do not.
e.   Used in the Sokol & Clarren FASD guidelines [5].

Issues to Consider

The following issues are important to consider as one assesses the strengths/limitations of the current FAS/D diagnostic guidelines.

Why are the criteria used to define the FAS facial phenotype so important to the medical validity of a FAS diagnosis? When one makes a diagnosis of FAS, one is stating implicitly that the individual has a syndrome caused by prenatal alcohol exposure [16]. One is also stating implicitly that the biological mother drank alcohol during pregnancy and, as a result, harmed her child. These are bold conclusions to draw and are not without medical and ethical consequences. How confident can one be when one infers a causal link between an individual's prenatal alcohol exposure and his or her syndromic features, especially when 2 of the 3 diagnostic features of this syndrome (growth deficiency and CNS damage/dysfunction) are not specific to (caused only by) prenatal alcohol exposure. The validity of the diagnosis rests solely on the specificity of the facial phenotype to the exposure (alcohol) and to the outcome (FAS). If a cluster of facial features is truly unique to prenatal alcohol exposure (e.g., alcohol is the only agent that can cause this facial phenotype) and is unique to the diagnosis of FAS (e.g., this exact phenotype is not present in any other medical condition), then one would expect to observe the following: (1) the face would be highly sensitive to FAS (e.g., individuals with FAS would have the FAS facial phenotype), (2) the face would be highly specific to FAS (e.g., individuals without FAS would not have the FAS facial phenotype), and (3) the face would be highly specific to prenatal alcohol exposure (e.g., individuals without prenatal alcohol exposure would not have the FAS facial phenotype). The rank 4 FAS facial phenotype, as defined by the 4-Digit Code, demonstrates all three of these qualities [7,9,16,20,39].

A highly specific FAS facial phenotype validates the FAS diagnosis, because the presence of the face confirms that an individual was affected, at least in part, by their prenatal alcohol exposure. The face also confirms the individual was exposed to alcohol. The latter is used to render a diagnosis of FAS in the absence of confirmed prenatal alcohol exposure. If the face is truly specific to alcohol, then individuals cannot have the face if they were not exposed to alcohol. This is why all diagnostic guidelines allow FAS to be diagnosed, even when prenatal alcohol exposure is unknown. When the face is confirmed to be highly specific to alcohol exposure, it can serve as a valid proxy measure for exposure. This is also why diagnostic guidelines cannot and do not allow ARND (or its equivalent) to be diagnosed when alcohol exposure is unknown. Since the FAS facial phenotype is not present in ARND, it cannot serve as a proxy measure for alcohol exposure. In the absence of a highly specific facial phenotype, the validity of the diagnostic process breaks down precipitously; an individual's outcome cannot be linked to their prenatal alcohol exposure, FAS becomes indistinguishable from ARND, and valid diagnoses cannot be made when alcohol exposure is unknown.

Considering the quintessential role the FAS facial phenotype plays in FAS diagnosis, its specificity cannot be assumed, it must be confirmed through properly designed empirical studies. The FAS facial criteria (Rank 4) used by the 4-Digit Code and Canadian Guidelines have confirmed high sensitivity and specificity (> 95%) [39]. The CDC and Hoyme guidelines have not reported the sensitivity and specificity of their relaxed facial criteria. When the Hoyme criteria were applied to a sample of normal to high functioning children with confirmed absence of prenatal alcohol exposure, 4 of the 16 met the Hoyme criteria for the full FAS facial phenotype [16]. This demonstrates the facial criteria have been relaxed too far.

Should an 'excessive' alcohol exposure be required for diagnoses under the umbrella of FASD? There remains no clear scientific consensus on what quantity, frequency, and duration of exposure is toxic to the fetus. There are a multitude of reasons for this. 1) As our tools for measuring outcome become more sensitive, our ability to identify adverse outcomes at lower exposures increases [53]. 2) Risk from alcohol exposure varies between fetuses, even between fraternal twins with ostensibly identical exposure [54, 55]. It is not uncommon for one fraternal twin to have full FAS, while the other appears unaffected. Identical twins are typically identically affected. 3) From a public health perspective, requiring excessive exposure implies lower levels of exposure are 'safe'. Safe for whom? 4) From a research perspective, artificially linking outcome to a threshold level of high exposure prevents assessing the true relationship between exposure and outcome. 5) Finally, from a clinical perspective, if an "excessive" exposure is required, it would be difficult to rationalize why an individual with all the features of FAS would receive a diagnosis of FAS if their exposure was unknown, but would fail to receive a diagnosis of FAS if their exposure was confirmed, but reportedly not excessive. This implies that practitioners have the ability to confirm the accuracy of exposure histories. They do not "Excessive" alcohol exposures should not be required for FASD diagnoses.

FAE and ARND: The field continues to struggle with what to label the condition characterized by prenatal alcohol exposure and CNS abnormalities when the FAS facial phenotype is absent. The problem with the diagnostic terms used to date Fetal Alcohol Effects (FAE) and Alcohol-Related Neurodevelopmental Disorder (ARND) is they imply that the patient's outcomes are *alcohol effects* or *alcohol-related* outcomes. They imply alcohol caused the patient's outcomes. But this presumption in an *individual* patient is medically invalid because CNS abnormalities are not specific to (caused only by) prenatal alcohol exposure. There are many other known or unknown risk factors that may be partly or even fully responsible for the patient's outcome. In the absence of the FAS facial phenotype, current medical technology has no ability to confirm or rule-out the etiologic role of alcohol in an *individual* patient.

The term FAE (or more accurately, possible FAE) was first introduced by Clarren and Smith in 1978 [4]. In 1995, Aase, Jones, and Clarren argued effectively that clinical use of the term FAE, with its implications of causation, should be abandoned [13]. In 1996, the IOM [1] acknowledged the concerns expressed by Aase and colleagues [13] and introduced ARND (and ARBD) to replace FAE. But ARND (and ARBD) presented with all the same limitations as FAE. In 1997, the 4-Digit Code introduced Static Encephalopathy/Alcohol Exposed (SE/AE)) and Neurobehavioral Disorder/Alcohol Exposed (NDAE) to replace ARND [35]. These new clinical classifications divided ARND into two subgroups; 1) individuals with severe dysfunction (CNS Rank 3) and 2) individuals with moderate dysfunction (CNS Rank 2). A recent MRI study confirmed SE/AE and ND/AE are distinct clinical subclassifications with clear evidence of CNS structural abnormality detectable by MRI volumetric analyses [9]. Importantly, the terms neither confirm nor rule-out the causal role of alcohol. In 2005, the Hoyme [19] and Canadian [37] guidelines also acknowledged the concern expressed by Aase and colleagues [13], but chose to continue the use of the term ARND. The Hoyme guidelines expressed the following reservations about the SE/AE and ND/AE terms introduced by the 4-Digit Code. They raised a number of important issues that warrant discussion.

"The Washington criteria place much emphasis on the encephalopathy and neurobehavioral disorder present among affected children. These 2 findings are not specifically defined and, as general terms, they are not unique to the prenatal effects of alcohol on fetal development. In addition, the family and genetic background of the child is not adequately integrated into the criteria. Because this highly structured system seems all-encompassing, there is the potential for over-diagnosis of alcohol-related disabilities; any child with a disability who has been exposed to alcohol prenatally can be assigned a diagnostic classification easily, even if the cause of the disability is genetic" (p. 41) [19].

To clarify, the 4-Digit Code cannot over-diagnose "alcohol-related" disabilities because the only "alcohol-related" diagnoses the 4-Digit Code generates are FAS and Partial FAS. The potential to over-diagnosis alcohol-related disabilities occurs with the use of the term Alcohol-Related Neurodevelopmental Disorder. The 4-Digit Code is the only FASD guideline that does not use this term. The 4-Digit Code does assign a diagnostic classification to all individuals who present with a disability. The classification reflects their disability; their *outcome* per se (e.g., FAS, PFAS, Static Encephalopathy, Neurobehavioral Disorder, etc). For example, if the individual presented with moderate impairment in memory and executive function, their disability would be classified as Neurodevelopmental Disorder. All children with or without a disability also have their prenatal alcohol exposure status reported. Their exposure is reported separate from their disability using the following naming convention: "disability/exposure" (eg., FAS / Alcohol Exposed, FAS / Alcohol Exposure Unknown, Neurobehavioral Disorder/ Confirmed Absence of Alcohol Exposure; No Sentinel Physical Findings or CNS Abnormalities Detected/Alcohol Exposed, etc). This naming convention neither implies nor rules-out a causal association between the outcome and the exposure in an individual patient. Hoyme and colleagues are correct in stating that static encephalopathy and neurobehavioral disorder are not unique to the prenatal effects of alcohol on fetal development. The same holds true for the neurodevelopmental disorder referenced in ARND. This is why it is so important that the nomenclature not assert the outcomes are unique (related) to the alcohol exposure. The use of a nomenclature that reports outcome separate from exposure is perhaps one of the most important features and strengths of the 4-Digit Code that distinguishes it from all other FASD diagnostic guidelines.

The 4-Digit Code was developed under the premise that a diagnosis should be based on verifiable facts, not supposition. The diagnostic nomenclature used by the 4-Digit Code reflects this. Growth deficiency and CNS damage/dysfunction are not specific to (caused only by) prenatal alcohol exposure. When an individual presents with prenatal alcohol exposure and CNS damage/ dysfunction, but does not have the FAS facial phenotype, the damage/dysfunction may be entirely attributable to the prenatal alcohol exposure, partially attributable to the prenatal alcohol exposure, or unrelated to the prenatal alcohol exposure. It is important to remember that even when a diagnosis of full FAS is rendered, one cannot necessarily attribute ALL of the individual's disabilities to their alcohol exposure. To the extent that other adverse risk factors are present, they too can, and likely will, contribute to the overall constellation of outcomes.

Current medical technology has no ability to confirm or rule-out the etiologic role of alcohol in an *individual* patient. This does not prevent one from effectively moving forward. An accurate diagnosis and effective intervention can proceed without confirming alcohol caused the person's disability. Access to services should be based on a person's disability, not on what caused their disability. Prevention can also proceed without linking outcome to exposure in an individual patient. In fact, on an empirical level, valid identification of causal associations requires exposures and outcomes to be documented separately.

When an individual presents with CNS damage/dysfunction and prenatal alcohol exposure, the 4-Digit Code calls it what it is: Static Encephalopathy/Alcohol Exposed if the CNS damage/dysfunction is severe or Neurobehavioral Disorder/Alcohol Exposed if the CSN dysfunction is moderate. The medical definition of static encephalopathy is *"any significant abnormal condition of the structure or function of brain tissue that is neither progressing nor regressing"* [56]. Including the phrase "Alcohol Exposed" in the diagnostic name serves to alert clinical providers that the individual was exposed to a teratogen and therefore is at risk for underlying brain damage. Knowledge of this risk is important, because the presence of underlying brain damage should influence a clinician's approach to ongoing care and intervention.

Aase and colleagues [13] urged "simple recording of the verifiable conclusions.... If prenatal alcohol exposure has taken place, but FAS cannot be substantiated, the exposure still should be indicated, and any nonspecific abnormalities or problems noted." (p. 49) This is the approach taken by the 4-Digit Code. The clinical summary templates for SE/AE and ND/AE include the following statement: "The diagnosis of Static Encephalopathy/Alcohol Exposed (or Neurobehavioral Disorder/Alcohol Exposed) does not mean that alcohol is the cause of the problem. A number of other factors could be contributing to the present issues, such as the patient's genetic background, other potential exposures or problems during pregnancy, and various experiences since birth" [14, 38]. The 4-Digit Code also devotes a chapter and 4-Digit ranking system to documentation of other prenatal (including genetic) and postnatal exposures and events that frequently occur with prenatal alcohol exposure and likely contribute to the outcomes observed for individuals [38]. In fact, the vast majority of the 1,400 patients with prenatal alcohol exposure diagnosed in the WA FAS DPN between 1993-2005 presented with multiple risk factors (93% were exposed to tobacco or illicit drugs in utero, 31% had no prenatal care, 36% had confirmed physical and/or sexual abuse, and 70% were in foster/ adoptive care) [50]. The impact of prenatal alcohol exposure is rarely if ever assessed in isolation from other risk factors.

The Hoyme guidelines [19] state, "FASD must always be a diagnosis of exclusion. Many genetic and malformation syndromes have some of the other clinical characteristics of FAS. If there is no indication of another genetic or malformation syndrome, then the revised IOM criteria can be applied to categorize a diagnosis within the FASD continuum" (quotes from pp. 45-46). Overlap between individual symptoms/anomalies is common throughout medicine. An astute clinician would not mistake FAS for William's syndrome simply because the two have some, but not all features in common. It is the constellation of features that distinguish the two syndromes. FAS is not a diagnosis of exclusion. Alcohol is a teratogen to all developing fetuses, including those with other genetic disorders or syndromes. It is worth noting that one child diagnosed with FAS in the WA FAS DPN also had Down syndrome. The child presented with growth deficiency below the 2nd percentile on a growth chart for children with Down syndrome. The child presented with the facial features of Down syndrome and FAS. The facial features of Down syndrome are distinct from the facial features of FAS. The two phenotypes were readily apparent and easily distinguished. The child presented with microcephaly (3 SDs below the mean for children with normal development, 1 SD below the mean for children with Down syndrome). The child presented with Bayley [57] Motor and Mental Index scores below 50; a level of developmental delay that can be observed in both Down syndrome and FAS. The birth mother was reported to have consumed alcohol daily throughout pregnancy. A FASD diagnostic team should consider alternative or co-occurring syndromic diagnoses and medical conditions at all times. The prevalence of other syndromes among 1,400 patients with prenatal alcohol exposure receiving a FASD diagnostic evaluation in a WA FAS DPN clinic is 1.8% [50].

Hoyme and colleagues [19] expressed concern that SE/AE and ND/AE are not specifically defined. The growth, face, CNS, and alcohol criteria are specifically defined for SE/AE and ND/AE (Table **3**). The CNS functional criteria specify which functional domains may be impaired, how many must be impaired, and how severely (in SDs) each must be impaired. Most of the current guidelines (4-Digit Code [38], CDC [36], and Canadian [37] now provide this enhanced level of detail when defining the CNS functional criteria for their FAS, PFAS and ARND classifications.

ARBD: The term Alcohol-Related Birth Defects (ARBD) was introduced by the IOM [1] with the caveat that "virtually every malformation has been described in some patient with FAS. The etiologic specificity of most of the anomalies to alcohol teratogenesis remains uncertain". This statement remains true today. For this reason, the 4-Digit Code [38] and Canadian [37] Guidelines do not include ARBD as a diagnostic classification. The 4-Digit Code and Canadian guidelines require the reporting of all birth defects; they simply do not support labeling them as ARBD. The Hoyme [19] guidelines do include ARBD as a diagnostic classification, but require the FAS facial phenotype to be present. Inclusion of the FAS facial phenotype may help increase the chance that the birth defect may be related to the alcohol exposure, but only if the etiologic specificity of the guideline's FAS facial criteria is confirmed to be high.

Are Lip-Philtrum Guides Needed for each Race? All guidelines published subsequent to the 4-Digit Code have adopted the use of the University of Washington Lip-Philtrum Guides for measuring philtrum smoothness and upper lip thinness (Fig. **3**). There are currently two Lip-Philtrum Guides; one normalized to Caucasians and one normalized to African Americans (Fig. **3**). The Guides are purposely labeled Guide 1 and Guide 2, respectively, for they were created for use on more than just Caucasian and African American individuals. Guide 1 is intended for use on all races (or racial combinations) that indigenously have lips similar in thickness to Caucasians. Guide 2 is intended for use on all races (or racial combinations) that indigenously have lips similar in thickness to African Americans. The Guide that best matches the indigenous phenotype of the patient's race(s) should be used. It is essential that the patient's medical record document which Guide was used for their diagnostic evaluation.

While it may seem obligatory to create a Lip-Philtrum Guide for every race, there are two fundamental reasons why this is neither feasible nor clinically necessary. First, racial categories are more a social-political construct than scientific or anthropological classifications. Racial categories are not sufficiently case-defined to classify individuals accurately into discrete groups and a large portion of the population is multiracial. Finally, race rarely translates into one homogeneous phenotype. For example, there is tremendous phenotypic variability between American Indian tribes, thus creation of an "American Indian" Lip-Philtrum Guide would be clinically invalid. Second, the magnitude of difference that would differentiate lips of the same rank across more than two "racially-normed" guides would become imperceptibly small. The magnitude of difference would become clinically irrelevant and below the level of accurate detection. To demonstrate this, look at how little difference there is between the Rank 5 lips on Guides 1 and 2 (Fig. **3**). Now imagine the Rank 5 lip on a Lip-Philtrum Guide for a race that falls between Guides 1 and 2.

Can an accurate diagnosis be rendered at any age? The answer depends on the diagnosis and the guidelines. If a diagnostic classification requires standardized psychometric evidence of *higher level* dysfunction across multiple domains like language, memory, executive function, and/or cognition, then a patient must be old enough to engage in this higher level assessment (generally > 7 years old) to confirm or rule-out dysfunction. This is not to say a diagnostic evaluation should be postponed until after age 7. There is tremendous benefit to early diagnosis and intervention [17,48,58]. The 4-Digit Code explicitly states that a diagnosis rendered at an early age could change (upgrade to a more severe classification) as the child ages and higher level cognitive impairments emerge. As an example, if a 10 year old child presented with the following features (growth deficiency, the FAS facial phenotype, a normal head size, severe dysfunction in memory, executive function, and attention, and prenatal alcohol exposure), she would receive a diagnosis of FAS (4-Digit Code 4434). If she had received a diagnostic evaluation at 1 year of age, her severe functional impairments would not yet be apparent. They may only manifest as moderate developmental delays on a Bayley Scales of Infant Development [57], resulting in a 4-Digit Code of 4424 (sentinel physical findings, neurobehavioral disorder, alcohol exposed). Her true diagnosis would be FAS, but at 1 year of age, she would not be old enough to reveal the true magnitude of her CNS dysfunction. She benefits nonetheless from her early diagnosis in two ways: 1) she receives early intervention, and 2) her high risk status is documented in her medical record with recommendations to monitor her closely over time. If and when she presents with more severe CNS dysfunction, she would receive a FASD diagnostic re-evaluation to upgrade her diagnostic classification appropriately.

Can an accurate diagnosis be rendered in an adult? Yes. Adults often present with more complex life histories and competing risks (traumatic head injury, their own alcohol and drug abuse, and mental health problems). Confirmation of exposure can also be more challenging. But the same diagnostic criteria and interdisciplinary approach are utilized. The interdisciplinary team will need expertise in adult psychological assessment and knowledge of community services available to adults. While adults will not have benefited from early intervention, an accurate diagnosis will lead to a better understanding of their disability and improved access to disability assistance and services.

Before leaving this topic, one additional question regarding age and diagnosis is often asked: **Does the face of FAS change with age?** Literature from the 80's and 90's [59-61] would lead one to believe that infants and adults are less likely to present with the full FAS facial phenotype than school-aged children. But the data were largely anecdotal and focused on facial features that are no longer regarded as diagnostic of the FAS facial phenotype [20]. Data from 1,400 patients evaluated for FASD in the WA FAS DPN document just the opposite. The proportion of subjects who presented with the full FAS facial phenotype (Rank 4) by age group was as follows: birth to 3.9 yrs (14%), 4 to 16.9 years (7.7%), and 17 to 53 years (9.5%). The age group with the highest prevalence of the FAS facial phenotype was infants under one year of age (23%) [50]. It is certainly possible for the facial features to change with age. Although, in our experience, when change occurs it has always been quite subtle. In the event that facial features do change over time, most diagnostic guidelines address this by stating that the features may be present at *any* age. For example, if an adult presents with some, but not all of the FAS facial features, but childhood photos document the full FAS facial phenotype, then the adult would meet the full FAS facial criteria based on their childhood photos.

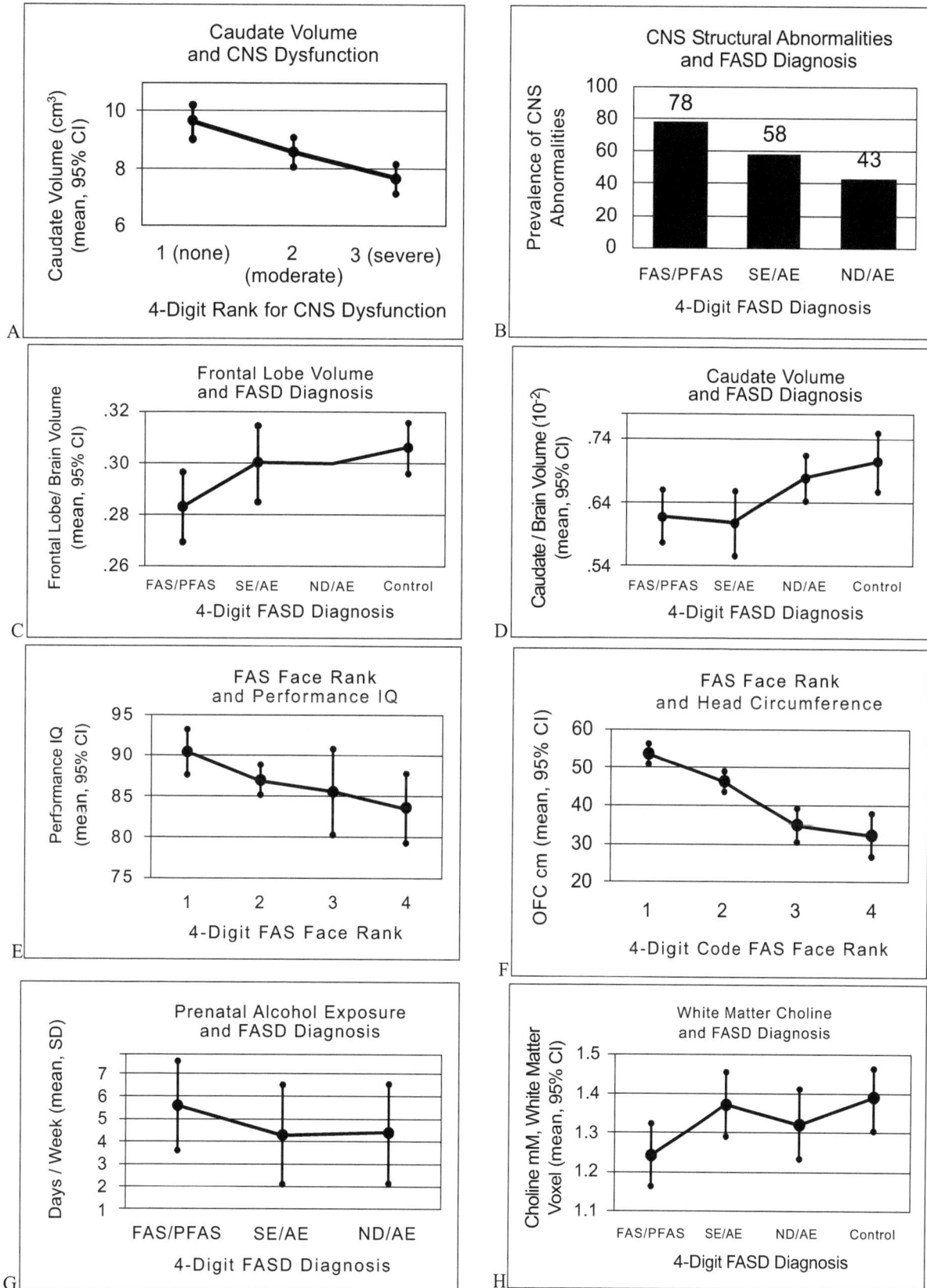

Figure 5: Examples of some of the many significant, empirical findings that serve to validate the performance of the FASD 4-Digit Diagnostic Code [9,10,50,63].

Overall, diagnostic evaluations for FASD can be conducted across the lifespan (newborn to adult). The diagnostic criteria do not change with age. The most accurate diagnosis can be rendered in childhood when the child is old enough to engage in all levels of assessment, but a diagnostic evaluation should not be postponed for this reason. Infants may require re-assessment. Adults present with unique challenges, but benefit nonetheless.

Validation of FASD Guidelines. It is imperative that the performance (reliability, accuracy, specificity, and validity) of diagnostic guidelines be confirmed through properly designed empirical studies [1]. A number of empirical studies have been published confirming the performance of the measurement tools, case-definitions, and diagnostic subclassifications used by the 4-Digit Code [7,9,10,14,16,20,21,39,50,62]. A recently completed MRI/fMRI/MRS study of children with FASD identified significant differences in neuropsychological outcomes [10], neurostructural outcomes [9], neuroactivation levels [21], and neurometabolite levels [63] between the FAS/PFAS, SE/AE and ND/AE clinical subgroups. Significant correlations were observed between size of brain regions and level of prenatal alcohol exposure, magnitude of FAS facial phenotype, and level of CNS dysfunction (Fig. 5). These findings confirm the 4-Digit Code produces three clinically distinct and increasingly more affected diagnostic subclassifications (FAS/PFAS, SE/AE, and ND/AE) under the umbrella of FASD.

Patient Examples that Exemplify Key Contrasts between the Guidelines

One practical method to assess the performance of the guidelines is to compare/contrast how they classify cases across the spectrum. Below are four hypothetical patient examples and the diagnostic classifications each would receive from the five most current FAS/D diagnostic guidelines [IOM [1], 4-Digit Code [38], Canadian [37], CDC [36], and Hoyme [19]]. These examples were selected to exemplify key contrasts between the guidelines. There are certainly many other examples that would result in identical diagnostic classifications across all five guidelines.

PATIENT EXAMPLE 1 (10 years old):

Growth: Hgt 10th percentile, wgt 95th percentile

Face: PFL 10th percentile;
Somewhat smooth philtrum, Rank 4;
Thick upper lip, Rank 1

CNS: OFC 10th percentile, FSIQ 120, No evidence of dysfunction.

Alcohol: Unknown

Diagnostic Classifications:

IOM: Unable to definitively classify. The IOM criteria are not sufficiently case-defined.

4-Digit Code: No sentinel physical findings or CNS abnormalities detected / Alcohol Unknown (4-Digit Code = 2212), Not FASD

Canadian: Not FASD

CDC: Not FAS

Hoyme: FAS / Alcohol Unknown

PATIENT EXAMPLE 2 (10 years old)

Growth: Hgt 2nd percentile, wgt 2nd percentile

Face: Small PFL, 2nd percentile,
Smooth philtrum, Rank 5,
Thin upper lip, Rank 5

CNS: OFC 30th percentile, No CNS structural/neurological abnormalities, FSIQ 50 (1st percentile). Severe dysfunction across all domains.

Alcohol: Intoxicated weekly throughout pregnancy

Diagnostic Classifications

      IOM: Partial FAS? (This diagnostic classification is in question because the IOM growth deficiency criteria are not strictly met)

4-Digit Code: FAS/Alcohol Exposed (Code = 4434)

    Canadian: FAS/Alcohol Exposed

        CDC: FAS/Alcohol Exposed

     Hoyme: Partial FAS/Alcohol Exposed

PATIENT EXAMPLE 3 (10 years old)

     Growth: Hgt 50th percentile, wgt 50th percentile

       Face: Normal PFL 50th percentile,
              Normal philtrum Rank 2,
              Normal upper lip Rank 2

       CNS: OFC 50th percentile, No CNS structural/neurological abnormalities. ADHD, Significant memory impairment, All other domains of function within normal range.

    Alcohol: One glass of wine nightly throughout pregnancy. No reports of binge drinking, intoxication, or problems with alcohol use.

Diagnostic Classifications:

      IOM: Not FASD

4-Digit Code: Neurobehavioral Disorder / Alcohol Exposed (Code = 1123)

    Canadian: Not FASD

        CDC: Not FAS.

     Hoyme: Not FASD

PATIENT EXAMPLE 4: (2 years old)

     Growth: Hgt 1st percentile, wgt 1st percentile

       Face: Small PFL 1st percentile,
               Smooth philtrum, Rank 5,
              Thin upper lip, Rank 5

       CNS: OFC 1st percentile, Bayley Scales of Infant Development outcomes within low-normal range.

    Alcohol: Intoxicated weekly throughout pregnancy

Diagnostic Classifications:

      IOM: Partial FAS? (This diagnosis is in question because the IOM growth deficiency criteria are not strictly met)

4-Digit Code: FAS/Alcohol Exposed (Code = 4444)

    Canadian: Not FASD

        CDC: FAS/Alcohol Exposed

     Hoyme: FAS/Alcohol Exposed

FUTURE DIRECTIONS

Without doubt, the one emerging arena that will have the greatest impact on the future of FASD diagnosis is brain imaging. All diagnostic guidelines include "evidence of abnormal brain structure (e.g., abnormal MRI, microcephaly)" as key diagnostic criteria for FAS, PFAS, and ARND (or its equivalent). Detection of abnormal structure currently relies on radiologist review (visual inspection) of brain images. But MRI technology can now produce accurate measures of size/shape/and tissue composition of brain regions that provide far more sensitive measures of structural abnormality [9, 64-66]. For example, in a recently completed FASD MRI study, none of the 23 children with ND/AE were identified as having an abnormal MRI by radiologist review, yet 43% of the subjects had one or more brain regions, two or more standard deviations below the mean size observed in the healthy Control group using MRI volumetric analysis [9]. Does this mean 43% of these children now meet the diagnostic criteria for having an "abnormal MRI"? Not necessarily. Norms for the size of brain regions, by gender and age, must be established using large, representative, population-based samples, rather than small, convenient research control samples. The National Institutes of Health MRI Study of Normal Brain Development [67, 68] is a landmark study that is documenting structural brain development and behavior longitudinally from birth to young adulthood in a large population-based sample of healthy children targeted to the United States 2000 census distribution. Thus, we will soon have "normal growth charts" for the size of brain regions, much like we have normal growth charts for height, weight, and head circumference. If microcephaly meets the FASD criteria for a structural brain abnormality, should a significantly small frontal lobe or caudate volume meet the criteria? The answer will likely depend, in part, on how size correlates with function. Decreasing head circumference is correlated with increasing severity of dysfunction [9, 69]. A rapidly growing literature documents similar correlations exist between regional brain volumes and function [9, 65,70] (Fig. **5A**). If brain imaging technology is adopted into the FASD diagnostic evaluation process, the prevalence of FAS/D will increase, simply by virtue of increased sensitivity to detect structural brain abnormality.

SUMMARY REMARKS

1. An FASD diagnostic evaluation is most accurately conducted by an interdisciplinary team.

2. The field should strive to adopt a single set of diagnostic guidelines for FASD.

3. Guidelines should undergo rigorous assessment of their accuracy, reliability, specificity, and validity to confirm their high performance, preferably before their release.

4. Use of the terms ARND and ARBD, like FAE, should be discontinued. They should be replaced by terminology that does not imply or rule-out a causal association between outcome and exposure in an individual patient.

5. Exposure and outcome should be assessed and reported separately.

6. The FAS facial phenotype must by highly specific to prenatal alcohol exposure and FAS to render a valid diagnosis of FAS, especially in the absence of a confirmed prenatal alcohol exposure. Specificity must be confirmed through properly designed empirical studies.

7. Diagnostic criteria should not require 'excessive' levels of alcohol exposure because a safe level of exposure has not been confirmed for all individuals and the accuracy of an exposure history can never be verified.

8. The report summarizing the outcome of an FASD diagnostic evaluation should report the FASD diagnostic classification, which diagnostic guidelines were used, all data required to confirm the diagnostic criteria were met and all recommendations documented.

9. Access to intervention services should be based on a patient's disability, not on what caused their disability.

CONCLUSIONS

Accurate, reliable, diagnoses across the full continuum of FASD have been available to families and clinicians for over a decade. As medical technology and our understanding of FASD advance, so must our diagnostic methods and tools. It is imperative that advancements in diagnostic methods be guided by an evidence base of rigorously designed, implemented, and peer-reviewed research. When a diagnosis under the umbrella of FASD is made, two individuals are affected directly; the child and the birth mother. The consequences of an incorrect diagnosis for both mother and child must be considered carefully. Diagnostic guidelines should guide professionals in rendering an accurate medical diagnosis. A diagnosis reflects the condition of a patient; however, because a diagnosis serves many purposes (eg, treatment, prevention, communication among specialists, and qualification for services), the process of rendering a diagnosis can sometimes be influenced by those different purposes. The only diagnosis that serves all purposes most effectively is a correct diagnosis. Access to services should be based on an individual's disabilities and not on what caused their disabilities. Therefore, services should be available for individuals across the full continuum of FASD and not just those with FAS.

REFERENCES

[1]   Stratton K, Howe C, Battaglia F. Fetal Alcohol Syndrome: Diagnosis Epidemiology Prevention and Treatment. Institute of Medicine. Washington D C National Academy Press; 1996.

[2]   Jones K, Smith D. Recognition of the fetal alcohol syndrome in early infancy. Lancet 1973; 2:999-1001.

[3]   Rosett H. A clinical perspective of the fetal alcohol syndrome. Alcohol Clin Exp Res 1980; 4(2): 119-22.

[4]   Clarren S, Smith D. The fetal alcohol syndrome. N Engl J Med 1978; 298(19): 1063-7.

[5]   Sokol R, Clarren S. Guidelines for use of terminology describing the impact of prenatal alcohol on the offspring. Alcohol Clin Exp Res 1989; 13: 597-8.

[6]   Abel E, Sokol R. Incidence of fetal alcohol syndrome and economic impact of FAS-related anomalies. Drug Alcohol Depend 1987; 19(1): 51-70.

[7]   Astley S, Stachowiak J, Clarren S, Clausen C. Application of the fetal alcohol syndrome facial photographic screening tool in a foster care population. J Pediatr 2002; 141(5): 712-7.

[8]   Astley S. Fetal alcohol syndrome prevention in Washington State: Evidence of success. Paediatr Perinat Epidemiol 2004; 18: 344-51.

[9]   Astley SJ, Aylward EH, Olson HC, Kerns K, Brooks A, Coggins TE. Magnetic resonance imaging outcomes from a comprehensive magnetic resonance study of children with fetal alcohol spectrum disorders. Alcohol Clin Exp Res 2009; 33(10):1-19.

[10]   Astley SJ, Olson HC, Kerns K, Brooks A, Aylward EH, Coggins TE. Neuropsychological and behavioral outcomes from a comprehensive magnetic resonance study of children with fetal alcohol spectrum disorders. Can J Clin Pharmacol 2009; 16(1): e178-e201.

[11]   Mattson SN, Schoenfeld AM, Riley EP. Teratogenic effects of alcohol on brain and behavior. Alcohol Res Health 2001; 25: 185-91.

[12]   Kodituwakku PW. Defining the behavioral phenotype in children with fetal alcohol spectrum disorders: a review. Neurosci Biobehav Rev 2007; 31(2): 192-201.

[13]   Aase JM, Jones KL, Clarren SK. Do we need the term "FAE"? Pediatrics 1995; 95: 428-30.

[14]   Astley SJ, Clarren SK. Diagnosing the full spectrum of fetal alcohol exposed individuals: Introducing the 4-Digit Diagnostic Code. Alcohol Alcohol 2000; 35: 400-10.

[15]   Chavez G, Cordero J, Becerra J. Leading major congenital malformations among minority groups in the United States, 1981-1986. Morbid Mortal Wkly Rep 1998; 37: 17-24.

[16]   Astley S. Comparison of the 4-Digit Diagnostic Code and the Hoyme diagnostic guidelines for fetal alcohol spectrum disorders. Pediatr Rev 2006; 118(4):1532-45.

[17]   Streissguth A, Kanton J. The Challenge of Fetal Alcohol Syndrome: Overcoming Secondary Disabilities Seattle WA University of Washington Press 1997.

[18]   Astley S, Bailey D, Talbot T, Clarren S. Fetal alcohol syndrome (FAS) primary prevention through FAS diagnosis: I. Identification of high-risk birth mothers through the diagnosis of their children. Alcohol Alcohol 2000; 35(5): 499-508.

[19]   Hoyme HE, May PA, Kalberg WO, *et al.* A practical clinical approach to diagnosis of fetal alcohol spectrum disorders: clarification of the 1996 Institute of Medicine criteria. Pediatrics 2005; 115: 39-47.

[20]   Astley SJ, Clarren SK. Measuring the facial phenotype of individuals with prenatal alcohol exposure: correlations with brain dysfunction. Alcohol Alcohol 2001; 36: 147-59

[21]   Astley SJ, Aylward EH, Olson HC, *et al.* Functional magnetic resonance imaging outcomes from a comprehensive magnetic resonance study of children with fetal alcohol spectrum disorders. J Neurodevelop Disord 2009; 1(1): 61-80.

[22]   Abel E. Was the fetal alcohol syndrome recognized by the Greeks and Romans? Alcohol Alcohol 1999; 34: 868-72.

[23]   Royal College of Physicians. Royal College of Physicians of London Annals 1726 p 253.

[24]   Goodacre K. Guide to the Middlesex Sessions Records 1549–1889. 1965.

[25]   Sullivan W. A note on the influence of maternal inebriety on the offspring. J Mental Sci 1899; 45: 489-503.

[26]   Lemoine P, Harousseau H, Borteyni J, Menuet J. Les enfants des parents alcoholiques: anomalies observees a propos de 127 cas [The children of alcoholic parents: anomalies observed in 127 cases]. Quest Med 1968; 8: 476-82.

[27] Ulleland C, Wennberg R, Igo R, Smith N, editors. The offspring of alcoholic mothers. American Pediatric Society and Society for Pediatric Research; 1970; Jersey City, New Jersey.

[28] Ulleland C. The offspring of alcoholic mothers. Ann N Y Acad Sci 1972; 197: 167-9.

[29] Jones K, Smith D, Ulleland C, Streissguth A. Pattern of malformation in offspring of chronic alcoholic mothers. Lancet 1973; 1: 1267-71.

[30] Astley S, Bailey D, Talbot T, Clarren S. Fetal alcohol syndrome (FAS) primary prevention through FAS diagnosis: II. A comprehensive profile of 80 birth mothers of children with FAS. Alcohol Alcohol 2000; 35(5): 509-19.

[31] Clarren S, Astley S. Development of the FAS Diagnostic and Prevention Network in Washington State. Streissguth A, Kanter J, editors. Seattle: University of Washington Press; 1997.

[32] Clarren S, Olson H, Clarren S, Astley S. A child with fetal alcohol syndrome. Guralnick M, editor. Baltimore: Paul H. Brookes Publishing Co; 2000.

[33] Astley S. FASD 4-Digit Code Online Course. www/fasd.org 2004.

[34] Astley S, Clarren S. Diagnostic guide for fetal alcohol syndrome and related conditions: the 4-Digit Diagnostic Code. 2 ed. Seattle: University of Washington Publication Services; 1999.

[35] Astley SJ, Clarren SK. Diagnostic Guide to FAS and Related Conditions: The 4-Digit Diagnostic Code 1st ed. Seattle: University of Washington Publication Services; 1997.

[36] Bertrand J, Floyd RL, Weber MK, *et al.* National Task Force on FAS/FAE Fetal Alcohol Syndrome: Guidelines for Referral and Diagnosis: Atlanta GA: Centers for Disease Control and Prevention 2004.

[37] Chudley AE, Conroy J, Cook JL, Loock C, Rosales T, LeBlanc N. Public Health Agency of Canada's National Advisory Committee on Fetal Alcohol Spectrum Disorder Fetal alcohol spectrum disorder: Canadian guidelines for diagnosis Can Med Assoc J 2005; 172: S1-S21.

[38] Astley SJ. Diagnostic Guide for Fetal Alcohol Spectrum Disorders: The 4-Digit Diagnostic Code. 3rd ed. Seattle WA: University of Washington Publication Services; 2004.

[39] Astley SJ, Clarren SK. A case definition and photographic screening tool for the facial phenotype of fetal alcohol syndrome. J Pediatr 1996; 129: 33-41.

[40] Cordero J, Floyd R, Martin M, Davis M, Hymbaugh K. Tracking the prevalence of FAS. Alcohol Health Res World 1994; 18: 82-5.

[41] Ernhart C, Greene T, Sokol R, Martier S, Boyd T, Ager J. Neonatal diagnosis of fetal alcohol syndrome: Not necessarily a hopeless prognosis. Alcohol Clin Exp Res 1995; 19(6): 1550-7.

[42] CDC. Birth certificates as a source for fetal alcohol syndrome case ascertainment-Georgia, 1989-1992. Morbid Mortal Wkly Rep 1995; 44(13): 712-7.

[43] CDC. Use of international classification of diseases coding to identify fetal alcohol syndrome-Indian Health Service facilities, 1981-1992. Morbid Mortal Wkly Rep 1995; 44(13): 253-5.

[44] Smith DW. The fetal alcohol syndrome Hosp Pract 1979; 14(10): 121-8.

[45] Astley S. FASD 4-Digit Code Short Form. [pdf] Seattle: University of Washington; 2008 [updated 2008 5/25/2008; cited 8/1/2009]; One-page electronically fillable pdf form.]. Available from: http://depts.washington.edu/fasdpn/pdfs/FASD-4digit-shortform-fillable-2004-052508.pdf.

[46] Astley S. Interdisciplinary Approach to FASD Diagnosis using the FASD 4-Digit Diagnostic Code: Training Programs. [website] Seattle: University of Washington; 2009 [updated 2009; cited 8/1/2009]; Available from: http://depts.washington.edu/fasdpn/htmls/training.htm.

[47] Bertrand J, Consortium F. Interventions for children with fetal alcohol spectrum disorders (FASDs): Overview of findings for five innovative research projects. Res Dev Disabil 2009; 30(5): 986-1006.

[48] Olson HC, Jirikowic T, Kartin D, Astley SJ. Responding to the challenge of early intervention for fetal alcohol spectrum disorders. Infants Young Child 2007; 20: 172-89.

[49] Clarren S, Astley S. Identification of children with fetal alcohol syndrome and opportunity for referral of their mothers for primary prevention - Washington, 1993-1997. Morbid Mortal Wkly Rep 1998; 47(40): 860-4.

[50] Astley S. profile of the first 1,400 patients receiving diagnostic evaluations for fetal alcohol spectrum disorder at the washington state fetal alcohol syndrome diagnostic & prevention network. Can J Clin Pharmacol Winter 2010; 17(1): e132-64.

[51] Last J. A dictionary of epidemiology. New York: Oxford University Press; 1988.

[52] Mosby. Mosby's Medical Dictionary. 8th ed.: Elsevier 2009.

[53] Sood B, Delaney-Black V, Covington C, *et al.* Prenatal alcohol exposure and childhood behavior at age 6 to 7 years: 1. dose-response effect. Pediatrics 2001; 108(2): 9.

[54] Streissguth A, Dehaene P. Fetal alcohol syndrome in twins of alcoholic mothers: concordance of diagnosis and IQ. Am J Med Genet 1993; 47(6): 857-61.

[55]   Chasnoff I. Fetal alcohol syndrome in twin pregnancy. Acta Genet. Med Gemellol (Roma) 1985; 34(3-4):229-32.

[56]   Mosby's Medical Nursing and Allied Health Dictionary, 6 ed. St. Louis; 2002.

[57]   Black M, Matula K. Essentials of Bayley Scales of Infant Development II Assessment. New York: John Wily; 1999.

[58]   Streissguth AP, Bookstein FL, Barr HM, Sampson PD, O'Malley K, Young JK. Risk factors for adverse life outcomes in fetal alcohol syndrome and fetal alcohol effects. J Dev Behav Pediatr 2004; 25(4):228- 38.

[59]   Majewski F. Alcohol embryopathy: Experience in 200 patients. Development Brain Dysfunction 1993; 6: 248-65.

[60]   Spohr H, Steinhausen H. Follow-up studies of children with fetal alcohol syndrome. Neuropediatrics 1987; 18:13-7.

[61]   Streissguth A, Clarren S, Jones K. Natural history of the fetal alcohol syndrome: A 10-year follow-up of 11 patients. Lancet 1985; 2:85-91.

[62]   Astley SJ. Fetal Alcohol Syndrome Facial Photograph Analysis Software. In: Astley SJ, editor. 1.0 ed. Seattle: University of Washington; 2003.

[63]   Astley SJ, Richards T, Aylward EH, *et al.* Magnetic resonance spectroscopy outcomes from a comprehensive magnetic resonance study of children with fetal alcohol spectrum disorders. Magn Reson Imaging 2009; 27: 760-78.

[64]   Riley EP, McGee CL, Sowell ER. Teratogenic effects of alcohol: A decade of brain imaging. Am J Med Genet 2004; 127C: 35-41.

[65]   Sowell E, Johnson A, Kan E, *et al.* Mapping white matter integrity and neurobehavioral correlates in children with fetal alcohol spectrum disorders. J Neurosci 2008; 28(6): 1313-9.

[66]   Archibald SL, Fennema-Notestine C, Ganst A, Riley EP, Mattson SN, Jernigan TL. Brain dysmorphology in individuals with severe prenatal alcohol exposure. Dev Med Child Neurol 2001; 43: 148-54.

[67]   Waber DP, Moor CD, Forbes PW, *et al.* The NIH MRI Study of Normal Brain Development: Performance of a Population Based Sample of Healthy Children Aged 6 to 18 Years on a Neuropsychological Battery. J Int Neuropsychol Soc 2007; 13: 1-18.

[68]   Almli C, Rivkin M, McKinstry R, Group BDC. The NIH MRI study of normal brain development Objective-2): Newborns, infants, toddlers, and preschoolers. Neuroimage 2007; 35: 308-25.

[69]   Dolk H. The predictive value of microcephaly during the first year of life for mental retardation at seven years. Dev Med Child Neurol 1991; 33: 974-83.

[70]   O'Hare ED, Kan E, Yoshii J, *et al.* Mapping cerebellar vermal morphology and cognitive correlates in prenatal alcohol exposure. Neuroreport 2005; 16: 1285-90.

CHAPTER 2

Interventions for Fetal Alcohol Spectrum Disorders: Implications from Basic Science Research

Jennifer D. Thomas* and Edward P. Riley

Center for Behavioral Teratology, San Diego State University, 6363 Alvarado Court, Suite 200, San Diego, CA 92120, USA

> *You cannot prevent the birds of sorrow from flying over your head, but you can prevent them from building nests in your hair*

Chinese Proverb

Abstract: Fetal Alcohol Spectrum Disorders (FASD) constitutes a serious worldwide health problem that persists, despite prevention efforts. This chapter examines preclinical research on methods to reduce the severity of FASD, either during the period of prenatal alcohol exposure or during postnatal development. Some prenatal treatments focus on directly blocking or minimizing alcohol's mechanisms of teratogenic action. The possibility that nutritional supplements during prenatal alcohol exposure may reduce the severity of FASD is also explored. Finally, treatments that may be effective even after the alcohol insult, during postnatal development are examined, including nutritional, pharmacological, and environmental/behavioral interventions. Many exciting and effective treatments for FASD have been identified and the challenge is now to translate these findings to clinical populations.

INTRODUCTION

Among the most common preventable developmental disorders are FAS and FASD, which may occur in over 1% of all live births [1]. Despite numerous and successful prevention efforts (see http://www.niaaa.nih.gov/AboutNIAAA/ Interagency/Reports/CurrentStudies.htm and http://www.fasdcenter.samhsa.gov /documents/WYNK Preventing FASD.pdf), recent data indicate that over 10% of women of child bearing age regularly engage in binge drinking [2] and 2% of pregnant women engage in risky levels of drinking [3] (Fig. **1**).

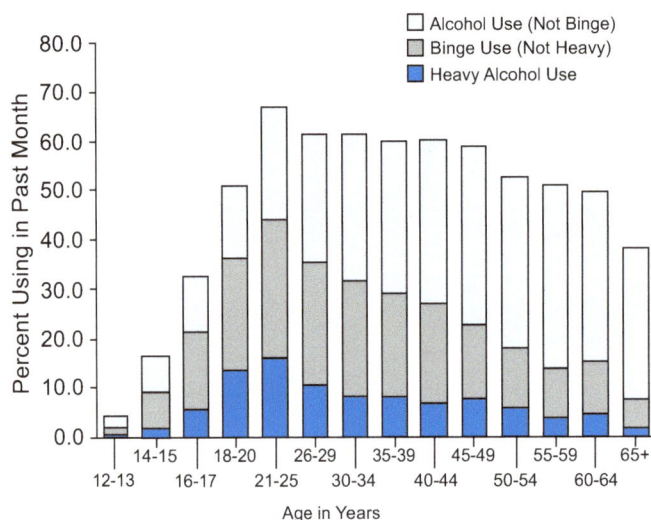

Figure 1: Among pregnant women aged 15 to 44 in 2002, 9.1 percent used alcohol and 3.1 percent reported binge drinking in the month prior to the survey. Reprinted from Substance Abuse and Mental Health Services Administration, (2003). Overview of Findings from the 2002 National Survey on Drug Use and Health (Office of Applied Studies, NHSDA Series H-21, DHHS Publication No. SMA 03-3774). Rockville, MD.

Address correspondence to Jennifer D. Thomas: Center for Behavioral Teratology, San Diego State University, 6363 Alvarado Court, Suite 200, San Diego, CA 92120, USA; E-mail: Thomas3@mail.sdsu.edu

Given these numbers and the resulting large public health implications, there is a need to identify means to either block or reduce ethanol's teratogenic effects during alcohol exposure or to intervene and reduce the impact of FASD after the exposure has occurred. Although a number of clinical studies have examined or are examining interventions in high risk women of child bearing age, pregnant women consuming alcohol, as well as in individuals with FASD, the review presented in this chapter focuses primarily on preclinical, basic science research. This research has identified a number of means to attenuate the physical and functional effects seen in FASD, although in many cases the translation to clinical practice is challenging for a variety of safety and practical concerns.

TREATMENTS DURING DEVELOPMENTAL ALCOHOL EXPOSURE

One possibility for intervening in FASD is to identify the mechanisms by which alcohol exposure might impact the developing embryo or fetus and to block those effects. Basic research has identified many potential mechanisms of ethanol teratogenesis (see **http://pubs.niaaa.nih.gov/publications/arh25-3/175-184.htm** [4]) and researchers are now basing some experimental therapeutics on these putative mechanisms. For example, ethanol has been postulated to damage the developing CNS via oxidative stress, increasing free radicals and reducing cellular antioxidant properties [5]. Numerous basic research studies in both cell cultures and whole animals have demonstrated that agents with antioxidant properties can block many of ethanol's teratogenic effects, including growth retardation, physical anomalies, and neuropathologies, including neuronal cell loss. These antioxidants include vitamin E [6], vitamin C [7], β-carotene [6], cyanidin-3-glucoside from blackberries [8], Pycnogenol© from pine bark [9], the superoxide-dismutase/catalase mimetic EUK-134 [10], and even the induction of Nrf2 protein which activates endogenous antioxidant enzymes [11].

However, demonstration of the effectiveness of antioxidants in animal models of FASD has not always been positive [12], and some studies show mixed results, especially regarding their effect on mitigating the behavioral outcomes following developmental alcohol exposure [13]. Of importance, a clinical study assessing vitamins C and E in mitigating the effects of prenatal alcohol exposure was terminated because of safety concerns (see **http://www.motherisk.org/JFAS documents/ JFAS7002 5 e3.pdf**) [14]. Nevertheless, given the large number of antioxidant agents, with varying qualities and potencies, it is possible that a different level or combination of antioxidants, or induction of inherent antioxidant machinery, may prove to be more effective and safe in clinical populations.

It is important to note that some of the agents described above may exert protective effects independent of that afforded by their antioxidant properties (e.g. [8]). For example, the vasoactive intestinal neuroprotective peptides NAPVSIPQ (NAP) and SALLFSIPA (SAL) (which are derived from activity-dependent neurotrophic factor (ADNF) and activity-dependent neuroprotective protein (ADNP)) also protect against oxidative stress. Administration of these agents can reduce prenatal alcohol-induced mortality and growth deficits [15]; physical effects, including neural tube defects [16]; neuropathology, including apoptotic cell loss [17]; loss of serotonergic neurons [18], and even spatial learning deficits [19] in mice. These neuroactive peptides, however, have not shown efficacy in protecting against neuronal cell death and behavioral alterations associated with 3rd trimester alcohol exposure in rats, suggesting that their protection may depend on other factors such as the developmental timing of administration. These neuroactive peptides may also be acting via other mechanisms besides anti-oxidation [20], including protection against alcohol's adverse effects on L1 cell adhesion molecules. NAP and SAL are currently undergoing development as neuroprotectants and for the treatment of various conditions including Alzheimer's disease.

Among the mechanisms of alcohol-induced teratogenesis is the action of alcohol on L1 cell adhesion molecules, which play a critical role in axon guidance and cell migration. Specifically, alcohol, at physiological doses, impairs the ability of cells to adhere or stick to one another, and this effect is antagonized by NAP and SAL [21]. 1-octanol also acts as an antagonist of ethanol inhibition of the L1 cell adhesion molecule and has been shown to protect against alcohol-induced apoptotic cell death and gross dysmorphology in the mouse (See Fig. **2** in **http://pubs.niaaa.nih.gov/publications/arh27-2/174-180.htm**) [22].

Further identification and development of targeted interventions that can protect against specific alcohol actions may prove to be fruitful.

Alcohol interacts with a number of neurotransmitter receptor sites, including the glutamatergic, N-methyl-d-aspartate (NMDA) receptor [23]. Acutely, alcohol inhibits NMDA receptors (it acts as an antagonist), which likely contributes to the sedative and intoxicating effects of alcohol (see http://pubs.niaaa.nih.gov/publications/arh314/310-339.htm [24]). This blockade may, by itself, induce apoptotic cell death [25]. In addition, as a consequence of this antagonism, neurocompensatory responses, such as increased glutamate release, release of modulators like polyamines, or receptor upregulation may occur, contributing to tolerance. This results in an overly sensitive glutamatergic system once the alcohol is removed. During periods of withdrawal, the NMDA receptor may become overactive leading to excitotoxic cell death, a mechanism of cell death that is believed to occur following a number of insults, including hypoxia, stroke/ischemia, Alzheimer's disease, and alcohol-related neuropathology [26]. The developing brain is rich in NMDA receptors, as these receptors play an important role during development (http://www.ncbi.nlm.nih.gov/bookshelf/br. fcgi?book=frnrec&part=ch1). However, because of this richness in receptors, it also presents a period when the brain may be more vulnerable to NMDA receptor-mediated excitotoxic cell death.

Consistent with this hypothesis, several studies have now shown that blockade of the NMDA receptor during withdrawal in the neonatal rat pup can protect against neuropathology and behavioral alterations associated with developmental alcohol exposure. The neonatal rat model is a model for human third trimester exposure, as brain development that occurs in the human fetus during the third trimester occurs in the rat during the first two weeks of life [27]. Exposure to alcohol during this period of time can produce a number of behavioral effects, including overactivity and spatial learning deficits. It has been found that MK-801, a noncompetitive antagonist of the NMDA receptor, reduces the severity of these behavioral effects, but only when administered at a period of time during ethanol withdrawal (as blood alcohol levels are approaching 0 mg/dl) [28]. MK-801's effects are dose-dependent, with lower doses (<0.5 mg/kg), but not a high dose (1.0 mg/kg), being effective [29], and time-dependent [30].

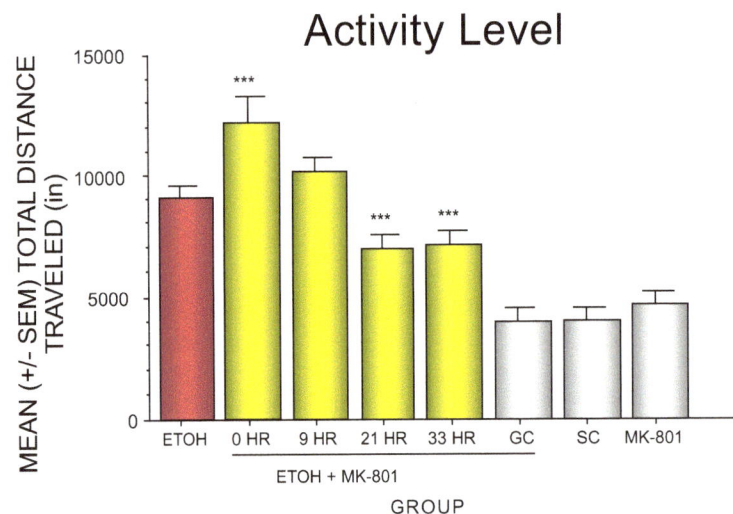

Figure 2: Alcohol exposure during early development significantly increased the total distance traveled in an automated open field (ETOH) compared to control groups (GC, SC). Administration of MK-801, an NMDA receptor antagonist exacerbated ethanol-related overactivity when administered at the same time as alcohol, but significantly attenuated ethanol-induced overactivity when administered during withdrawal (21 and 33 hr post-ethanol). MK-801 by itself did not significantly affect activity level. ***= significantly different from other groups.

As can be seen in Fig. **2**, if MK-801 is administered at the same time as the alcohol or while the blood alcohol levels are still high, it exacerbates the effects of the alcohol exposure, but if it is administered during withdrawal, it protects against alcohol-related behavioral alterations. Such characteristics limit the clinical use of MK-801; nevertheless, other NMDA receptor antagonists may be more suitable candidates for intervening in pregnant women or for neonates undergoing withdrawal. For example, ethanol targets NMDA receptors that contain 2B subunits (each NMDA receptor comprises a 1 subunit and a combination of four various 2 subunits (a-d), the same receptors that are modulated by polyamines). The administration of eliprodil, which antagonizes the NMDA receptor at the polyamine modulatory site, during developmental alcohol withdrawal, has also been shown to reduce the severity of spatial reversal learning deficits [31] (see Fig. **3**). Similarly, blockade of the NMDA receptor polyamine modulatory site with agmatine during withdrawal also protects against cerebellar-related motor deficits, indicating that antagonism of NMDA receptors may protect against a wide variety of neuropathology and behavioral alterations [32].

Reversal Learning
Total Errors

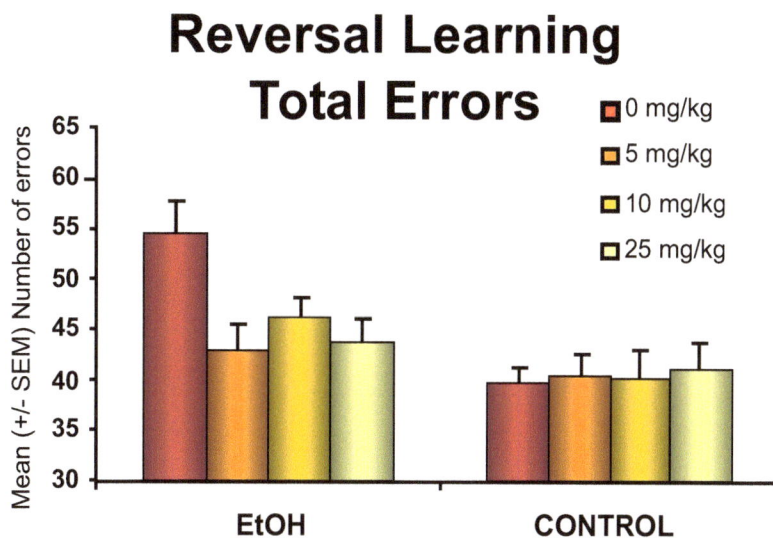

Figure 3: Alcohol exposure during development impairs performance on a spatial reversal learning task. Administration of various doses of eliprodil, an NMDA receptor antagonist that acts on the polyamine modulatory site significantly mitigates ethanol-related learning deficits, without affecting performance of controls.

Finally, administration of memantine, an NMDA receptor antagonist that is currently used clinically for the treatment of Alzheimer's disease, also reduces the behavioral effects resulting from neonatal alcohol exposure. Interestingly, memantine has potent effects in mitigating the effects on motor coordination resulting from prenatal alcohol exposure and protects against cerebellar Purkinje cell loss (the cerebellum is intimately related to motor coordination), more so than on having an effect on cognitive performance. Similarly, in vitro studies indicate that administration of memantine can also protect against hippocampal cell loss associated with developmental alcohol exposure [33].

Serotonergic neurons are also among the systems adversely affected by prenatal alcohol exposure. Given that serotonin possesses trophic properties (properties that promote neuronal growth), loss of serotonin can produce a consequent cascade of neuropathology. A number of studies have shown that administration of serotonin agonists can protect against alcohol-induced neuropathologies. Specifically, administration of buspirone or ipsapirone, drugs that act as serotonin (5-HT) 1A receptor agonists, protect against prenatal alcohol induced cell death of serotonergic and other rhombencephalic (hindbrain) neurons [34], and alcohol-induced alterations in serotonergic functioning [35, 36].

Prenatal alcohol exposure can also interfere with neurotrophic factors, which are chemicals that promote growth. Administration of a number of such growth factors, including brain-derived neurotrophic factor (BDNF), glial-derived neurotrophic factor (GDNF), fibroblast growth factor (FGF-2), nerve growth factor (NGF), and insulin-like growth factor (IGF-1), has been shown to reduce fetal alcohol effects. Many *in vitro* studies have shown that neurotrophic factors can reduce the severity of neuropathology [37-42]. One of the challenges is administering growth factors to influence desired targets without affecting non-targeted developmental processes, although there are now *in vivo* studies showing beneficial effects as well [43] (see Fig. **4**).

Prenatal alcohol also is associated with nutritional deficiencies, in part because individuals who are drinking heavily are not consuming adequate levels of nutrients, but also because alcohol can impair nutrient uptake and utilization [44]. Early animal studies investigated whether nutritional status interacted with alcohol exposure [45]. This work showed that the effects of prenatal alcohol were frequently exacerbated by concomitant nutritional deficiencies. For example, when protein level of the diet was varied, animals receiving suboptimal levels of protein had offspring more severely affected than those on normal levels of protein [46]. Animal studies have shown that the teratogenic effects of alcohol, including low birth weight [46], physical anomalies [47], brain damage [48] and reduced IGF levels [49], are more severe when consumed with suboptimal nutrition; however, the exacerbation was often related to increased peak blood alcohol levels among malnourished subjects. Despite the effects of alcohol on nutritional status, and the early basic science studies showing how prenatal alcohol could influence the nutritional status of the offspring, it is surprising that more work has not been done on examining the influence of nutritional supplements in the mother and/or offspring.

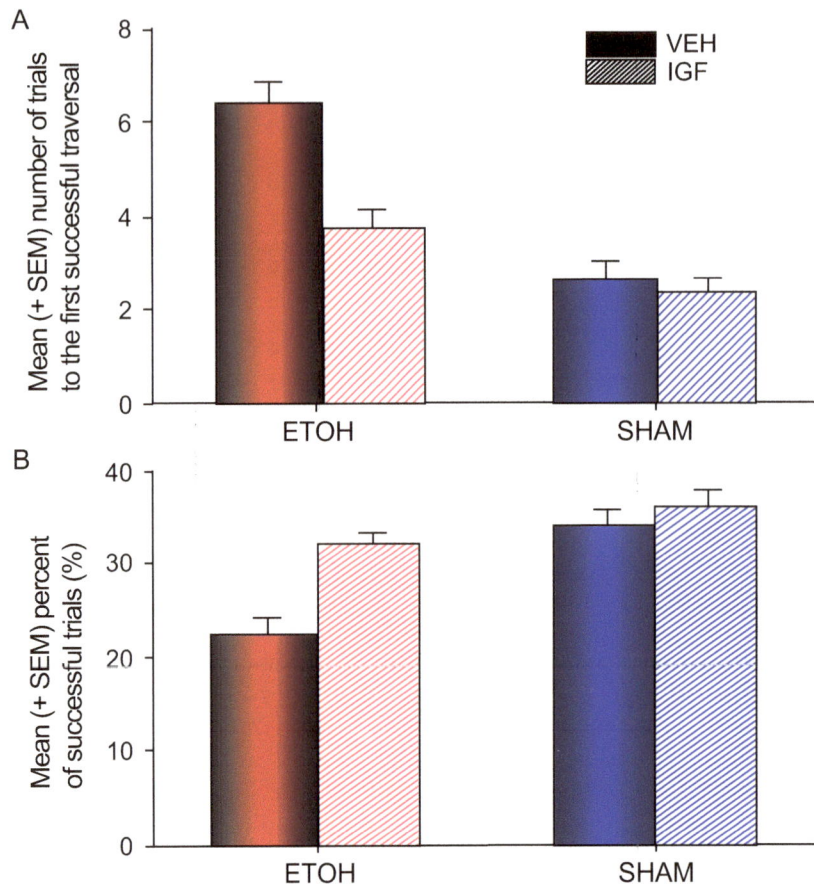

Figure 4: Insulin-like growth factor (IGF-I) administered shortly after developmental alcohol exposure attenuates ethanol-related deficits in motor coordination. Panel A shows the number of trials to success on a parallel bar motor coordination task. Ethanol-exposed subjects treated with vehicle (VEH) took longer to be successful compared to all other groups. Similarly, the percent of successful trials was significantly reduced in ethanol-exposed subjects treated with vehicle compared to all other groups, including the ethanol-exposed subjects treated with IGF-I.

A recent line of research that has garnered much interest is the recent work on choline supplementation and choline deficiency. It has been demonstrated that prenatal choline supplementation in the pregnant rat at the same time as alcohol exposure (gestational days 5-20) reduces the severity of alcohol-related body weight reductions and normalizes many alcohol-induced alterations in reflex development [50]. Importantly, choline did not significantly affect blood alcohol levels or food intake. Further discussion on choline is found below.

Another potential nutritional intervention is zinc. Zinc supplementation during ethanol exposure on GD 8 in mice has been shown to reduce physical abnormalities [51], as well as spatial learning memory deficits [52]. In contrast, zinc was not successful in attenuating the cerebellar Purkinje cell loss associated with 3rd trimester equivalent alcohol exposure [53], although there were no alcohol-related reductions in zinc. It is not clear if zinc supplementation is effective only among certain cell populations or only at particular times of development, nor is it known whether zinc is effective only when replenishing a zinc deficiency or via a different mechanism.

Another nutrient, nicotinamide (an amide of vitamin B3), has been shown to protect against alcohol-related apoptotic cell death. Specifically, nicotinamide inhibited activation of caspase-3, severity of neuronal cell death, overactivity and contextual fear conditioning deficits associated with alcohol exposure on postnatal day 7 in mice, a period of development equivalent to a portion of the third trimester in humans [54]. These findings are very intriguing, although it should be noted that the doses of nicotinamide used translate to much higher doses than are used clinically in humans.

Finally, there is some indication that folic acid supplementation, particularly when administered with vitamin B12, may have some beneficial effects against alcohol's teratogenic effects [55]. In summary, there are a number of potential nutritional interventions that may be useful in mitigating prenatal alcohol effects. Given the potential interactions of alcohol and nutrients, the benefits of nutritional supplementation have not been adequately explored. Large scale clinical studies that examine nutritional status of pregnant alcohol-drinking women and determine the potential efficacy of nutritional interventions are needed.

The challenge with agents that block or reduce ethanol's teratogenic effects is that they must be present during the alcohol exposure if they are to be effective, which may not be feasible since it is unlikely that an individual will be able to intervene at the time of intoxication. Also, many women who are drinking heavily may not be seeking prenatal care on a regular basis. More likely the individual who has been exposed to alcohol prenatally and is already exhibiting signs of FASD would be the target of intervention. Early diagnosis is key, as interventions administered early in development may be more effective. Nevertheless, treatments that are effective even during later periods of development are critical, as the first populations diagnosed with FAS are now in young adulthood. At this point, the challenge is to determine how much plasticity the nervous system maintains and to capitalize on ways that will allow the alcohol-exposed CNS to improve function and compensate for regional deficits.

EFFECTIVE TREATMENTS AFTER PRENATAL ALCOHOL EXPOSURE

The potential of a dietary intervention, choline, in reducing the severity of fetal alcohol effects is currently being investigated. Choline is a vital nutrient that is necessary for normal development, including CNS development. Choline acts as a precursor to the neurotransmitter acetylcholine, as a methyl donor, and as a precursor to components of cellular membranes; thus, its actions on brain development are varied. The high demand for choline during development is demonstrated by the high levels in breast milk [56,57] and it is now recommended that pregnant women consume 550 mg of choline/day. Animal studies have shown that perinatal choline supplementation influences neuronal morphology, electrophysiology, and the neurochemistry of the hippocampus and cortex (areas of the brain involved in learning and memory) [58-60]. Consistent with these CNS changes, perinatal choline supplementation leads to long-lasting enhancements in spatial learning and memory, attention, and temporal memory [58, 59]. Since it is known that developmental alcohol exposure disrupts development of the hippocampus and cortex, leading to alterations in cholinergic functioning, it is hypothesized that choline could mitigate some of ethanol's adverse effects on development, even when administered after alcohol exposure.

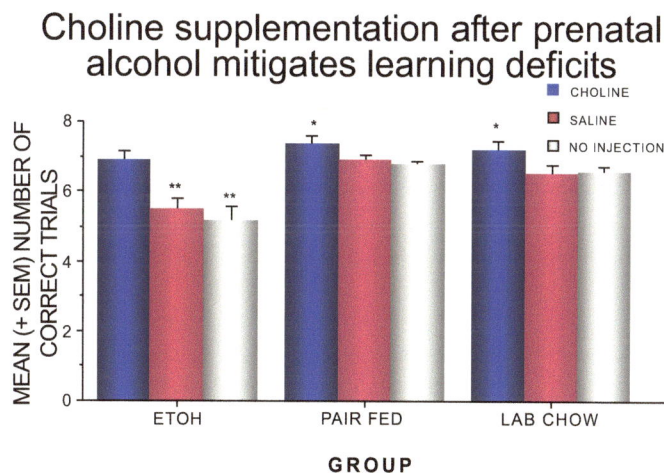

Figure 5: Prenatal ethanol exposure impaired performance on a working memory task, significantly reducing the number of correct trials achieved in adult rats, compared to pair-fed and lab chow controls. Cognitive deficits were mitigated with administration of choline from PD 2-21 (shown in blue). In fact, ethanol-exposed subjects treated with choline performed at levels similar to those of controls.

The first study demonstrated that choline supplementation from postnatal days (PD) 1-21 could reduce the severity of working memory deficits in adult rats exposed to alcohol prenatally (see Fig. **5**) [61]. That is, exposure to choline for the first three weeks postnatally in the rat, mitigated effects on a memory task when that animal was tested as an adult. It was subsequently demonstrated that choline is effective in attenuating open field activity and reversal learning deficits when administered during and after 3rd trimester equivalent alcohol exposure (PD 4-30) (see Fig. **6**) [62].

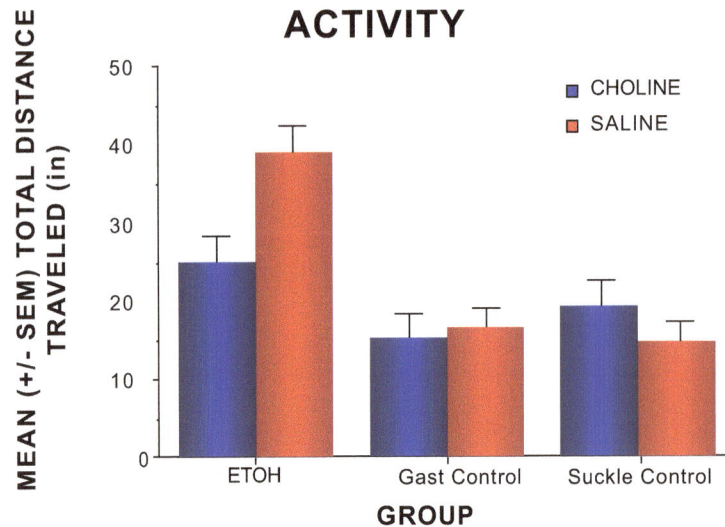

Figure 6: Alcohol exposure during the 3rd trimester equivalent led to increases in locomotor activity in an automated open field chamber. Choline supplementation significantly reduced the severity of alcohol-related hyperactivity. In fact, activity levels of ethanol-exposed subjects treated with choline did not differ significantly from that of controls.

Similar effects were observed by Wagner and Hunt (2006) [63] who demonstrated that an identical choline treatment reduces the severity of alcohol-related trace fear conditioning deficits. In trace conditioning, there is a period of time between the offset of the conditioned stimulus (tone) and the onset of the unconditioned stimulus (shock) and this paradigm requires the hippocampus to maintain the memory (memory trace) of the conditioned stimulus. As mentioned previously, the first few postnatal weeks in the rat may be akin to the third trimester in humans.

To further determine if choline was effective when administered later in development, subjects were given choline from PD 10-30. In humans this would be equivalent to administering choline to the young child. Choline supplementation mitigated ethanol-related deficits in spatial learning that were evident at PD 180. So, choline was effective in reducing the severity of fetal alcohol-related learning deficits when administered after the 3rd trimester equivalent and during a period of development equivalent to postnatal development in humans, as well [64]. In fact, choline supplementation during either PD 11-20, 21-30, or 11-30 reduced the severity of spatial learning and memory deficits [65], suggesting that choline could be administered even in later childhood and improve some cognitive abilities. Moreover, administration of choline from PD 40-60 in the rat reduced the severity of working memory deficits [66], but not overactivity or simple spatial learning deficits, suggesting that administration during adolescence or young adulthood may have an impact on prefrontal cortical functioning. In sum, choline shows promise as a treatment that can be administered to individuals after prenatal alcohol exposure.

Other pharmacologic agents may also reduce the severity of FASD, even when administered later in life. For example, Medina and colleagues have shown that the cognitive enhancer vinpocetine (a phsophodiesterase (PDE) 1 inhibitor, which increases cAMP over cGMP) enhances sensory-related cortical plasticity. Specifically, administration of vinpocetine on PD 40-50 in the ferret restored plasticity of ocular dominance columns in the visual cortex [67], which were impacted by prenatal alcohol exposure. Whether such agents have similar effects in other brain regions, like the hippocampus, and effects on behaviors like learning and memory, is not known; nevertheless, cognitive enhancers may have the potential to effectively reduce deficits among individuals with FASD, even when administered during adolescence or adulthood.

ENVIRONMENTAL/BEHAVIORAL INTERVENTIONS

Much can be learned from what is known of factors that influence typical development. Experience-dependent plasticity is maintained throughout the lifespan of the nervous system, not only allowing an individual's environment and own behavior to shape the structure and function of the CNS, but also facilitate recovery from damage. That does not necessarily mean, however, that the alcohol-exposed brain maintains the same degree of plasticity [68] or that the experiences that are best suited for typically developing individuals are identical for those who are compromised. Some amount of creativity may be needed to tailor the appropriate experience for the individual with FASD. Nevertheless, current data are encouraging (see [69] for review).

A large animal literature indicates that environmental enrichment, whether experienced early or later in life, can have long-lasting benefits on CNS development and behavior [70,71]. The typical enriched environment includes social, motor, and sensory stimulation, by including stimulation such as peers, running wheels and toys in the environment (see video below).

An obvious question is whether the CNS that has been exposed to alcohol prenatally responds similarly to this type of experience. Hannigan *et al.,* [72] illustrated that environmental enrichment mitigated ethanol-related deficits in gait in prenatally alcohol-exposed rats. Animals that had been exposed to alcohol and then reared in standard cages showed narrow gaits indicative of problems with balance. However, when these animals were reared in stimulating environments, they showed normal gaits. The enriched environment also improved performance on a spatial learning task in both controls and prenatally alcohol-exposed subjects, an effect that is still observable weeks after the environmental enrichment experience [69], although it should be noted that there were no adverse effects of prenatal alcohol in several studies [72, 73].

Communal rearing also can attenuate ethanol-related deficits in conditioned taste aversion [74]. Even handling has been shown to attenuate some fetal alcohol effects (see [69, 75] for reviews).

In contrast, others have reported that postnatal plasticity following developmental alcohol exposure is compromised. For example, Choi *et al.,* [76] reported that environmental enrichment increases adult neurogenesis (the formation of new neurons) in controls, but not among subjects exposed to alcohol prenatally. Similarly, environmental enrichment failed to attenuate ethanol-related reductions in cortical thickness [73] and dendritic spine densities [77].

Other more specific experiences have also shown promise in reducing the severity of FASD. Motor rehabilitation and enhanced cerebellar and motor cortical plasticity can be achieved with an acrobatic motor training regimen (an obstacle course that requires climbing, balancing, and other motor challenges (see video here).

Twenty days of complex motor training in adult rats improved overall motor performance among both controls and subjects exposed to alcohol during development [78] and increased cerebellar synaptogenesis [79]. Importantly, increased plasticity in the cerebellum translates into improved performance on other cerebellar-related tasks, such as classical conditioning of the eyeblink response, suggesting that the plasticity gained with one experience can affect domains outside that experience. Even exercise has been shown to enhance plasticity. Recently, Christie and colleagues illustrated that simple physical exercise (running wheel experience) in mice exposed to alcohol prenatally may enhance electrophysiological activity in the hippocampus, spatial memory performance [80], and cytogenesis [81]. Similarly, exercise reduces spatial learning deficits and overactivity in the open field associated with developmental alcohol exposure in rats, even weeks after the exercise wheel is no longer available (see Fig. 7) [82].

These preclinical studies are exciting because they do suggest that environmental and behavioral interventions can be effective. Such studies are now supported by clinical studies illustrating that specialized training can improve social skills [83], behavioral problems [84] and math skills [84]. These data suggest that the CNS can respond to environmental interventions even after a developmental alcohol insult. Again, the challenge is to identify the optimal characteristics of the training that best suits individuals with FASD.

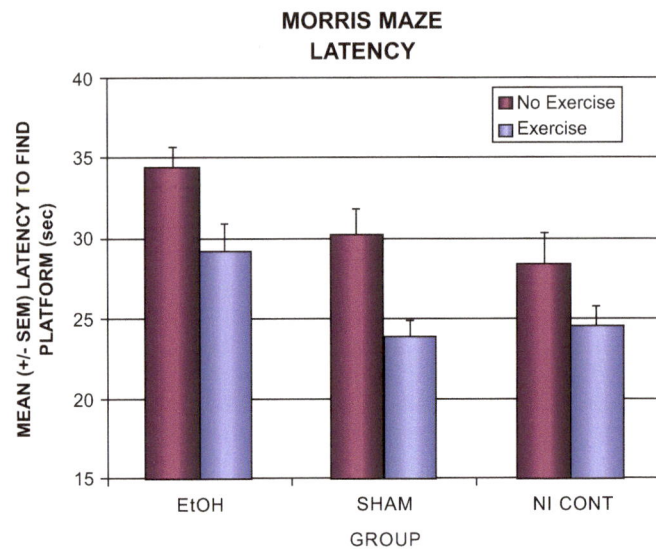

Figure. 7: Ethanol exposure during development led to impairments in spatial learning, as seen as an increase in the latency to find a hidden platform based on spatial cues. Exercise, however, improved performance among ethanol-exposed and control groups, illustrating that exercise enhances cognitive abilities.

IMPLICATIONS

Current research suggests a number of promising treatment strategies that might be applied to pregnant women who are drinking or for individuals with FASD. Currently, most children with FASD are treated for specific symptoms. For example, if they exhibit ADHD they are medicated with stimulants [85], although no large scale studies have been conducted to determine the most effective medications for treating ADHD [86]. In addition, many symptoms that may contribute to additional learning and attentional problems, such as sensory deficits, sleep disturbances and mood disorders, also should be directly treated.

Many positive effects can be achieved outside of medications and the studies described in this chapter suggest that a variety of nutritional and environmental factors may improve outcome. Capitalizing on the CNS plasticity that remains after a developmental alcohol insult may be key. Maintenance of plasticity in the alcohol-exposed CNS is exciting, as it affords the opportunity to enhance behavioral functioning. On the flip side, it also suggests that the alcohol-exposed CNS can be adversely affected by negative experiences. For example, early social stress exacerbates ethanol's adverse effects on cognitive performance [87]; thus, preventing environments known to put the individual at risk is also key to intervention. Clinical studies have shown that stable home environments are associated with a better outcome than unstable, stressful environments [88], so part of the treatment may include minimizing stress and instability in the environment of the individuals with FASD.

In summary, a variety of pharmacological, nutritional, educational, and social factors may modify the expression of FASD. It is likely that a combination of approaches may be optimal and the goal now is to identify those effective combinations and implement them on a large scale.

REFERENCES

[1] Sampson PD, Streissguth AP, Bookstein FL, *et al.* Incidence of fetal alcohol syndrome and prevalence of alcohol-related neurodevelopmental disorder. Teratology 1997 Nov; 56(5): 317-26.

[2] Tsai J, Floyd RL, O'Connor MJ, Velasquez MM. Alcohol use and serious psychological distress among women of childbearing age. Addict Behav 2009 Feb; 34(2): 146-53.

[3] Alcohol use among pregnant and nonpregnant women of childbearing age - United States, 1991-2005. MMWR Morb Mortal Wkly Rep 2009 May 22; 58(19): 529-32.

[4] Charles R. Goodlett KHH. Mechanisms of Alcohol-Induced Damage to the Developing Nervous System. Alcohol Res Health 2001; 25(3): 175-84.

[5] Cohen-Kerem R, Koren G. Antioxidants and fetal protection against ethanol teratogenicity. I. Review of the experimental data and implications to humans. Neurotoxicol Teratol 2003 Jan-Feb; 25(1): 1-9.

[6] Mitchell JJ, Paiva M, Heaton MB. The antioxidants vitamin E and beta-carotene protect against ethanol-induced neurotoxicity in embryonic rat hippocampal cultures. Alcohol 1999 Feb; 17(2): 163-8.

[7] Peng Y, Kwok KH, Yang PH, *et al.* Ascorbic acid inhibits ROS production, NF-kappa B activation and prevents ethanol-induced growth retardation and microencephaly. Neuropharmacology 2005 Mar; 48(3): 426-34.

[8] Chen G, Bower KA, Xu M, *et al.* Cyanidin-3-glucoside reverses ethanol-induced inhibition of neurite outgrowth: role of glycogen synthase kinase 3 Beta. Neurotox Res 2009 May; 15(4): 321-31.

[9] Siler-Marsiglio KI, Shaw G, Heaton MB. Pycnogenol and vitamin E inhibit ethanol-induced apoptosis in rat cerebellar granule cells. J Neurobiol 2004 Jun; 59(3): 261-71.

[10] Chen SY, Dehart DB, Sulik KK. Protection from ethanol-induced limb malformations by the superoxide dismutase/catalase mimetic, EUK-134. FASEB J 2004 Aug; 18(11): 1234-6.

[11] Dong J, Sulik KK, Chen SY. Nrf2-mediated transcriptional induction of antioxidant response in mouse embryos exposed to ethanol *in vivo*: implications for the prevention of fetal alcohol spectrum disorders. Antioxid Redox Signal 2008 Dec;10(12): 2023-33.

[12] Tanaka H, Iwasaki S, Nakazawa K, Inomata K. Fetal alcohol syndrome in rats: conditions for improvement of ethanol effects on fetal cerebral development with supplementary agents. Biol Neonate 1988; 54(6): 320-9.

[13] Tran TD, Jackson HD, Horn KH, Goodlett CR. Vitamin E does not protect against neonatal ethanol-induced cerebellar damage or deficits in eyeblink classical conditioning in rats. Alcohol Clin Exp Res 2005 Jan; 29(1):117-29.

[14] Y Ingrid Goh WU, Joanne Rovet, Gideon Koren. Mega-Dose Vitamin C and E in Preventing FASD: The Decision to Terminate the Study Prematurely. J FAS Int 2007 4/3/2007 [cited; Available from: http://www.motherisk.org/JFAS_documents/JFAS7002_5_e3.pdf

[15] Spong CY, Abebe DT, Gozes I, Brenneman DE, Hill JM. Prevention of fetal demise and growth restriction in a mouse model of fetal alcohol syndrome. J Pharmacol Exp Ther 2001 May; 297(2):7 74-9.

[16] Chen SY, Charness ME, Wilkemeyer MF, Sulik KK. Peptide-mediated protection from ethanol-induced neural tube defects. Dev Neurosci 2005 Jan-Feb;27(1): 13-9.

[17] Sari Y. Activity-dependent neuroprotective protein-derived peptide, NAP, preventing alcohol-induced apoptosis in fetal brain of C57BL/6 mouse. Neuroscience 2009 Feb 18; 158(4): 1426-35.

[18] Zhou FC, Fang Y, Goodlett C. Peptidergic agonists of activity-dependent neurotrophic factor protect against prenatal alcohol-induced neural tube defects and serotonin neuron loss. Alcohol Clin Exp Res 2008 Aug; 32(8): 1361-71.

[19] Vink J, Auth J, Abebe DT, Brenneman DE, Spong CY. Novel peptides prevent alcohol-induced spatial learning deficits and proinflammatory cytokine release in a mouse model of fetal alcohol syndrome. Am J Obstet Gynecol 2005 Sep; 193(3 Pt 1): 825-9.

[20] Sari Y, Gozes I. Brain deficits associated with fetal alcohol exposure may be protected, in part, by peptides derived from activity-dependent neurotrophic factor and activity-dependent neuroprotective protein. Brain Res Brain Res Rev 2006 Aug 30; 52(1): 107-18.

[21] Wilkemeyer MF, Menkari CE, Spong CY, Charness ME. Peptide antagonists of ethanol inhibition of l1-mediated cell-cell adhesion. J Pharm Exp Ther 2002; 303(1): 110-6.

[22] Chen SY, Wilkemeyer MF, Sulik KK, Charness ME. Octanol antagonism of ethanol teratogenesis. FASEB J 2001 Jul; 15(9): 1649-51.

[23]   Lovinger DM, White G, Weight FF. Ethanol inhibits NMDA-activated ion current in hippocampal neurons. Science 1989; 243: 1721-4.

[24]   Peter Clapp SVB, and Paula L. Hoffman. How Adaptation of the Brain to Alcohol Leads to Dependance: A Pharmacological Perspective. Alcohol Res Health 2008; 31(4): 310-39.

[25]   Ikonomidou C, Bittigau P, Ishimaru MJ, *et al.* Ethanol-induced apoptotic neurodegeneration and fetal alcohol syndrome. Science 2000 Feb 11; 287(5455): 1056-60.

[26]   Rothman SM, Olney JW. Excitotoxicity and the NMDA receptor--still lethal after eight years. Trends Neurosci 1995 Feb;18(2):57-8.

[27]   Dobbing J, Sands J. Comparative aspects of the brain growth spurt. Early Hum Dev 1979 Mar; 3(1): 79-83.

[28]   Thomas JD, Weinert SP, Sharif S, Riley EP. MK-801 administration during ethanol withdrawal in neonatal rat pups attenuates ethanol-induced behavioral deficits. Alcohol Clin Exp Res 1997; 21: 1218-25.

[29]   Thomas JD, Fleming SL, Riley EP. Administration of low doses of MK-801 during ethanol withdrawal in the developing rat pup attenuates alcohol's teratogenic effects. Alcohol Clin Exp Res 2002 Aug; 26(8) :1307-13.

[30]   Thomas JD, Fleming And SL, Riley EP. MK-801 can exacerbate or attenuate behavioral alterations associated with neonatal alcohol exposure in the rat, depending on the timing of administration. Alcohol Clin Exp Res 2001 May; 25(5): 764-73.

[31]   Thomas JD, Garcia GG, Dominguez HD, Riley EP. Administration of eliprodil during ethanol withdrawal in the neonatal rat attenuates ethanol-induced learning deficits. Psychopharmacology 2004;175:189-95.

[32]   Lewis B, Wellmann KA, Barron S. Agmatine reduces balance deficits in a rat model of third trimester binge-like ethanol exposure. Pharmacol Biochem Behav 2007 Nov; 88(1): 114-21.

[33]   Stepanyan TD, Farook JM, Kowalski A, Kaplan E, Barron S, Littleton JM. Alcohol withdrawal-induced hippocampal neurotoxicity *in vitro* and seizures *in vivo* are both reduced by memantine. Alcohol Clin Exp Res 2008 Dec; 32(12): 2128-35.

[34]   Druse MJ, Tajuddin NF, Gillespie RA, *et al.* The serotonin-1A agonist ipsapirone prevents ethanol-associated death of total rhombencephalic neurons and prevents the reduction of fetal serotonin neurons. Brain Res Dev Brain Res 2004 Jun 21; 150(2): 79-88.

[35]   Tajuddin NF, Druse MJ. Treatment of pregnant alcohol-consuming rats with buspirone: effects on serotonin and 5-hydroxyindoleacetic acid content in offspring. Alcohol Clin Exp Res 1993 Feb; 17(1): 110-4.

[36]   Kim JA, Druse MJ. Protective effects of maternal buspirone treatment on serotonin reuptake sites in ethanol-exposed offspring. Brain Res Dev Brain Res 1996 Apr 30; 92(2): 190-8.

[37]   Barclay DC, Hallbergson AF, Montague JR, Mudd LM. Reversal of ethanol toxicity in embryonic neurons with growth factors and estrogen. Brain Res Bull 2005 Nov 30; 67(6): 459-65.

[38]   Bonthius DJ, Karacay B, Dai D, Pantazis NJ. FGF-2, NGF and IGF-1, but not BDNF, utilize a nitric oxide pathway to signal neurotrophic and neuroprotective effects against alcohol toxicity in cerebellar granule cell cultures. Brain Res Dev Brain Res 2003 Jan 10; 140(1): 15-28.

[39]   Endres M, Toso L, Roberson R, *et al.* Prevention of alcohol-induced developmental delays and learning abnormalities in a model of fetal alcohol syndrome. Am J Obstet Gynecol 2005 Sep; 193(3 Pt 2): 1028-34.

[40]   Heaton MB, Paiva M, Swanson DJ, Walker DW. Modulation of ethanol neurotoxicity by nerve growth factor. Brain Res 1993 Aug 20; 620(1): 78-85.

[41]   Heaton MB, Mitchell JJ, Paiva M. Overexpression of NGF ameliorates ethanol neurotoxicity in the developing cerebellum. J Neurobiol 2000 Nov 5; 45(2): 95-104.

[42]   McAlhany RE, Jr., West JR, Miranda RC. Glial-derived neurotrophic factor (GDNF) prevents ethanol-induced apoptosis and JUN kinase phosphorylation. Brain Res Dev Brain Res 2000 Feb 7; 119(2): 209-16.

[43]   McGough NN, Thomas JD, Dominguez HD, Riley EP. Insulin-like growth factor-I mitigates motor coordination deficits associated with neonatal alcohol exposure in rats. Neurotoxicol Teratol 2009 Jan-Feb; 1(1): 40-8.

[44]   Dreosti IE. Nutritional factors underlying the expression of the fetal alcohol syndrome. Ann N Y Acad Sci1993 Mar 15; 678: 193-204.

[45]   Abel EL, Hannigan JH. Maternal risk factors in fetal alcohol syndrome: provocative and permissive influences. Neurotoxicol Teratol 1995 Jul-Aug; 17(4): 445-62.

[46]   Wiener SG, Shoemaker WJ, Koda LY, Bloom FE. Interaction of ethanol and nutrition during gestation: influence on maternal and offspring development in the rat. J Pharmacol Exp Ther 1981 Mar; 216(3):572-9.

[47]   Weinberg J, D'Alquen G, Bezio S. Interactive effects of ethanol intake and maternal nutritional status on skeletal development of fetal rats. Alcohol 1990 Sep-Oct; 7(5): 383-8.

[48]   Wainwright P, Fritz G. Effect of moderate prenatal ethanol exposure on postnatal brain and behavioral development in BALB/c mice. Exp Neurol 1985 Jul; 89(1): 237-49.

[49]   Shankar K, Hidestrand M, Liu X, *et al.* Physiologic and genomic analyses of nutrition-ethanol interactions during gestation: Implications for fetal ethanol toxicity. Exp Biol Med (Maywood) 2006 Sep;231(8):1379-97.

[50]   Thomas JD, Abou EJ, Dominguez HD. Prenatal choline supplementation mitigates the adverse effects of prenatal alcohol exposure on development in rats. Neurotox Teratol 2009 Sep-Oct; 31(5): 303-11.

[51]   Carey LC, Coyle P, Philcox JC, Rofe AM. Zinc supplementation at the time of ethanol exposure ameliorates teratogenicity in mice. Alcohol Clin Exp Res 2003 Jan; 27(1): 107-10.

[52]   Summers BL, Rofe AM, Coyle P. Prenatal zinc treatment at the time of acute ethanol exposure limits spatial memory impairments in mouse offspring. Pediatr Res 2006 Jan; 59(1): 66-71.

[53]   Chen WJ, Berryhill EC, West JR. Zinc supplementation does not attenuate alcohol-induced cerebellar Purkinje cell loss during the brain growth spurt period. Alcohol Clin Exp Res 2001 Apr; 25(4): 600-5.

[54]   Ieraci A, Herrera DG. Nicotinamide protects against ethanol-induced apoptotic neurodegeneration in the developing mouse brain. PLoS Med 2006 Apr; 3(4): e101.

[55]   Xu Y, Li Y, Tang Y, *et al.* The maternal combined supplementation of folic acid and Vitamin B(12) suppresses ethanol-induced developmental toxicity in mouse fetuses. Reprod Toxicol 2006 Jul; 22(1): 56-61.

[56]   Ilcol YO, Ozbek R, Hamurtekin E, Ulus IH. Choline status in newborns, infants, children, breast-feeding women, breast-fed infants and human breast milk. J Nutr Biochem 2005 Aug; 16(8): 489-99.

[57]   Zeisel SH. Dietary choline: biochemistry, physiology, and pharmacology. Annu Rev Nutr 1981; 1: 95-121.

[58]   McCann JC, Hudes M, Ames BN. An overview of evidence for a causal relationship between dietary availability of choline during development and cognitive function in offspring. Neurosci Biobehav Rev 2006; 30(5): 696-712.

[59]   Meck WH, Williams CL. Metabolic imprinting of choline by its availability during gestation: implications for memory and attentional processing across the lifespan. Neurosci Biobehav Rev 2003; 27:385-99.

[60]   Meck WH, Smith RA, Williams CL. Organizational changes in cholinergic activity and enhanced visuospatial memory as a function of choline administered prenatally or postnatally or both. Behav Neurosci 1989 Dec; 103(6): 1234-41.

[61]   Thomas JD, La Fiette MH, Quinn VR, Riley EP. Neonatal choline supplementation ameliorates the effects of prenatal alcohol exposure on a discrimination learning task in rats. Neurotoxicol Teratol 2000 Sep-Oct; 22(5): 03-11.

[62]   Thomas JD, Garrison M, O'Neill TM. Perinatal choline supplementation attenuates behavioral alterations associated with neonatal alcohol exposure in rats. Neurotoxicol Teratol 2004 Jan-Feb; 26(1): 35-45.

[63]   Wagner AF, Hunt PS. Impaired trace fear conditioning following neonatal ethanol: reversal by choline. Behav Neurosci 2006 Apr; 120(2): 482-7.

[64]   Thomas JD, Biane JS, O'Bryan KA, O'Neill TM, Dominguez HD. Choline supplementation following third-trimester-equivalent alcohol exposure attenuates behavioral alterations in rats. Behav Neurosci 2007 Feb; 121(1): 120-30.

[65]   Ryan SH, Williams JK, Thomas JD. Choline supplementation attenuates learning deficits associated with neonatal alcohol exposure in the rat: Effects of varying the timing of choline administration. Brain Res 2008 Oct 27; 1237: 91-100.

[66]   Schneider R, Dominguez HD, Thomas JD. Postnatal choline supplementation reduces working memory deficits in rats exposed to alcohol during development. Alcohol Clinic Exp Res 2008; 32: 138A.

[67]   Medina AE, Krahe TE, Ramoa AS. Restoration of neuronal plasticity by a phosphodiesterase type 1 inhibitor in a model of fetal alcohol exposure. J Neurosci 2006 Jan 18; 26(3): 1057-60.

[68]   Medina AE, Krahe TE. Neocortical plasticity deficits in fetal alcohol spectrum disorders: lessons from barrel and visual cortex. J Neurosci Res 2008 Feb 1; 86(2): 256-63.

[69]   Hannigan JH, O'Leary-Moore SK, Berman RF. Postnatal environmental or experiential amelioration of neurobehavioral effects of perinatal alcohol exposure in rats. Neurosci Biobehav Rev 2007; 31(2): 202-11.

[70]   Rosenzweig MR, Bennett EL. Psychobiology of plasticity: effects of training and experience on brain and behavior. Behav Brain Res 1996 Jun;78(1):57-65.

[71]   Sale A, Berardi N, Maffei L. Enrich the environment to empower the brain. Trends Neurosci 2009 Apr; 32(4): 233-9.

[72]   Hannigan JH, Berman RF, Zajac CS. Environmental enrichment and the behavioral effects of prenatal exposure to alcohol in rats. Neurotoxicol Teratol 1993; 15: 261-6.

[73]   Wainwright PE, Levesque S, Krempulee L, Bulman-Fleming B, McCutcheon D. Effects of environmental enrichment on cortical depth and Morris-maze performance in B6D2F2 mice exposed prenatally to ethanol. Neurotoxicol Teratol 1993; 15: 11-20.

[74]   Opitz B, Mothes HK, Clausing P. Effects of prenatal ethanol exposure and early experience on radial maze performance and conditioned taste aversion in mice. Neurotoxicol Teratol 1997 May-Jun; 19(3): 185-90.

[75]   Clausing P, Mothes HK, Opitz B. Preweaning experience as a modifier of prenatal drug effects in rats and mice--a review. Neurotoxicol Teratol 2000 Jan-Feb; 22(1): 113-23.

[76]   Choi IY, Allan AM, Cunningham LA. Moderate fetal alcohol exposure impairs the neurogenic response to an enriched environment in adult mice. Alcohol Clin Exp Res 2005 Nov; 29(11): 2053-62.

[77]   Berman RF, Hannigan JH, Sperry MA, Zajac CS. Prenatal alcohol exposure and the effects of environmental enrichment on hippocampal dendritic spine density. Alcohol 1996 Mar-Apr; 13(2): 209-16.

[78]   Klintsova AY, Cowell RM, Swain RA, Napper RM, Goodlett CR, Greenough WT. Therapeutic effects of complex motor training on motor performance deficits induced by neonatal binge-like alcohol exposure in rats. I. Behavioral results. Brain Res 1998 Jul 27; 800(1) :48-61.

[79]   Klintsova AY, Scamra C, Hoffman M, Napper RM, Goodlett CR, Greenough WT. Therapeutic effects of complex motor training on motor performance deficits induced by neonatal binge-like alcohol exposure in rats: II. A quantitative stereological study of synaptic plasticity in female rat cerebellum. Brain Res 2002 May 24; 937(1-2): 3-93.

[80]   Christie BR, Swann SE, Fox CJ, *et al.* Voluntary exercise rescues deficits in spatial memory and long-term potentiation in prenatal ethanol-exposed male rats. Eur J Neurosci 2005 Mar; 21(6): 1719-26.

[81]   Redila VA, Olson AK, Swann SE, *et al.* Hippocampal cell proliferation is reduced following prenatal ethanol exposure but can be rescued with voluntary exercise. Hippocampus 2006; 16(3): 305-11.

[82]   Thomas JD, Sather TM, Whinery LA. Voluntary exercise influences behavioral development in rats exposed to alcohol during the neonatal brain growth spurt. Behav Neurosci 2008 Dec; 122(6): 1264-73.

[83]   O'Connor MJ, Frankel F, Paley B, *et al.* A controlled social skills training for children with fetal alcohol spectrum disorders. J Consult Clin Psychol 2006 Aug; 74(4): 639-48.

[84]   Kable JA, Coles CD, Taddeo E. Socio-cognitive habilitation using the math interactive learning experience program for alcohol-affected children. Alcohol Clinic Exp Res 2007; 31(8): 1425-2434.

[85]   O'Malley KD. Pathophysiology of ADHD in patients with ADHD and fetal alcohol spectrum disorders: The role of medication in ADHD and Fetal Alcohol Spectrum Disorders (FASD): Nova Science Publishers 2007.

[86]   Burd L, Christensen T. Treatment of fetal alcohol spectrum disorders: are we ready yet? J Clinic Psychopharmacol 2009 Feb; 29(1): 1-4.

[87]   Zimmerberg B, Weston IIE. Postnatal stress of early weaning exacerbates behavioral outcome in prenatal alcohol-exposed juvenile rats. Pharmacol Biochem Behav 2002 Aug; 73(1): 45-52.

[88]   Streissguth AP, Barr HM, Kogan J, Bookstein FL. Understanding the Occurrence of Secondary Disabilities in Clients with Fetal Alcohol Syndrome (FAS) and Fetal Alcohol Effects (FAE). Seattle: University of Washington, Fetal Alcohol & Drug Unit; 1996 August 1996. Report No.: 96-06.

CHAPTER 3

FASD: Diagnostic Dilemmas and Challenges for a Modern Transgenerational Management Approach

Natalie Novick Brown[1,*], Kieran O'Malley[2] and Ann P. Streissguth[1]

[1]Fetal Alcohol and Drug Unit, Department of Psychiatry and Behavioral Sciences School of Medicine, University of Washington, Box 359112, Seattle, Washington, 98195-9112, USA and [2]Lucena Clinic, Child Adolescent Mental Health Service (CAMHS), Exchange Hall, Tallaght, Dublin 24, Ireland

> *May the enduring spirit of Michael Dorris light the evolution of our understanding*
>
> **Kieran O'Malley**

Abstract: For approximately 40 years, Fetal Alcohol Spectrum Disorders (FASD) has been defined consistently in terms of three diagnostic features in the presence of prenatal alcohol exposure: two physical criteria (*i.e.,* dysmorphic face and growth deficits) and central nervous system dysfunction (structural, neurological, and/or functional). Despite this relatively long and intact diagnostic history, identifying FASD has been difficult historically due to the complexity of presenting symptoms, varied handling by different diagnostic schemes, need for multidisciplinary assessment, and the masking of neurodevelopmental symptoms behind psychiatric diagnoses ("co-occurring disorders"). The objectives of this chapter are threefold: (1) to summarize diagnostic schema and characteristics of children and adults with FASD; (2) to increase awareness of some of the diagnostic challenges that currently exist in FASD assessment, particularly in terms of co-occurring disorders; and (3) to recommend a model standard of multidisciplinary assessment and multimodal treatment that may be useful to professionals in the clinical setting.

HISTORICAL OVERVIEW

Fetal Alcohol Syndrome (FAS) was initially described by Lemoine and colleagues in a regional French medical publication [1]. It was independently re-discovered in Seattle, Washington [2,3], by medical researchers who reported similar physical and growth anomalies and central nervous system (CNS) disorders in a small group of children born to alcoholic mothers. The early diagnoses were made by dysmorphologists who were experts in birth defects and physical anomalies, many of which had genetic origins, but some also derived from environmental etiologies [4]. Early on, FAS was identified by characteristic physical anomalies (particularly of the face), growth deficiency, and some central nervous system deficits. Shortly before his death, David W. Smith made a plea for recognition of a wider spectrum of offspring damage caused by prenatal alcohol exposure, which he termed "Fetal Alcohol Effects" (FAE) [5]. Sixteen years later, the Institute of Medicine (IOM) studied FAS and came up with a new term "Alcohol Related Neurodevelopmental Disorders" (ARND) to describe persons who did not have the full FAS but had behaviors shown to be associated with prenatal alcohol exposure that could have been caused by prenatal alcohol exposure [6]. More recently, the term "Fetal Alcohol Spectrum Disorders" (FASD) was designated as an umbrella term describing the range of effects than can occur in an individual whose mother drank alcohol during pregnancy. These effects may include physical, mental, behavioral, and/or learning disabilities with possible lifelong implications. The term FASD is not intended for use as a clinical diagnosis, according to the "Consensus Statement on FASD" (April 7, 2004) agreed upon by representatives of the lead agencies in the field (National Institute on Alcohol Abuse & Alcoholism (NIAAA); Centers for Disease Control and Prevention (CDC); National Organization on Fetal Alcohol Syndrome (NOFAS); Substance Abuse and Mental Health Services Administration (SAMHSA), including Center for Substance Abuse Prevention (CSAP); and several FAS scientists) [7]. (The term FASD had been used earlier by Streissguth and colleagues) [8]. The term "Partial Fetal Alcohol Syndrome" (PFAS) has been used more recently by dysmorphologists to identify children in epidemiologic studies [9], as has a similar term: "incomplete Fetal Alcohol Syndrome" [10].

*****Address correspondence to Natalie Novick Brown:** Dept. of Psychiatry & Behavioral Sciences, Box 359112, University of Washington, Seattle, Washington, 98195, USA; E-mail: fstnat@yahoo.com

Susan A. Adubato and Deborah E. Cohen (Eds)

The dysmorphology approach to identifying FAS has been effective in clinical settings where there are adequate numbers of dysmorphologists, geneticists, and specially trained pediatricians, as well as in epidemiological studies where experienced dysmorphologists trained local pediatricians to diagnose FAS (eg, South Africa [11], Italy [12], Russia [13], and with Native Americans [14]). Hoyme and colleagues [15] expanded the IOM guidelines by setting specific criteria for the facial features, growth deficiency, and brain/head circumference criteria in FAS and Partial FAS, as well as defining ARND from a practical standpoint. The intent was that these proposed revisions would provide criteria useful for clinical pediatric practice. However, the lack of adequate dysmorphology/genetic coverage for identifying and diagnosing patients with FASD of various ages led to another diagnostic system, which presumably could train teams of evaluators to evaluate and make recommendations for patients with FASD conditions within a given community using a 4-digit code [16]. Currently, both systems are in use, but to this date, many children with FAS still are never identified, and they and their communities suffer as a result.

As more children and adults with FASD were identified, it became apparent that there was a very wide range of intellectual functioning among patients with this diagnosis [17] and that, in general, there was a relationship between severity of physical findings and intellectual deficiency.

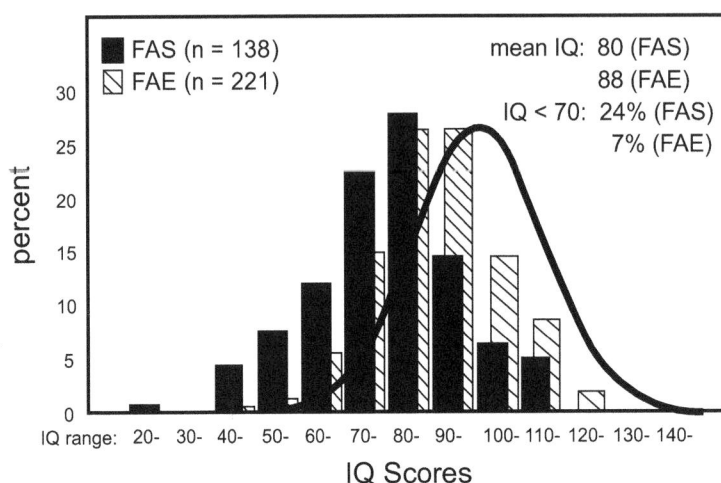

Figure 1: IQ scores in FASD from Streissguth *et al.* 2004 (JDBP).

Fig. **1** [17] shows an IQ distribution of 359 patients diagnosed with FAS or FAE by dysmorphologists. As shown, patients identified with FAE had somewhat higher IQ scores in general than those identified as FAS (FAE mean IQ=88 vs. FAS mean IQ=80), but the overlap was considerable. As the usual cutoff score for developmental disability services is an IQ < 70 in conjunction with other deficits in adaptive functioning, it is clear that only 24% of this large group of patients diagnosed by dysmorphologists with full FAS would easily obtain services in their communities based on their intellectual disability, and only 7% of those with FAE would so qualify. Despite their apparent developmental disabilities, it is clear that patients with FASD are not, as a group, distinguishable by their intellectual disability.

Despite the utility of dysmorphological signs and IQ tests as a means of describing patients with FAS, these two "yardsticks" have seldom served as a basis for understanding the full impact of prenatal alcohol on the developing offspring, particularly across the age span. The first large scale study of 61 adolescents and adults with FASD [17] found that the faces were less distinctive after puberty, but the patients tended to remain short and microcephalic, although their weight became somewhat closer to the mean with increasing age, and a few were frankly obese. Average intellectual functioning was at the second-to fourth-grade level, with arithmetic deficits the most characteristic learning disability. Maladaptive behaviors such as poor judgment, distractibility, and difficulty perceiving social cues were common. Family environments were remarkably unstable: 69% of the birth mothers were known to be deceased. Of the many behavioral adjustment scales evaluated, the Vineland Adaptive Behavior Scales (VABS) was most effective in terms of measuring FASD functional deficits. The 24 diagnosed patients who received the VABS had a mean chronological age of 17 years and were functioning in general at the 7-year old level. This first study of adolescents and adults with FAS concluded that "Fetal Alcohol Syndrome is not just a childhood disorder: there is a predictable long-term progression of the disorder into adulthood, in which maladaptive behaviors present the greatest challenge to management" [17].

CO-OCCURRING DISORDERS

In a larger study focused on "secondary disabilities" (problems that presumably patients were not born with but appeared as life course problems as they matured), 415 patients with FAS/FAE were examined, (median IQ = 86, IQ range from 29-126) [18,19]. Life span prevalence of "Disrupted school experiences" was 61%; "Trouble with the law" was 60%; "Confinement in detention, jail, prison, or a psychiatric or alcohol/drug inpatient setting" was 50%; "Repeated inappropriate sexual behaviors" was 49%; and "Alcohol/drug problems" was 35%. Over 90% of these patients displayed co-occurring mental health disorders. The home lives of these patients were not stellar: 80% were not raised by their biological mothers, and 72% were reported to have experienced sexual or physical abuse. In this large study, the patients ranged in age from children to adults. Those with FAS had an average IQ of 78, while their average Composite standard score on the VABS Adaptive Behavior Scale was 61. A similar discrepancy held for those with FAE: average IQ was 90, but average Adaptive Behavior Composite was 67. The Adaptive Behavior Composite score is often a better predictor of life course outcomes than the IQ score. Recent follow-up studies of patients with FASD in Germany describe adolescents and adults not unlike ours but who display almost a total absence of "Trouble with the law", presumably due to the stronger social net, and better training programs and living situations that are available for persons with disabilities [20,21]. In one of the first studies of FAS among youth in the criminal justice system, Fast and colleagues in British Columbia found that 23% could be diagnosed with FASD [22].

Secondary disabilities and co-occurring disorders in patients with FASD should be considered in light of not only the brain damage caused by the prenatal alcohol which are documented in many studies [23-29] but also the environmental circumstances often accompanying female alcoholism. In one large study by Streissguth and colleagues [18,19,30] in which mothers, parents, or caretakers of 415 patients with FAS/FAE were queried about a variety of behavioral problems, by far the most prevalent problems reported were mental health conditions. Over 90% of these 415 patients diagnosed with FAS or FAE had been to a mental health provider for help, with the proportion remaining the same across three age groups: children, adolescents and adults. Attention deficit problems were the most prevalent condition among children and adolescents (60%), while Depression was the most prevalent mental health disorder among adults (52%).

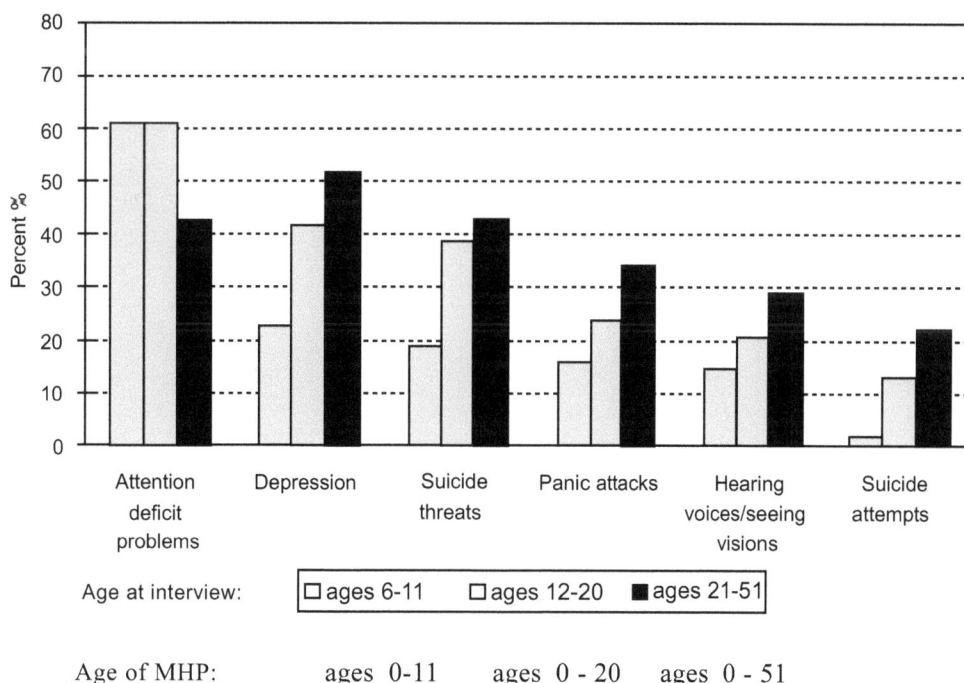

Figure 2: From Streissguth *et al.* 1996 Secondary Disabilities Report to the CDC.

Fig. **2** [18] shows the most prevalent mental health problems for each of the three age groups [18,31] found a similarly high rate of mental health disorders among 62 adults with FASD: 92% had a mental health diagnosis, including 65% with ADHD, 45% with depression, and 21% with panic disorder. This preponderance of mental health problems among adult patients with FAS was first reported by Lemoine [32] in their remarkable 30-year follow-up of Lemoine's original child patients. As adults, these former patients were not located in their familial homes or in institutions for the intellectually disabled but were found most characteristically in psychiatric residential care facilities.

As part of the first "secondary disabilities" study [18], data were obtained on 90 adults who were at least 21 years of age (median age: 26 years) at the time of the study. Only seven of these 90 lived independently and without employment problems. Adults with FAE had as high a rate of "Dependent Living" as those with FAS, despite having generally higher IQ scores. However, those with FAE had a lower rate of "Problems with Employment", which may reflect their higher IQ level. Caregivers reported that over 80% of these adults with FAS/FAE had difficulty managing money, and over 80% had "poor judgment." Nearly 80% had difficulty making decisions, approximately 80% had poor organizational skills, and around 55% had trouble with interpersonal relations. All of these impairments involve deficient executive functioning.

In these long-term studies of large numbers of diagnosed patients with FASD, it is clear that co-occurring disorders, particularly those involving mental illness, present great obstacles to appropriate treatment. For example, as psychiatric disorders are more readily diagnosed than FASD, the most likely scenario is that the psychiatric diagnosis is observed and diagnosed and thus becomes the primary diagnosis in determining treatment. However, as patients with FASD are likely to have more significant problems with adaptive behaviors than psychiatric patients without FASD, failure to consider their FASD can be a major detriment to effective treatment, particularly in the adolescent and adult years. Even for children, recognition of their FASD is important, as more effective family-based interventions can be implemented during the early years (see Carmichael Olson and Montague chapter). Regardless of the patient's age, failure of psychiatric treatment to take into account the FASD condition can easily result in treatment failures and lost opportunities.

Although longitudinal studies suggest that individuals with FASD are at high risk for adverse life course outcomes such as mental health problems and poor social adjustment, the long-term effects of FASD are not well known outside the research community. Mental health professionals are not routinely trained in FASD, and medical students receive only superficial training unless they specialize in pediatrics, gynecology/obstetrics, dysmorphology, or genetics. The situation is worse in the lay population. Many women continue to drink alcohol during pregnancy or when they might become pregnant despite a long-standing public health advisory urging them to abstain. In fact, recent national survey data found that 10 percent of pregnant women reported alcohol consumption at some point during their pregnancy, with 2 percent reporting binge drinking or frequent use of alcohol [33]. Each year, more than 40,000 infants continue to be born with FASD, which is equivalent to 1 percent of all live births [34]. Total annual cost to the U.S. economy for FAS alone is estimated at $3.6 billion, and annual lifetime cost per affected individual due to health, social, and justice system costs plus indirect costs (lost productivity due to mortality, morbidity, disability, and/or incarceration/career crime) is estimated at $2 million or more [35]. Reports suggest that individuals with FASD are over-represented in psychiatric samples [36] and in juvenile detention and correctional settings [22,37].

DIAGNOSTIC DILEMMAS

Despite the enormous personal and societal costs of FASD, the effects of prenatal alcohol exposure have been very difficult and expensive to diagnose and treat. Because the broad cognitive-behavioral sequelae of FASD are not well understood, FASD symptoms may be overlooked and misdiagnosed as one or more co-occurring disorders. For example, in childhood the attention deficits and hyperkinetic activity often associated with FASD may be diagnosed by medical doctors as Attention-Deficit/Hyperactivity Disorder (ADHD) and treated with standard stimulant medications, often with only modest success. Mood dysregulation due to FASD-associated deficits in self-soothing ability may result in a Bipolar Disorder diagnosis that gets treated with mood stabilizers, typically with little beneficial result. Although progress has been made in terms of measuring the physical manifestations of FASD (e.g., 2-D and 3-D facial modeling, brain imaging), and research is currently underway to detect biomarkers, relatively little effort has focused on refining diagnostic assessment of co-occurring conditions that frequently mask the underlying medical condition. This is especially problematic for ARND, which may have as severe an impact on neurodevelopmental and adaptive functioning as FAS and PFAS [8,18] but which lacks the overt physical markers that provide an etiological clue to the FAS. In fact, even in FAS, with its characteristic face and growth deficit and almost 40 years of research and thousands of publications in medical journals, only 62 percent of pediatricians recently felt prepared to identify the condition, 50 percent felt prepared to diagnose it, and only 34 percent felt prepared to manage and coordinate the treatment of children with FASD [38].

The diagnosis and, ultimately, treatment and management of people affected by prenatal alcohol exposure have been complicated for many years by the lack of appropriate neuropsychiatric diagnostic formulation. In fact, some have described this state of affairs as a "crisis" [8]. Although as noted above, FASD tended to be diagnosed in the past by medical specialists trained in diagnosing childhood dysmorphic conditions, the process began to change in the late 1990s following the IOM's publication of an FASD diagnostic manual [6], which specified neurodevelopmental and neurocognitive deficits as well as the familiar physical abnormalities. Thus, it became evident with this publication that FASD diagnosis should involve mental health as well as medical practitioners. A medical doctor is necessary to assess the physical manifestations of FASD (including structural brain damage and associated neurological dysfunction as well as facial abnormalities and growth deficit) and rule out other diagnostic possibilities, and mental health expertise is necessary to assess central nervous system dysfunction (*i.e.*, functional deficits). Ideally for children, multidisciplinary teams should include other developmental specialties as well (e.g., speech and language, social work, occupational and physical therapy, family and behavioral therapy, education).

As noted earlier in this chapter, FASD nomenclature has long been a source of lay confusion. Until the IOM's diagnostic publication in the mid-1990s, FASD conditions that did not meet criteria for FAS were called Fetal Alcohol Effect(s), Possible or Partial FAS, or sometimes, static encephalopathy/alcohol exposed. With the identification by the IOM of five discrete conditions under the FASD umbrella, specific terminology was introduced (and one could say, "standardized") for two conditions that met some but not all of the physical criteria for FAS (*i.e.*, Partial FAS and ARND). It is noteworthy that the IOM did not distinguish between these two conditions and FAS in terms of severity of central nervous system dysfunction, which was consistent with the research. [8,18] Although the IOM criteria were an improvement, they contained only general parameters regarding diagnosis in each category. For example, exact parameters for the growth deficit and dysmorphic facial features were not defined for each diagnostic category. In addition, a specific cognitive-behavioral phenotype associated with the central nervous system dysfunction was not provided except for the general notation of a "complex pattern of behavioral or cognitive difficulties." Finally, there were no guidelines for assessment of family and genetic history as well as maternal drinking.

In response to the above diagnostic ambiguities, Astley and Clarren [16] developed a more objective set of diagnostic criteria, commonly referred to as either the "4-Digit Code" (because of the measurement system) or the "Washington criteria" (because they were formulated through reviews of the medical records of 1014 children with FAS in the Washington State Fetal Alcohol Syndrome Diagnostic and Prevention Network). (See Astley chapter.) Although the 4-Digit Code is extremely precise in that it places a child into an FASD diagnostic category based on a specific measurement metric, the myriad diagnostic categories (256 in number) are thought by some to be confusing, even for FASD professionals and therefore impractical for use in clinical practice [15], although the system is routinely used to diagnose patients in the FAS Diagnostic and Prevention Network in Washington State (**http://depts.washington.edu/fasdpn/htmls/4-digit-code.htm**). One of the most positive and important aspects of the 4-Digit Code is its objective definition and quantification of diagnostic criteria, including the facial phenotype [39], which goes far beyond previous "gestalt" methods. Another benefit in terms of diagnostic accuracy is the 4-Digit Code also requires that all other adverse prenatal and postnatal events be documented as they are additional risk factors which must be taken into consideration when developing diagnostic and intervention plans.

A problem with the 4 Digit-Digit Code as well as the IOM protocol and other diagnostic guidelines that have been developed is their focus on only three specific dysmorphic conditions of the face, while for many years patients with FAS have been described as having many other dysmorphic and dysfunctional conditions of the body as well. For example in a diagnostic method used to screen grade school children in Africa, Italy, and a few towns in the U.S. for "active case ascertainment," an experienced dysmorphologist has trained local pediatricians to diagnose children using a more traditional exam including hands, arms, ears, and heart as well as face. Training has reportedly not only been quite simple and accurate but produces a far higher rate of children with FAS or PFAS compared to the clinical case method [40]. Following a similar training program in Russian orphanages and boarding schools, Jones [41] concluded that after a 2-day training session with two dysmorphologists, the four pediatricians were "reasonably accurate in diagnosing FAS on the basis of physical features and in recognizing most of the selected specific features associated with the disorder."

Eventually, the diagnostic process for FAS was refined in 2004 by the CDC [33], which published precise criteria and recommended multidisciplinary assessment. However, diagnostic specifications were excluded in this publication for conditions that did not meet the full facial and growth criteria for FAS (*i.e.*, PFAS and ARND). These omissions left the IOM publication in 1996 as the only government-endorsed guidelines in the United States that specifically addressed PFAS and ARND. To further confuse (or perhaps improve?) the situation, another set of guidelines [42] was published in Canada a year after the CDC guidelines were issued. The Canadian guidelines also advocated multidisciplinary diagnosis and covered the full spectrum of FASD disorders, but they included more stringent criteria for the medical definition of "abnormal" (*i.e.*, a threshold of 2 or more standard deviations below the mean rather than 1 or the 10th percentile), similar to the 4-Digit Code.

Ultimately, the CDC publication may have affected the standard of care in the United States with respect to diagnosing PFAS and ARND as well as FAS since it is unknown at the outset of an FASD assessment whether the individual will eventually meet criteria for full FAS or for another condition under the FASD umbrella. Thus, best practice in the United States is now considered multidisciplinary assessment using either the diagnostic classifications and general criteria described in 1996 by the IOM [15,43], further informed by the specific measurement guidelines for FAS described by the CDC [33] or the 4-Digit Code. The benefit from using the CDC guidelines with *any* FASD diagnosis under the IOM classification scheme is their improved clarification for all four of the diagnostic criteria, regardless of the ultimate FASD diagnosis. The benefit from using the 4-Digit Code is a greater degree of clarity and diagnostic precision across all potential FASD conditions.

With the publication of FASD criteria in two government publications that illuminate the cognitive-behavioral as well as the physical aspects of FASD along with a diagnostic standard of care involving a multidisciplinary team, the next issue is how to communicate the diagnosis and associated co-occurring disorders within the medical and mental health communities. Two diagnostic treatises are commonly used to communicate diagnostic findings: International Classification of Diseases (ICD), published by the World Health Organization [44], and the Diagnostic and Statistical Manual (DSM), published by the American Psychiatric Association. The ICD is now in its tenth edition (ICD-10), and the DSM is now in its fourth edition with a Text Revision (DSM-IV-TR) [45]. The international manual is used for both medical and mental health diagnoses; the DSM-IV-TR is used solely for mental health diagnoses. Both are necessary for communicating the complex deficits and conditions associated with FASD, but these classification systems present problems with respect to FASD diagnosis because they are outdated.

The ICD-10, published in 1992, lists "Fetal Alcohol Syndrome (dysmorphic)" (Q86.0) as a specific medical diagnosis under a section on congenital malformations. Thus, there is no dispute that an FAS diagnosis is a medical condition that belongs with other medical conditions on axis III in a complete diagnostic formulation. However, the ICD-10 is silent on PFAS and ARND. Since both of these conditions are also associated with brain damage and CNS structural, neurological, and functional problems, it is common practice to diagnose these conditions on axis III as with FAS.

DIAGNOSING CO-OCCURRING DISORDERS

Because of multiple deficits in basic abilities necessary for effective adaptive functioning, children and adults with FASD do best in settings where life is predictable and structured, expectations are clear and reasonable, and they have appropriate role models and are treated with respect and understanding [8]. In fact, it is well established that the quality and stability of the childhood home environment is the single most important factor in the ultimate outcome of those with FASD [43]. When children with FASD are not in such settings, they can easily develop co-occurring mental disorders as well as other secondary disabilities because of primary deficits in skills (*i.e.*, adaptive and executive functioning) that affect ability to self-regulate and cope. For example, in a classic resiliency study beginning in infancy, children who were found to be the least resilient across their lifetimes were those born to alcoholic mothers [46]. Such children experience both the prenatal and the postnatal consequences of the mother's alcohol problems.

Adverse environmental conditions may interact with central nervous system dysfunction in FASD to produce "secondary" disabilities or negative outcomes of significant proportions, including mental health problems [8,18]. This interaction between FASD and negative environment has been called a "double jeopardy" effect by Olson and colleagues [43]. Capable diagnostic protocol involves identifying both the underlying medical condition and the residual effects of environmental influences from the individual's past (e.g., malnutrition, maltreatment, stress and fear, neglect, abuse), which may have triggered enduring biological changes and cognitive-behavioral sequelae of their own [47] that are superimposed on whatever brain damage the individual was born with due to prenatal alcohol exposure.

Because they are medical conditions, FASD is not included in the DSM-IV-TR, and since FASD conditions are not listed as psychiatric diagnoses, they are often ignored by mental health professionals [8]. Moreover, the symptom presentations of individuals with FASD appear similar to what is seen in a number of psychiatric disorders. These problems are compounded by the high prevalence of mental disorders in the FASD population plus a variety of cognitive-behavioral phenotypes where deficits are not always apparent. Other than noting the importance of underlying general medical conditions in differential diagnosis, the DSM-IV-TR does not specifically note prenatal alcohol exposure as an etiological possibility for many of the mental health disorders associated with FASD except for Learning Disorders. This omission of the mental health sequelae of FASD in the DSM has long been decried by professionals in the field [8,43].

It is particularly noteworthy that the DSM-IV-TR's differential diagnostic guidelines omit specific reference to prenatal alcohol exposure as an etiological possibility in "Cognitive Disorder Not Otherwise Specified (NOS)," which besides learning disorders and Attention-Deficit/Hyperactivity Disorder is the condition that best captures some of the core co-occurring mental conditions often associated with FASD. Thus, the only way to achieve diagnostic clarity with respect to mental health conditions associated with prenatal alcohol exposure is for well-trained diagnosticians to note specifically the underlying medical condition if an FASD has been diagnosed (e.g., Cognitive Disorder NOS, secondary to FAS) or confirmed exposure itself if an FASD has not been diagnosed (e.g., Cognitive Disorder NOS, alcohol exposed). Although the DSM-IV-TR does not provide explicit decision-tree guidelines for each and every mental health diagnosis in the manual, it does clarify a differential diagnosis process to be used prior to making *any* mental health diagnosis from the DSM-IV-TR when an underlying medical condition may account for the mental health symptoms:

> "When a Mental Disorder Due to a General Medical Condition or a Substance-Abuse Induced Disorder is responsible for the symptoms, it preempts the diagnosis of the corresponding primary disorder with the same symptoms" [45p.6].

Among the most common misdiagnoses and co-occurring mental conditions in children with FASD are the following:

- Attention-Deficit/Hyperactivity Disorder
- Autistic Disorder
- Asperger's Disorder
- substance use disorders
- psychotic disorders
- Major Depressive Disorder
- Bipolar Disorder
- Generalized Anxiety Disorder
- Separation Anxiety Disorder
- Reactive Attachment Disorder
- Posttraumatic Stress Disorder
- Traumatic Brain Injury
- Intermittent Explosive Disorder
- Conduct Disorder
- Oppositional Defiant Disorder.

In adults with FASD, some of the most frequently seen misdiagnoses include:

- mood conditions

- psychotic disorders

- personality disorders (e.g., Antisocial Personality Disorder, Borderline Personality Disorder, Personality Disorder Not Otherwise Specified).

Because of the virtual absence of FASD training in medical schools and graduate programs, the behavioral problems commonly associated with FASD confuse even the most meticulous diagnosticians. Even if genetic endowment plays a role in symptom expression, social service and mental health professionals are trained to view the parenting and social environments as the most likely source of "bad" or atypical behavior, with the individual (child or adult) having some degree of self-control over his or her conduct and mental health. Often overlooked are the broad underlying central nervous system deficits that may diminish personal competence. However, as the charts below indicate, even though behavior may superficially resemble symptom presentation, the underlying dynamics that prompted the behavior may stem from something entirely different.

Diagnosing FASD, ADHD, and Conduct Disorder

FASD	ADHD	Conduct Disorder
Steals ■ Boundary confusion	Steals ■ Acting on urge	Steals ■ Entitlement
Hits others ■ Someone told him to ■ Misinterpreted other's behavior ■ Modeling caregiver's abuse	Hits others ■ Impulsive act	Hits others ■ Intentional act
Takes risks ■ Doesn't perceive danger	Takes risks ■ Minimizes danger	Takes risks ■ Feels omnipotent

Treating FASD, ADHD, and Conduct Disorder

FASD	ADHD	Conduct Disorder
Provide case management, mentor, systematic behavioral modifcation (e.g, repetitive role playing)	Behavioral approaches, medication	Targeted psychotherapy, environmental modification

Figure 3: Differential Diagnosis and Treatment: FASD, ADHD, Conduct Disorder.

As depicted in Fig. **3**, etiology is very important. In the case of FASD, etiology may have a significant impact on treatment planning, course, and ultimately, prognosis [8,48]. In fact, using a superficial approach to symptom identification while ignoring etiology and differential diagnosis may have far-reaching ramifications, such as unemployment, psychiatric hospitalization, loss of family, homelessness, criminal conduct, incarceration, or death (by suicide, accident, murder, untreated physical illness, or jury verdict). Consequently, best practice in terms of diagnosis involves investigating the confluence of both biological and environmental factors in an individual's clinical presentation [49,50] and noting the underlying medical condition (or likely condition, if one is suspected) whenever there are deficits in basic primary abilities such as attention, learning, cognition, self-soothing, and adaptive and executive functioning. As noted in the DSM-IV-TR (p. 6), for disorders that may involve interactions between cognitive-behavioral abilities and environmental traumas (e.g., child conduct disorders, impulse control disorders, and adult personality disorders), an FASD may even *preempt* an Axis I or II diagnosis, especially in cases where environmental problems are minimal or nonexistent [45]. Alternatively, FASD (with its impairments in adaptive and executive functioning) may *compound and escalate* the negative effects that a bad environment has on an individual's behavior, due to biologically-created resiliency deficits. For example, with respect to the large numbers of individuals with FASD who have trouble with the law, a number of researchers [22,51,52] suggest that this problem may stem in large part from an interaction between an adverse environment and FASD-associated primary disabilities in learning, socialization and executive functioning. In other words, the presence of primary disabilities *beyond the individual's control* undermines his or her ability to withstand negative environmental influences, thereby diminishing personal culpability for bad acts. Obviously, accurate differential diagnosis in such situations requires careful attention to environmental antecedents as well as the underlying medical condition and other etiological factors.

Many if not most co-occurring mental health problems stem from impairments in primary neurocognitive abilities. For example, deficient self-regulation may first emerge in affected infants as a biological deficit in emotion modulation. Later, this deficit may manifest as the child's inability to calm herself when frustrated. Still later, she may develop what appear to be anxiety or mood symptoms in adolescence or adulthood. Although the outward symptoms may be identical to those listed in the DSM-IV-TR for anxiety and mood disorder diagnoses, she may fail to respond well to standard medications and psychotherapy treatment because structural brain damage underlies her symptoms. Another example is a child with hyperkinesis who is unable to sit still in class and focus on his teacher. While he may appear to meet criteria for ADHD, the fact that his symptoms are due to FASD-associated deficits in sensory integration and self-regulation abilities may be very relevant to his treatment and prognosis as well as his diagnosis.

If the co-occurring mental health conditions in individuals with FASD are due to multiple neurodevelopmental deficits as well as environmental stressors, it might be expected that they would be phenotypically different than those without FASD. For example, in a study of children with ADHD, those who also had FASD demonstrated significantly weaker social cognition and emotion-processing ability than those without FASD [53]. These researchers reported a distinct behavioral profile for children with FASD and concluded that problems in social cognition and emotion processing may contribute to the higher incidence of social behavioral problems in children with both ADHD and FASD.

If children with FASD are not diagnosed accurately in early childhood and subsequently provided with positive, structured, and nurturing environments where their deficits are addressed with consistent and coordinated supportive services and behavior modification, it is *predictable* as they progress through life that they will develop one or more co-occurring mental health disorders [8,18,19]. Often, by the time a child with an undiagnosed FASD reaches adulthood, he or she has a history of multiple diagnoses, many of which may be inaccurate or incomplete. Not only is development of co-occurring mental health problems in FASD predictable, it also is *sequential*. Brain damage impairs basic neurocognitive abilities which are seen during school years as deficits in attention, information processing, cognition, learning, and memory (*i.e.*, primary disabilities). Normally in adolescence, as external environmental structure (e.g., family, school) diminishes, internal executive and adaptive abilities become increasingly important for successful, pro-social transition to adulthood. However, those with behavior control problems, such as individuals with an undiagnosed FASD, often receive mental health diagnoses that connote *volitional* self-control problems (e.g., conduct disorders, impulse control disorders). By adulthood, individuals with FASD may be diagnosed with one or more personality disorders because their behavioral abnormalities and maladjustment are seen as characterological as well as volitional.

In general, if there are impairments in multiple primary abilities, there is an inadequate foundation for resiliency and ability to cope adequately with negative life experiences. It is little wonder that children with FASD who experience traumatic environmental experiences are less able than unimpaired peers to deal effectively with those traumas. In fact, youth with undiagnosed FASD and inaccurately or incompletely diagnosed co-occurring disorders not only have "double jeopardy" [43] due to an interaction between their FASD condition and adverse childhood environment, they also have a triple handicap when their FASD and co-occurring disorders have not been correctly identified and addressed. By adulthood, these individuals have had to tackle developmental challenges within the framework of multiple cognitive-behavioral impairments with no supportive services to assist or buffer them, and they also must deal with misattributions (and perhaps misdiagnoses) by professionals that suggest they are wholly or mostly to blame for their secondary disabilities. Since many individuals with FASD often pass through the trials and tribulations of life without an accurate diagnosis, they enter adulthood and even parenthood without an appreciation of their underlying medical condition and their psychiatric disorders and socialization deficits. This situation is confusing and often overwhelming to the 70 to 75% of patients with FASD who have normal IQs [8,18,50,54]. "Oh, is THAT what I have?"; gasped an adolescent girl with obvious relief, when we discussed her FAS diagnosis with her for the first time.

IMPORTANCE OF EARLY NURTURING ENVIRONMENT

Infants born with prenatal exposure to alcohol come from differing social environments that modulate the effects of that exposure. For example, infants born to mothers who are depressed and also drink during pregnancy have vulnerability for psychiatric disorders which begin with an immediate impairment of primary attachment. This maternal depression may be due to biological/familial or environmental reasons (such as previous physical or sexual abuse) and should be monitored by a mental health professional. These infants and young children not only show a legacy of organic brain damage from prenatal alcohol but may enter an emotionally disconnected world as well due to familial mental illness where a parent is emotionally unavailable for active parenting.

One patient, a 28-year-old married Caucasian mother ("ZK") suffering from depression drank steadily throughout pregnancy. She could not cope with her infant who had ARND (quantified by structural brain anomalies on cranial ultrasound). The infant presented with a "Difficult to Settle Temperament" including many problems in sensory integration. The mother could not breast feed because the infant had a poor sucking reflex. However, it was explained to her that this was not "her fault" but rather a recognized neurological consequence of prenatal alcohol exposure. She was actively managed by a combination of adult mental health support, health visitor (public health nurse) support, and child psychiatric consultation which included parent/infant dyad therapy.

Some alcohol-exposed infants may develop in utero within a violent, disorganized home setting. Sometimes this is reflective of the transgenerational cognitive legacy of alcohol, which impairs maternal and paternal organizational and emotional regulation abilities. Other times, it is simply the prevalence of domestic violence. Prenatal stress or PTSD in the pregnant mother has its own emotional and neurochemical sequelae on HPA axis function, which in turn has an impact on fetal brain development [55]. These are the situations where a referral to child protection services during pregnancy would be a safety and prophylactic measure for both mother and infant. Additionally, referral to long-term support services for mothers and babies, like the Parent Child Assistance Program (PCAP), headquartered in Seattle [56], have been shown to be effective in safeguarding infants and facilitating appropriate mother/child interactions.

A pregnant 18-year-old Caucasian teenager ("CD") binge drank during the first and second trimesters of pregnancy. When she entered Adolescent Psychiatric services in mid-pregnancy because she was feeling suicidal and had one serious self-harm cutting episode, she was diagnosed with ARND. CD had a clear history of prenatal alcohol exposure when she was born, with well-documented cognitive testing and school records attesting to a complex learning disability. Her pre-pregnancy personality involved a combination of ADHD and autistic-type features that had not responded to individual insight-orientated psychotherapy. She was estranged from the father of her baby, an illegal immigrant who had physically threatened and abused her in early pregnancy. Child protection services were contacted by the consulting Adolescent Psychiatrist, and they obtained a "No Contact Order" and informed the Government Asylum Seeking Agency, which provided information on the father's previous convictions for drug and violence offences in his home country. He was deported, and CD gave birth to an infant with no immediate features of FASD but with a health care team in support. CD did not know how to measure the milk for infant feeding nor how to store it but was trained by the Health Visitor (Public Health Nurse) in these basic mother-baby skills.

All alcohol-exposed infants are subsequently reared in environments that have a modulating effect one way or other on clinical expression of the neurotoxic effects of that exposure. In particular, a mother who drinks during pregnancy *and* suffers postpartum depression creates an immediate challenge to parent/infant bonding.

"EG" was a single Caucasian professional mother who gave birth to her first child at 35 years of age. Her boyfriend had abandoned her during early pregnancy, and she hid her weekend binge drinking from friends and family. Her obstetrician was not aware she was drinking during her pregnancy as assessment of prenatal drinking history was not part of standard clinical inquiry for patients of a certain social class. Her infant had problems in the neonatal period, and a full clinical evaluation showed FAS features. Later, the mother required hospitalization for acute Postpartum Depression which included some psychotic features.

She was carefully managed by an Adult Hospital Psychiatrist, but her child with FAS was taken into care because she was deemed an unfit mother due to her continuing alcohol abuse, and her child was seen as "at risk." The removal of her child precipitated a suicide attempt. Three years later, she was still trying to obtain custody of her child.

The above scenario is more common than one might believe and illustrates the unfortunate disconnect among adult and child services in the medical, social service and psychiatric fields. Scales such as the Edinburgh Postpartum Depression Scale are useful, and measures such the Parenting Stress Index may provide a global sense of early parent/infant dyadic problems which are driven by the parent's functioning [57,58]. Unfortunately, few programs exist that employ advocates who provide advocacy and supportive services to vulnerable mothers and infants. Washington State's Parent Child Assistance Program (PCAP) developed is an exception [56].

Among the Postnatal and Early Childhood vulnerabilities in FASD is a tendency for infants and young children to experience multiple placements before the fifth birthday due to their difficult and unpredictable behaviors, including the possibility of being reared in settings with little stimulation. The latter situation often occurs with children from Eastern Europe who may be adopted later in life into places such as the UK, Ireland, or USA. These children suffer the effects of early emotional deprivation as well as organic brain damage from their FASD condition. This can lead to challenging, but not untreatable, "Insecure Attachment" profiles such as Ambivalent Resistant or Avoidant Resistant patterns. Not infrequently, the history of these children's prenatal alcohol exposure is either minimized or not even noted in pre-adoption papers and only comes to light after placement when behavioral problems emerge. It is important to acknowledge that many children from these environments become very attached to their adoptive or foster parents. In these situations, especially when the new family environment is protective and nurturing, the challenging behaviors are most likely caused by deficient adaptive, social and executive functioning stemming from the organic brain damage [59].

A BROADER APPROACH TO ASSESSMENT

Multiple Generations

A transgenerational perspective is recommended in order to address effectively the social as well as the biological factors that influence FASD. The rule of thumb in the transgenerational management of FASD should be: "Always think multi-generations, multi-system and multi-modal and remember that alcohol is at the core of the problem." Clinicians who see FASD patients are not dealing simply with the so-called "identified patient." Alcohol dependence and abuse weave their way through different races, cultures and generations, so patients presenting in the clinician's office frequently bring the legacy of previous generations with them and are a harbinger of generations to come. Documentation of these intergenerational alcohol and offspring characteristics has recently been reported from northern France [60].

The idea that alcohol craving and subsequent abuse or dependence in adolescents and adults with FASD may have their origins in prenatal alcohol exposure has been demonstrated by animal researchers and later human researchers [61-63]. Alcohol use during pregnancy is at the very heart of FASD, and so effective management should involve general acceptance that maternal drinking may not be just an inherited genetic condition but may reflect a biochemical craving for alcohol due to the effect of prenatal exposure on the developing brain, especially the Nucleus Accumbens. Already, longitudinal studies using standardized psychiatric assessment instruments such as the Structured Clinical Interview for the DSM-IV (SCID) I and II have shown the prevalence of alcohol dependence and abuse in young adults prenatally exposed to alcohol [64]. Alcohol counselling for birth mothers is a key therapeutic approach, but it needs to be acknowledged that this form of psychotherapy and motivational interviewing does not always connect with patients who have cognitive impairment in fundamental cause and effect reasoning. At least with cocaine addiction, psychopharmacology has been used successfully [65] in blocking the central nervous system craving. Agents such as Naltrexone or Acamprasate also have been used successfully in patients with FASD but still require rigorous scientific testing, especially for use during pregnancy [66,67].

Transgenerational management of alcohol abuse and dependence requires health and social service systems to collaborate across traditional age-divides (e.g. child/adolescent/adult). For example, obstetricians and midwives need to become sensitive to implicit risks in the developing fetus from alcohol use in *any* trimester of pregnancy. Although teenage pregnancy has been acknowledged as a risk for both pregnancy and delivery, co-occurring alcohol or substance abuse is too often simply accepted rather than seen as a warning sign for the health of the infant [68,69]. Until such time that all of the professionals managing and delivering pregnant women who drink really believe that any amount of alcohol is unsafe, the ongoing clinical management of FASD will be with us.

A seven-year-old Italian boy ("AB") received many services since birth but still was unmanageable. Numerous specialists had administered countless tests in an effort to determine the cause of his problems. In addition to being short and underweight, he had a small head, absent corpus callosum, ventricular septal defect and a mixed neurocognitive picture with clear deficits in all areas as well as profound expressive and receptive language problems. No syndrome could capture what ailed him, but a supplementary dysmorphological examination revealed full FAS facial abnormalities. It was a social worker who alerted the child psychiatrist in the case to assess the patient for an FASD because of his small stature and "funny looking face." The 25-year-old mother ("NA") was overwhelmed but not surprised by the diagnostic frame used to explain the multiple disparate clinical findings in her son. She had never been asked about her alcohol use during pregnancy but now freely admitted to binge drinking in the first trimester. As the story unfolded, NA's 44-year-old mother had severe mental illness and was an alcoholic who drank throughout her pregnancy with NA. So, NA had a neurotoxin-created craving for alcohol from an early age as well as a significant risk for alcohol abuse and possible later addiction due to the possible effects of prenatal alcohol exposure in utero on her developing liver. Except for the alert social worker who noticed AB's unusual face, at no time during either of NA's pregnancies (or those of her mother) or follow-up of their children did medical and social service professionals consider prenatal alcohol exposure, let alone transgenerational alcohol exposure, to be a problem.

Now what if AB in the clinical case example above had been a girl rather than a boy – a girl who started craving alcohol at 10 years of age and drifted into binge drinking, unprotected sex, and pregnancy at 15 years of age? Another cycle in this family's sad legacy would have repeated itself.

Current clinical experience in Ireland and the UK as well as recent studies in France [70] provide more than their fair share of these types of transgenerational alcohol stories [71]. For example, in a recent clinical consultation case, the grandmother of three children had become their primary parent. One of the grandchildren had an FASD, the mother of a second grandchild had died prematurely in her 30's of alcohol related causes, and the mother of the third grandchild had been admitted to hospital with cirrhosis of the liver. In contrast to the situation in Europe where there a greater tendency for extended family to step into primary parenting roles in situations such as the ones in the preceding example, in the USA and Canada, 70-80% of children with FASD are brought up in structured non-alcoholic foster or adoptive homes [18,72].

Multiple Systems

Pediatricians, General Practitioners and Health Visitors (Public Health Nurses) need to be better educated in the immediate and long-term clinical features of FASD and more aware of the potential effects of prenatal alcohol on the developing child. Medical practitioners, regardless of specialty, should be aware that infants born to mothers who drink alcohol not only may have dysmorphic external features but internal physical abnormalities as well, including brain damage and the complicated neurodevelopmental sequelae that accompany that brain damage. Unfortunately, clinical medicine still tends to be no better than the old maxim: "what you look for, you will see." This is an enduring clinical diagnostic dilemma for practitioners who examine these infants and children. Even if FAS is diagnosed in childhood, the diagnosis does not always bring the medical and other services that these children need because conventional wisdom still sees these infants and children as COAs (children of alcoholics) who merely reflect the chaotic alcoholic environment they were born into.

In many European countries, the profound, long-lasting developmental neuropsychiatric effects of prenatal alcohol as a legacy of central nervous system disruption, is typically below the professional radar. Although parts of the USA, Canada and France are many years ahead of the rest of Europe in the integrated understanding of these issues, they still have much to learn as well. For example, despite a recent prevalence study among school-age children in Italy in which 2-5.5% of first grade children with FASD were documented, [12,40] there still is no government pronouncement warning women to refrain from alcohol use during pregnancy [73]. In particular, clinical scientific neurological and neuropsychiatric studies are needed to quantify ARND, which is much more common than FAS. There also needs to be a diagnostic blending of the concepts of developmental impairment of executive function, developmental impairment of social cognition and communication (adaptive functioning), and developmental impairment of sensory integration (described earlier in this chapter) -- all the kernel of ARND as well as FAS [66,74-76].

One of the confusing clinical issues in diagnosis and management of FASD is that the developmental impairments do not appear at uniform times. For example, according to the Regulatory Disorders Guidelines in the Zero-to-Three

Classification of Mental Health Disorders [77], sensory integration problems are identifiable in infancy, while social cognition and communication problems are more easily identified during the toddler years, and developmental executive function problems most commonly surface in the school setting under the guise of ADHD or behavior problems and Learning Disabilities [74]. These co-occurring clinical issues that are the "functional face" of children with FASD often become a diagnostic stew of "ADHD with autistic features" or "ADHD with behavior problems," frequently in combination with "unpredictable mood instability." (This combination of symptoms is reminiscent of some children with traumatic brain injury.)

The characteristic growth and facial features in classic FAS sensitize the clinician to explore and quantify the complex learning disabilities, which are a legacy of prenatal alcohol's effects on the developing central nervous system. However, the dysmorphic characteristics account for only 10 to 15% of patients affected by prenatal alcohol exposure. While ARND is far more prevalent, because it is more difficult to diagnose, it presents the ultimate challenge to clinicians in terms of diagnosis and management. Management begins with the ability to form a diagnostic or working hypothesis, which is how medical and mental health professionals should begin to approach the clinical presentation of a possible FASD (or any diagnosis, for that matter). As noted earlier in this chapter, the essential clinical component is the presence of a developmental neuropsychiatric disorder, and the etiology being sought is either genetic or acquired.

The initial step in establishing a diagnostic FASD hypothesis is to acquire a detailed drinking and drug use history from every pregnant or recently delivered woman, which is still not routinely done in many places despite the relative ease of adding quick screens to pre- and postnatal examinations. It is important to mention that, while some women may acknowledge cocaine or other drug use, use of drugs seldom occurs without alcohol use as well. Early efforts at quantifying alcohol consumption during pregnancy, as well as the Binge Alcohol Rating Criterion (BARC) and the Frequency-Binge Aggregate Score (F-BAS) have been found to be effective, found in Barr [78], Little [79], and Rosett [80]. These should be routinely administered upon admission to delivering women in the hospital in order to facilitate getting the information directly into the infant's and mother's medical records. Although scientists are testing biochemical markers for alcohol abuse in pregnancy (e.g., FAEE in meconium, acetaldehyde adduct in the mother's blood, fetal movement, or cranial ultrasound), no definitive marker has yet been established [66, 81-83]. In addition, genetic testing in newborns and young infants presenting with dysmorphic and growth features is recommended in cases involving confirmed prenatal alcohol exposure to rule out an FASD.

Beyond infancy, additional diagnostic steps for children and adults might include the following procedures:

(1) review obstetric, birth, and childhood medical records as well as school and social service records to look for indications of alcohol (or drug) use by the mother (traffic violations; drunken driving charges, alcohol treatment programs, etc.,) and signs of early developmental problems in the infant (e.g., poor suck, difficult temperament, attachment issues, slow development, growth deficit, cognitive-behavioral deficits and "problems");

(2) administer neuropsychological and other standardized testing to assess for the presence of at least three of the many neurodevelopmental deficits that typically comprise the complex pattern of primary disabilities seen in individuals with FASD (e.g., deficits in attention, speech and language, learning, motor skills, memory, sensory integration, socialization, executive functioning, adaptive functioning, and cognition), keeping in mind that deficits in cognition rarely fall as low as an IQ of 70;

(3) examine the face for dysmorphic features;

(4) assess for evidence of neurological damage upon medical examination and/or evidence of structural damage (e.g., corpus callosum) through brain imaging;

(5) determine if the patient displays the characteristic "adaptive/executive functioning deficit profile" as measured by standardized scales such as the Vineland Adaptive Behavior Scale; and

(6) assess for the presence of the classic cognitive-behavioral "downward" seen in most individuals with FASD (*i.e.*, a pattern involving a decline from Full Scale IQ score to achievement test results, with the latter higher yet than adaptive composite) (see Fig **4**):

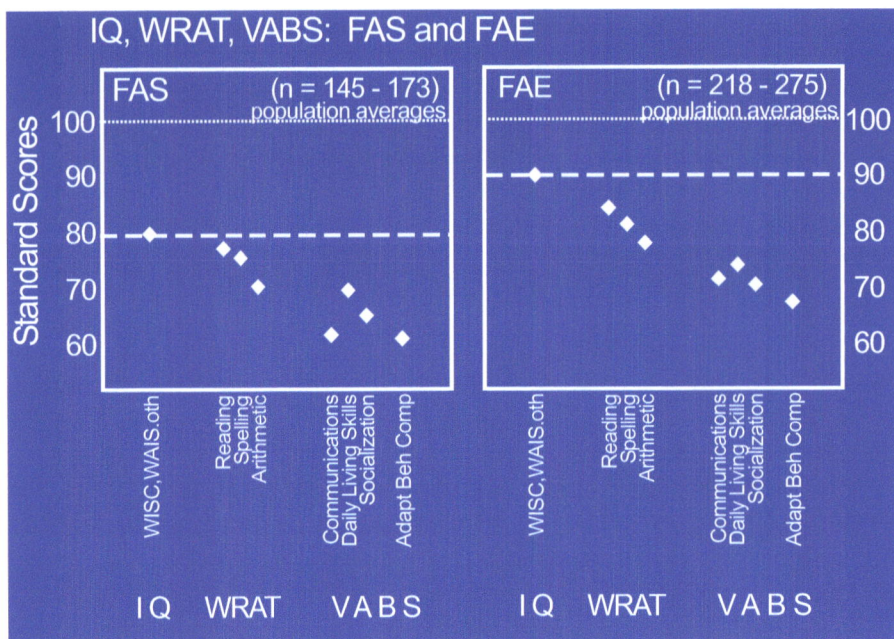

Figure 4: Characteristic downward decline in IQ-achievement-adaptive scores from Streissguth *et al.* 1996 Secondary Disabilities Report to the CDC.

From Streissguth, *et al.,* 1996 [18] shows this characteristic linear decline, regardless of FASD diagnosis, with adaptive composite scores falling below 70 – the traditional standard score threshold for Intellectual Disability.

Regardless of age, assessment of a possible FASD should include differential diagnosis to rule out competing etiological possibilities (e.g., toluene or other teratogenic exposure in utero, genetic or inherited conditions, post-natal trauma or injury).

A BROADER APPROACH TO MANAGEMENT

Ultimately, the guiding principle at the core of effective clinical management of FASD is the construction of a "scaffolding containment" system around the patient. Regardless of patient age, clinicians need to adopt a family-based systemic approach that identifies key environmental supports and stressors in the patient's environment [43,66,76, 84]. If diagnosis is missed in early childhood, then the next opportunity for identification often is the school environment.

Academic Services

School-based assessment typically focuses on learning disabilities plus any classroom behaviors that may be affecting a child's learning progress. However, standard school testing is often limited and misses the multiple functional impairments associated in FASD with failure to learn. IQ level is typically the yardstick: if a child underperforms on achievement tests compared to IQ-based expectation, "learning disability" is the conclusion, which triggers a search for the "reason" as well as educational supports. If the child displays attention problems and disruptive behaviors in the classroom, an attention deficit disorder is often the presumed etiology, and a recommendation may be made for a medication assessment. However, as noted previously, medication has little impact on dysfunctional behaviors arising from CNS impairment. Moreover, if Attention-Deficit/Hyperactivity Disorder or some other mental health condition is determined to be the source of the learning problem, this presumption shuts off further inquiry and, perhaps, more comprehensive assessment. As children enter their middle and high school years, academic failure and ultimately disinterest are assumed to be increasingly volitional in nature, and the search for a "reason" ends with a conclusion that the problem is the child's lack of motivation. Unfortunately, because so few children with FASD are diagnosed in early childhood, their underlying medical condition is missed, which precludes the wide array of extra-curricular interventions necessary to promote academic success and reduce secondary disabilities. In addition to a significant difference between IQ and achievement test scores, the following additional discrepancies indicate the possibility of an underlying CNS condition and, consequently, the need for comprehensive neuropsychological testing: a significant split between Verbal and Performance IQ in standardized IQ testing and a 15-point or more difference between IQ and adaptive behavior composite standard score.

Social and Psychological Services

As learned in the large government-sponsored secondary disability study at the University of Washington [18], prevention of co-occurring mental health disorders and other negative life course outcomes in individuals with FASD depends on early childhood diagnosis and an array of developmental disabilities services as well as a nurturing, protective home environment. The objective of service provision is not only to maximize whatever learning potential children with FASD have but also to create an external, structured network to protect these vulnerable individuals.

The foundation of effective service provision is lifelong case management and regular multidisciplinary team monitoring. Key to building this foundation is the acquisition of developmental disability services as soon in life as possible, which typically requires a diagnosis as well as deficient cognitive and adaptive test results. Specific services provided in childhood may include speech and language therapy and occupational therapy during the elementary school years, physical therapy if indicated, baseline neuropsychological testing and ongoing re-testing to monitor progress, systematic behavioral modification and social skills training, sensory integration therapy, family systems therapy and behavioral training, regular educational testing and supportive school-based services, mentoring, and medication if appropriate. Most important in this service delivery process is long-term case management to assure consistent overview and monitoring of treatment needs and effectiveness.

Few evidence-based mental health interventions have been shown to work in FASD populations. According to a review by Bertrand [85], several interventions show promise. Important elements in these interventions include parent education or training and teach children specific social and executive function skills that children typically learn through observation or abstraction. Another promising aspect of these interventions was their integration into existing mental health treatment systems.

Because neuropsychological impairments in FASD tend to be lifelong, it is clear that as youth with FASD mature into adulthood, case management should continue indefinitely. Most adults with FASD are unable to live independently and support themselves. Thus, the vast majority need residential assistance (ideally, a structured living environment) and assistance with adaptive tasks (e.g., nutrition, shopping, transportation, money management, time management, leisure activities and socialization, job coaching, acquisition of medical and dental care). Since many adults with FASD who are *not* living in structured, supervised living environments have trouble with the law, structured living situations that involve some form of supervision and staff assistance will enhance their chances of success.

Medication Management

Current research in epigenetics is beginning to help professionals unravel the contradictory clinical presentations of patients with FASD [76,86-88]. Animal research has implicated the short allele of the Serotonin Transporter Gene (5HTT) as being affected by prenatal alcohol and influencing the appearance of anxiety disorders through its action in increasing HPA axis (Hypothalamic Pituitary Adrenal Axis) activation [89]. Furthermore, animal research has identified the effect of prenatal alcohol exposure on Dopamine 2 Receptors (D2R) as a key biochemical factor in the development of sensory under or over-responsiveness [90].

Although medication, and especially polydrug therapy, is used extensively in co-occurring psychiatric disorders associated with FASD, this is done without FDA (Food and Drug Administration of the United States) or NICE (National Institute of Clinical Excellence in the United Kingdom) approval. In fact, there is no medium- or large-scale scientific drug industry or government-sponsored randomized clinical studies in any age group of this patient population [67]. However, co-occurring mood disorders present in almost all children and adults with FASD. Presentation in childhood is commonly coupled with physical symptoms such as disruptive behavioral problems, chronic headaches, abdominal pain or unspecified pain. This somatic expression and externalization are due to the common inability of children with FASD to express their emotional distress in words. For example, in the language disability Alexithymia [91,92], patients somaticize their emotional pain and present physical pain as the focus of their distress. Mood disorders must always be assessed in the context of the family, as environmental factors (e.g. abuse, recent losses or separations, change in family constellation such as arrival of a new sibling, or illness in a parent) may have a profound kindling, or synergistic effect, on the appearance or severity of the mood disorder.

Mood disorders range from deep depressive feelings to uncontrollable mood instability which mimics a rapid cycling bipolar disorder. In FASD, a mood disorder is really emotional dysregulation caused by the effects of prenatal exposure on developing neurotransmitters. Patients with co-occurring mood disorders may present with what is called "emotional incontinence," or unprovoked cascades of crying or laughing. Carbamazepine, valproic acid or even GABA agents such as gabapentin can be effective in treating these symptoms [93]. If these agents are used, there must be awareness of potential teratogenic problems if the bipolar patient becomes pregnant. Fetal valproate syndrome, for example, has many of the physical and some of the CNS hallmarks seen in FASD. Coupled with an appreciation that early childhood regulation disorders are often a disturbance of attention, behavior, and mood, recent interest in early onset bipolar disorder (EOBD) in the USA is beginning to offer clinical insights into the understanding of the initial psychiatric presentation of FASD [94,95].

Medications that are useful for mood disorders include fluoxetine in liquid or tablet form, sertraline, and citalopram. However, the tricyclic antidepressants increase the risk of cardio-toxicity in a patient population known to have potential cardiac problems from their prenatal alcohol exposure [66,67,96,97]. Therefore, it is best to start with low dosage fluoxetine and build slowly, being especially aware of an activation effect in the first week which may bring forth increased agitation or even increased suicidality. If tricyclic antidepressants are used, and the patient becomes pregnant, dosage needs to be monitored carefully as neonatal neurobehavioral effects have been described in infants who have been exposed to SSRIs during pregnancy [98,99]. Oberlander and his Canadian research group noted that the clinical challenge is to unravel the effects of the prenatal Selective Serotonin Reuptake inhibitors (SSRI) exposure on the infant from the impact of the mother's depressive disorder.

Attention and concentration deficits, often with hyperactivity and impulsivity, are the most common mental health presentation of both children and adults with FASD [18,66,96,100]. Medications such as psychostimulants do have an ameliorating role, and clinical studies have shown that Dextroamphetamine seems more efficacious than methylphenidate. Long-acting biphasic or bimodal (in USA) agents such as Concerta (USA), Equasym, and Medikinet (UK) may be helpful and can increase medication compliance. However, proper double-blind placebo studies are yet to be performed in patients with FASD. Compared to other co-occurring mental health disorders, there is a greater recognition of the prevalence of ADHD in FASD [101]. In addition, prenatal exposure to nicotine also has been identified as a synergistic biochemical agent that kindles ADHD [102-104]. Long-acting guanfacine (which is not available in the UK) may be useful in such cases, as is the short-acting version, but this needs to be studied in this patient population [105].

Significant conduct problems are seen in children who come from family environments where there is a transgenerational history of disorganized or even absent parenting. FASD tends to run through multiple generations in a family, and recent clinical work in the UK and Ireland has focused on the risk of conduct disorders when FASD affects several generations within a family. Conduct Disorders frequently include aggressive/explosive episodes and may progress to fire setting or even cruelty to animals. A Sleep Deprived EEG may rule out a Complex Partial Seizure Disorder, and a supplementary examination may uncover sexual or physical abuse. Medications such as carbamazepine and valproic acid are useful, especially if mood instability is present with the conduct disorder. Also, fluoxetine in liquid form for young children and tablet form for adolescents (20 mg tablet only available in UK) may help if there has been a traumatic history, as it has an antidepressant quality.

Chronic anxiety often co-occurs in children and adults with FASD, partly due to a chronic inability to self-soothe. A combination of psychostimulant and guanfacine or clonidine has been effective in the treatment of such symptoms, if they are present in the context of ADHD with co-occurring anxiety disorder. It is important to check blood pressure and pulse and do an ECG prior to prescribing these medications due to their possible cardio toxicity when used in combination. If the anxiety disorder is the primary psychiatric presentation, it also is essential to unravel the environmental stressors in the history as individual non-verbal play therapy may be better than medication as the first option in young children. If medication is indicated, then buspirone or lorazepam may be helpful [97].

Psychotic symptoms may be quite difficult to spot as patients with FASD and average or higher IQs may concoct fantastical stories that are not delusional but rather only a way to "fill in the blanks" due to severe deficits in working memory, social cognition and communication. Newer atypical agents are used in such cases but are still unpredictable. For example, Risperidone can precipitate a manic switch due to its differential effect on the 5HT receptor. Clinically, Olanzepine seems to be most effective if the patient is displaying acute mania features.

Some symptoms on the autistic spectrum are invariably coupled with FASD, with its developmental impairments in executive function and sensory integration. It is developmental impairments in social cognition and communication that appear to bring the most secondary psychiatric issues such as anxiety disorders and possible psychotic disorders. Psychostimulants might be used with caution as they can precipitate a schizoid personality change, sometimes described as "zombie" type states in the USA, or increase perseveration due to enhancing focus. Atomoxetine seems to be a good fit in some patients [67,76].

As emphasized above, if medication management is selected for patients with FASD, it needs to be embedded in an array of services for both the child and his/her family. The risks of combined pharmacotherapy in children and adolescents have been highlighted recently, and patients with FASD have had no studies of single medications, let alone combinations of medications [106]. Family therapy and support are essential. Moreover, medication may improve the participation of FASD patients in other important treatment modalities such as nonverbal play therapy, speech and language therapy or sensory integration therapy [66,107].

SUMMARY

Historical overview of the diagnostic dilemmas described in this chapter serves a salutary function by demonstrating that health care professionals have failed to appreciate appropriately the broad implications of FASD. As long as diagnostic treatises fail to acknowledge FAS and ARND as functional disabilities with multiple developmental and co-occurring psychiatric problems, then it will not be possible to conduct scientific research on outcome or management. Notwithstanding these constraints, it is becoming increasingly obvious that a transgenerational management perspective with alcohol abuse at the core of understanding is the only effective way to approach FASD. The family-centered, transgenerational approach spans all age groups and is, by its nature, multi-modal and multi-systemic as it encompasses every discipline involved in FASD assessment and management: medicine, education, social welfare, psychology, occupational and language therapy, and legal advocacy. Although this new perspective may seem rather daunting in its scope, ultimately the goal is to produce a scaffolding containment system for the affected child and his or her family that achieves a balance between over-ambitious parenting and "good enough" parenting [108].

ACKNOWLEDGEMENTS

The authors wish to thank Richard Adler, MD, of FASD Experts for his review and consultation in the development of this chapter and Kristi Pimental of the University of Washington Fetal Alcohol and Drug Unit for her editing assistance.

REFERENCES

[1]   Lemoine P, Harousseau H, Borteyru JP, Menuet JC. Children of alcoholic parents: Abnormalities observed in 127 cases. Selected Translations of International Alcoholism Research (STIAR). Rockville, MD: National Institute on Alcohol Abuse and Alcoholism 1968. [Translation from the French of: Les enfants de parents alcooliques: Anomalies observées, à propos de 127 cas. Ouest Medical (Paris) 1968; 21: 476-82.

[2]   Jones KL, Smith DW, Ulleland CN, Streissguth AP. Pattern of malformation in offspring of chronic alcoholic mothers. Lancet 1973; 1: 1267-71.

[3]   Jones KL, Smith DW. Recognition of the fetal alcohol syndrome in early infancy. Lancet 1973; 2: 999-1001.

[4]   Smith DW. Recognizable patterns of human malformation; genetic, embryologic, and clinical aspects. 1st ed. Philadelphia: WB Saunders 1970.

[5]   Smith DW. Fetal alcohol syndrome and fetal alcohol effects. Neurobehav Toxicol Teratol 1981; 3: 127.

[6]   Stratton K, Howe C, Battaglia F, Eds. (Institute of Medicine) Fetal alcohol syndrome: diagnosis, epidemiology, prevention, and treatment. Washington, D.C.: National Academy Press 1996.

[7]   Warren K, Floyd L, Calhoun F, *et al.* Consensus Statement on FASD. Washington, DC: National Organization on Fetal Alcohol Syndrome, April 7, 2004.

[8]   Streissguth AP, O'Malley KD. Neuropsychiatric implications and long-term consequences of fetal alcohol spectrum disorders. Seminars Clin Neuropsychiatry 2000; 5: 177-90.

[9]   May PA, Gossage JP, Marais AS, *et al.* The epidemiology of fetal alcohol syndrome and partial FAS in a South African community. Drug Alc Dep 2007; 88: 259-271.

[10]   Kvigne VL, Leonardson GR, Borzelleca J, Neff-Smith M, Welty TK. Characteristics of children whose siblings have fetal alcohol syndrome or incomplete fetal alcohol syndrome. Pediatrics 2009; 123: e526-33.

[11]   May PA, Brook L, Gossage JP, *et al.* Epidemiology of fetal alcohol syndrome in a South African community In the Western Cape Province. Am J Public Health 2000; 90: 1905-12.

[12]   May PA, Fiorentino D, Gossage JP, *et al.* Epidemiology of FASD in a province in Italy: prevalence and characteristics of children in a random sample of schools Alc Clin Exp Res 2006; 30: 1562-75.

[13]   Jones KL, Robinson LK, Bakhireva LN, *et al.* Accuracy of the diagnosis of physical features of fetal alcohol syndrome by pediatricians after specialized training. Pediatrics 2006; 118: e1734-8.

[14]   May PA, McCloskey J, Gossage, JP. Fetal alcohol syndrome among American Indians: epidemiology, issues, and research. In Mail PD, Heurtin-Roberts S, Martin SE, Howard J, eds. Alcohol use among American Indians: multiple perspectives on a complex problem. National Institute on Alcohol Abuse and Alcoholism Research Monograph No. 37. Bethesda, MD: National Institute on Alcohol Abuse and Alcoholism, 2002.

[15]   Hoyme HE, May PA, Kalberg MA, *et al.* A practical clinical approach to diagnosis of fetal alcohol spectrum disorders: clarification of the 1996 Institute of Medicine criteria. Pediatrics 2005; 115: 39-47.

[16]   Astley SH, Clarren SK. Diagnosing the full spectrum of fetal alcohol exposed individuals: introducing the 4-digit diagnostic code. Alcohol Alcohol 2000; 35: 400-410.

[17]   Streissguth AP, Aase JM, Clarren SK, Randels SP, LaDue RA, Smith DF. Fetal alcohol syndrome in adolescents and adults. JAMA 1991; 265: 1961-7.

[18]   Streissguth AP, Barr HM, Kogan J, Bookstein FL. Understanding the occurrence of secondary disabilities in clients with fetal alcohol syndrome (FAS) and fetal alcohol effects (FAE). Final report to the Centers for Disease Control and Prevention (CDC). Seattle: University of Washington 1996.

[19]   Streissguth AP, Bookstein FL, Barr HM, *et al.* Risk factors for adverse life outcomes in fetal alcohol syndrome and fetal alcohol effects. J Dev Behav Ped 2004; 25: 228-38.

[20]   Löser H, Bierstedt T, Blum A. Fetal alcohol syndrome in adults: Long-term observations on 52 patients. (Alkoholembryopathie im erwachsenenalter: Eine langzeituntersuchung). Deutsche Medizinische Wochenschrift 1999; 124: 412-8.

[21]   Spohr HL, Willms J, Steinhausen HC. Fetal alcohol spectrum disorders in young adulthood. J Pediatr 2007; 150: 175-9.

[22]   Fast DK, Conry J, Loock CA. Identifying fetal alcohol syndrome among youth in the criminal justice system. J Dev Behav Pediatr 1999; 20: 370-2.

[23]   Archibald SL, Fennema-Notestine, C, Ganst, A, Riley, EP, Mattson, SN, Jernigan, TL. Brain dysmorphology in individuals with severe prenatal alcohol exposure. Dev Med Child Neurol 2001; 43: 148-154.

[24]   Bookstein FL, Sampson PD, Connor PD, Streissguth AP. Midline corpus callosum is a neuroanatomical focus of fetal alcohol damage. Anat Rec 2002; 269: 162-174.

[25]   Mattson SN, Riley EP, Sowell ER, Jernigan TL, Sobel DF, Jones KL. A decrease in the size of the basal ganglia in children with FAS. Alcohol Clin Exp Res 1996; 20: 1088-1093.

[26]   Riley EP, Mattson SN, Sowell ER, Jernigan TL, Sobel DF, Jones KL. Abnormalities of the corpus callosum in children prenatally exposed to alcohol. Alcohol Clin Exp Res 1995; 19: 1198-1202.

[27]   Sowell ER, Thompson PM, Mattson SN, *et al.* Voxel-based morphometric analyses of the brain in children and adolescents prenatally exposed to alcohol. Neuroreport 2001; 12: 515-523.

[28]   Sowell ER, Lu LH, O'Hare ED, *et al.* Functional magnetic resonance imaging of verbal learning in children with heavy prenatal alcohol exposure. Neuroreport 2007; 18: 636-639.

[29]   Sowell E, Johnson A, Kan E, *et al.* Mapping white matter integrity and neurobehavioral correlates in children with fetal alcohol spectrum disorders. J Neurosci 2008; 28(6): 1313-1319.

[30]   Streissguth A, Barr H, Kogan J, Bookstein F. In: Streissguth, AP, Kanter J, eds. The challenge of fetal alcohol syndrome: Overcoming secondary disabilities. Seattle, University of Washington Press 1997: 25-39.

[31]   Clark E, Lutke J, Minnes P, Ouellette-Kuntz H. Secondary disabilities among adults with fetal alcohol spectrum disorder in British Columbia. J FAS 2004; 2: 1-12.

[32]   Lemoine P, Lemoine PH. Avenir des enfants de mères alcooliques (Étude de 105 cas retrouvés à l'âge adulte) et quelques constatations d'intérêt prophylactique [Outcome in the offspring of alcoholic mothers (study of one hundred five adults) and considerations with a view to prophylaxis]. Ann Pediatr (Paris) 1992; 39: 226-35.

[33]   Centers for Disease Control (CDC). Fetal Alcohol Syndrome: Guidelines for referral and diagnosis. In coordination with National Task Force on Fetal Alcohol Syndrome and Fetal Alcohol Effect, American Academy of Pediatrics, American College of Obstetricians and Gynecologists, March of Dimes, and National Organization on Fetal Alcohol Syndrome (NOFAS). 2004.

[34]   Fetal Alcohol Spectrum Disorders Center for Excellence, Substance Abuse and Mental Health Services Administration (SAMHSA). Fetal Alcohol Spectrum Disorders by the Numbers. March 6, 2010. www.samhsa.org

[35]   Lupton C, Burd L, Harwood R. Cost of fetal alcohol spectrum disorders. Am J Med Genet 2004; 127C:42-50.

[36]   O'Connor MJ, McCracken J, Best A. Under recognition of prenatal alcohol exposure in a child inpatient psychiatric setting. Mental Health Aspects Devel Disabil 2006; 9: 105-8.

[37]   Burd L, Selfridge R, Klug M, Bakko S. Fetal alcohol syndrome in the United States corrections system. Addict Biol 2004; 9: 177-8.

[38]   Gahagan S, Sharpe TT, Brimacombe M, *et al.* Pediatricians' knowledge, training, and experience in the care of children with fetal alcohol syndrome. Pediatrics 2006; 118: 657-68.

[39]   Astley SJ, Clarren SK. Measuring the facial phenotype of individuals with prenatal alcohol exposure: Correlations with brain dysfunction. Alcohol Alcohol 2001; 36: 47-59.

[40]   May PA, Gossage JP, Kalberg WO, *et al.* Prevalence and epidemiologic characteristics of FASD from various research methods with an emphasis on recent in-school studies. Dev Dis Res Rev 2009; 15: 176-192.

[41]   Jones KL, Robinson LK, Bakhireva LN, *et al* Accuracy of the diagnosis of physical features of fetal Alcohol Syndrome by pediatricians after specialized training. Pediatrics 2009; 118: 1734-1739.

[42]   Chudley AE, Conry J, Cook JL, Loock C, Rosales T, LeBlanc N. Fetal alcohol spectrum disorder: Canadian guidelines for diagnosis. Can Med Assoc J 2005; 172: s1-s21.

[43]   Olson HC, Ohlemiller MM, O'Connor MJ, *et al.* A call to action: Advancing essential services and research on fetal alcohol spectrum disorders. A report of the national task force on fetal alcohol syndrome and fetal alcohol effects. March 2009.

[44]   World Health Organization. International statistical classification of diseases and related health problems 10th revision. Geneva Switzerland; 1992.

[45]   American Psychiatric Association. Diagnostic and statistical manual of mental disorders, 4th ed, text revision. Washington, DC; 2000.

[46]   Werner EE. Resilient offspring of alcoholics: A longitudinal study from birth to age 18. J Studies Alcohol 1986; 47: 34-40.

[47]   Child Welfare Information Gateway. Understanding the effects of maltreatment on early brain development. Bulletin for professionals. US Department of Health and Human Services, Administration on Children, Youth, and Families, Children's Bureau. October 2001.

[48]   O'Connor MJ, Paley B. Psychiatric conditions associated with prenatal alcohol exposure. Devel Disabil 2009; 15: 225-34.

[49]   Streissguth AP. Fetal alcohol syndrome: A guide for families and communities. Baltimore: Brooks Publishing Co 1997.

[50]   Streissguth AP, Kanter J, Eds. The challenge of fetal alcohol syndrome: Overcoming secondary disabilities. Seattle: University of Washington Press 1997 (edited book).

[51]   Baumbach J. Some implications of prenatal alcohol exposure for the treatment of adolescents with sexual offending behaviors. Sexual Abuse 2002; 14: 313-27.

[52]   Moore TE, Green M. Fetal alcohol spectrum disorder: A need for closer examination by the criminal justice system. Crim Reports 2004; 19: 99-108.

[53]   Greenbaum RL, Stevens SA, Nash K, Koren G, Rovet J. Social cognitive and emotion processing abilities of children with fetal alcohol spectrum disorders: A comparison with attention deficit hyperactivity disorder. Alc Clin Exp Res 2009; 33: 1656-70.

[54]   Mukherjee RAS, Holinis S, Turk J. Fetal Alcohol Spectrum Disorder. J Royal Society Med 2008; 99: 298-302.

[55]   Meewise ML, Reitsma JB, De Vries GJ, Gersons BPR, Olff M. Cortisol and post traumatic stress disorder in adults: Systematic review and meta-analysis. Br J Psychiatry 2007; 191: 387-92.

[56]   Grant T, Youngblood Pedersen J, Whitney N, Ernst C. In O'Malley KD, ed. ADHD and fetal alcohol spectrum disorders (FASD), 2nd printing, Nova Science Publishers, New York, 2008; pp.69-93.

[57] Cox JL, Holden JM, Sagovsky R. Detection of postnatal depression. Development of the 10-item Edinburgh Postnatal Depression Scale. Br J Psychiatry 1987; 150: 782-6.

[58] Abidin RR. Parenting Stress Index Manual. 2nd ed. Charlottesville: Pediatric Psychology Press 1986.

[59] O'Connor TG, Rutter M. Attachment disorder behavior following early severe deprivation: extension and longitudinal follow up. J Am Acad Child Adol Psychiatry 2000; 38: 703-12.

[60] Handley Ed, Chassin L. Intergenerational transmission of alcohol expectancies in a high-risk sample. JSAD 2009; 709: 675.

[61] Bond NW, Di Gusto EL. Effects of prenatal alcohol exposure on open field behavior and alcohol preference in rats. Psychopharmacologia 1976; 46: 163-5.

[62] Reyes E, Garcia KD, Jones BC. Effects of maternal consumption of alcohol on alcohol selection in rats. Alcohol 1985; 2: 323-6.

[63] Baer JS, Sampson PD, Barr HM, Connor PD, Streissguth AP. A 21-year longitudinal analyses of the effects of prenatal alcohol exposure on young adult drinking. Arch Gen Psychiatry 2003; 60: 377-85.

[64] Barr HM, Bookstein FL, O'Malley KD, Connor PD, Huggins J, Streissguth AP. Binge drinking during pregnancy as a predictor of psychiatric disorders on the Structured Clinical Interview for DSM-IV in young adult offspring. Am J Psychiatry 2006; 163: 1061-5.

[65] Sinha R, O'Malley SS. Craving for alcohol: Findings from the clinic and the laboratory. Alcohol Alcohol 1999; 34: 223-30.

[66] O'Malley KD. In: O'Malley KD, ed. ADHD and fetal alcohol spectrum disorders (FASD). 2nd Printing. New York: Nova Science publishers 2008; pp.1-23.

[67] O'Malley KD. In: Stolerman IP, ed, Encyclopedia of psychopharmacology. Berlin Heidelberg, Springer-Verlag 2010a; 1-5.

[68] O'Malley KD. In: Pumariega AJ, Winters NC, Eds. The handbook of child and adolescent systems of care, The new community psychiatry. Jossey-Bass 2003; 276-315.

[69] Henshaw C, Cox J, Barton J. Modern management of perinatal psychiatric disorders. London: Royal College of Psychiatrists Publications 2009.

[70] Dumaret, A-C, Cousin, M, Titran, M. Two generations of maternal alcohol abuse: impact on cognitive levels in mothers and their children. Early Child Dev Care 2009; 1-11.

[71] Orakwue N, Mc Nicholas F, O'Malley KD. Not a drop, fetal alcohol spectrum disorders. The Irish perspective. Irish J Psychological Med 2010; Submitted.

[72] Koren G, Nulman J, Chudley A, Locke C. Fetal alcohol spectrum disorder. Can Med Assoc J 2003; 169: 1181-5.

[73] Ceccanti M, Spagnolo PR, Tarani L, et al. Clinical delineation of fetal alcohol spectrum disorders (FASD) in Italian children: Comparison and contrast with other racial/ethnic groups and implications for diagnosis and prevention. Neurosci Biobehav Rev 2007; 31: 270-7.

[74] Brown TE, ed. ADHD comorbidities. Handbook for ADHD complications in children and adults. Arlington: American Psychiatric Press 2009.

[75] Brown TE. A new model of understanding ADHD: Implications for patient care, 2010, January 29TH, Lilly National Meeting on Topics in Psychiatry, Westbury Hotel, Dublin, Ireland

[76] O'Malley KD. In: Howlin, P Charman T and Ghazziuddin M, Eds. The Sage Handbook of Developmental Disorders. Chapter 24, UK/Amazon, 2011: In Press.

[77] DC: 0 to 3R classification. Washington DC: Zero To Three Press 2005.

[78] Barr HM, Streissguth AP. Identifying maternal self-reported alcohol use associated with Fetal Alcohol Spectrum Disorders. Alcoholism: Clin Exp Res 2001; 25: 283-7.

[79] Little RE, Streissguth AP, Guzinski GM, et al. An evaluation of the pregnancy and health program: Alcohol Health Res World 1985; 10: 44-53, 75.

[80] Rosett HL, Weiner L, Edelin KC. Treatment experience with pregnant problem drinkers. J Am Med Assoc 198: 249; 2029-33.

[81] Bearer CF. Markers to detecting drinking during pregnancy. Alcohol Res Health 2001; 25: 210-8.

[82] Dreosti IE. Nutritional factors underlying the expression of fetal alcohol syndrome. Ann NY Acad Sci 1993; 678: 193-204.

[83] Little JF, Hepper PG, Dornan JC. Maternal alcohol consumption during pregnancy and fetal startle behaviour. Physiol Beh 2002; 76: 691-4.

[84] Grant TM, Huggins JE, Sampson PD, Ernst CC, Barr HM, Streissguth AP. Alcohol use before and during pregnancy in western Washington, 1989-2004: Implications for the prevention of fetal alcohol spectrum disorders. Am J Obstet Gynecol, Online Extra; 25 November 2008eExtra.

[85] Bertrand J. Interventions for children with fetal alcohol spectrum disorders (FASD): Overview of findings for five innovative research projects. Res Dev Dis 2009; 30: 986-1006.

[86] Pembrey ME. Time to take epigenetic inheritance seriously. Europ J Hum Genet 2002; 10: 669-71.

[87]   Tchurikov NA. Molecular mechanisms of epigenetics. Biochemistry (Moscow) 2006; 70: 406-23.

[88]   Haycock PC. Fetal alcohol spectrum disorders: the epigenetic perspective. Biol Reprod 2009; 81: 607-17.

[89]   Kraemer GW, Moore CF, Newman TK, Barr CS, Schneider ML. Moderate fetal alcohol exposure and serotonin transporter gene promoter polymorphism effect neonatal temperament and limbic-hypothalamic-pituitary-adrenal axis regulation in monkeys. Biologic Psychiatry 2008; 63: 317-24.

[90]   Screiber ML, Moore CF, Gajewski LL, *et al.* Sensory processing disorder in primate model: evidence from a longitudinal study of prenatal alcohol and prenatal stress effects. Child Dev 2008; 79: 100-13.

[91]   Coggins TE, Timler GR, Olswang LB. In O'Malley KD, ed. ADHD and fetal alcohol spectrum disorders (FASD), 2nd printing, Nova Science Publishers, New York, 2008; 161-78.

[92]   Sullivan A. In O'Malley KD, ed. ADHD and fetal alcohol spectrum disorders (FASD), 2nd printing, Nova Science Publishers, New York, 2008; 215-45.

[93]   Wozniak J, Biederman J. A pharmacological approach to the quagmire of comorbidity in juvenile mania. J Am Acad Child Adol Psychiatry 1996; 35: 826-8.

[94]   Carlson GA, Findling RL, Post RM, *et al.* AACAP 2006 Research forum-advancing research in early-onset bipolar disorder: Barriers and suggestions. J Child Adolesc Psychopharmacol 2009; 19: 3-12.

[95]   Althoff RR. Dysregulated children reconsidered. J Am Acad Child Adolesc Psychiatry 2010; 49: 302-4.

[96]   Hagerman RJ. Neurodevelopmental disorders: Diagnosis and treatment. New York: Oxford University Press 1999; 3-59.

[97]   Byrne C. Psychopharmacology basics for FASD. Workshop Presentation, 3rd National biennial conference on adolescents and adults with Fetal Alcohol Spectrum Disorder, April 98th -12th, 2008; Vancouver, BC, Canada.

[98]   Lattmore Keri A, Donn SM, Kaciroti N, Kemper AR, Neal CR, Vazquez DM. Selective serotonin reuptake inhibitors (SSRI) use during pregnancy and effects on the fetus and newborn: A metal analysis. J Perinatol 2005; 25: 595-603.

[99]   Oberlander TF, Gingrich JA, Ansorge MS. Sustained neurobehavioral effects of exposure to SSRI antidepressants during development: Molecular to clinical evidence. Clin Pharmacol Therap 2009; 86: 672-7.

[100] O'Malley KD, Nanson, J. Clinical implications of a link between fetal alcohol spectrum disorder and attention -deficit hyperactivity disorder. Can J Psychiatry 2002; 4: 349-54.

[101] Turk J. Behavioural phenotypes: Their applicability to children and young people who have learning disabilities. Adv Mental Health Learn Dis 2007; 1: 4-13.

[102] Milberger S, Biederman J, Farone SV, Chen L, Jones J. Is maternal smoking during pregnancy a risk factor for attention deficit hyperactivity disorder in children? Am J Psychiatry 1996; 153: 1138-42.

[103] Mick E, Biederman J, Farone S, Sayer J, Kleinman S. Case-control study of ADHD and maternal smoking, alcohol use and drug use during pregnancy. J Acad Child Adolesc Psychiatry 2002; 41: 378-85.

[104] Altink ME, Slaate-Willense DIE, Ronnelse NNJ, *et al.* Effects of maternal and paternal smoking on attentional control in children with and without ADHD. Eur Child Adolesc Psychiatry 2009: 18; 465-75.

[105] Salee FR, Lyne A, Wigal T, McGough JJ. Long term safety and efficacy of guanfacine extended release in children and adolescents with attention-deficit/hyperactivity disorder. J Child Adolesc Psychopharmacol 2009; 19: 215-26.

[106] Wilens TE. Combined pharmacotherapy in pediatric psychopharmacology: Friend or foe? J Child Adolesc Psychopharmacol 2009; 19: 483-4.

[107] O'Malley KD. Medication therapy's role for FAS. Iceberg, 1997: 7; 1-4.

[108] Winnicott DW. In: Lomas P, ed. The predicament of the family: A psychoanalytical symposium. London, Hogarth Press 1967: 26-33.

CHAPTER 4

An Innovative Look at Early Intervention for Children Affected by Prenatal Alcohol Exposure

Heather Carmichael Olson[1,*] and Rachel A. Montague[2]

[1]*Department of Psychiatry and Behavioral Sciences, University of Washington School of Medicine, Seattle Children's Hospital Child Psychiatry Outpatient Clinic, Fetal Alcohol Syndrome Diagnostic and Prevention Network, Families Moving Forward Research Program, Seattle, WA, USA and* [2]*Seattle Pacific University, Department of Clinical Psychology, USA*

From Parents of Children with FASD:

"That's the whole idea… early intervention so we can catch the problems in those [first] difficult years…."

"So, when our kids are little and we have an [intervention] program, then we would have structure and know the way to handle things right from the start."

Abstract: Early intervention is vital for children born affected by prenatal alcohol exposure, and may take advantage of 'plasticity' in the developing brain. Early diagnosis is associated with more positive life outcomes among those with FASD. Early intervention leads to better child and family outcomes in populations with similar challenges and, in initial research, to improved outcomes among those with prenatal alcohol exposure. This chapter begins with a 'neurodevelopmental viewpoint,' central to thinking about early intervention with this population. This viewpoint emphasizes 'brain-based difficulties' arising from alcohol's teratogenic effects, and the need to reduce risks and increase protective factors. Current research on child and family strengths and deficits, and the necessary step of early identification, are reviewed. Treatment recommendations from expert professional opinion and the collective family wisdom, and findings from the few studies of early intervention in this population, are provided. To spark research progress in the field, a variety of promising existing early interventions are discussed, including ideas for needed adaptations. Links are provided to websites, parent support information, training topics for early intervention providers, and new data on behavior regulation in young children with FASD. Early intervention is an exciting research direction for the field of FASD.

INTRODUCTION

A Real-Life Scene Between a Young Boy with FASD and His Mother:

His mom asks: *"What should people know about working with kids like you?"*

The boy groans and says: *"We have to have another talk about how my brain works?"*

His mom explains there is a book being written about kids like him and that people interested in FASD will read this book. He jumps up on the bed with his arms outstretched and head thrown back, and yells: *"This is FANTASTIC mom!"*

The boy says: *"They should know how to help our brains work really hard. It would be like I told them a secret of how to help and they got it!… We need to be working together to make things better for me and other people…"*

They talk more, and then the boy says: *"I feel like I am in the center of the world and I am part of the world. I am happy to be me!"*

–Ian, age 8

*Address correspondence to Heather Carmichael Olson: 2001 Eighth Avenue, Suite 400, Seattle, Washington, 98121, USA; Fax: (206) 884-7801: E-mail: heather.carmichael_olson@seattlechildrens.org; quiddity@u.washington.edu

Sending this to the Authors, the Mom Writes About Her Son:

"[This conversation] reaffirmed to me how truly insightful he is about himself and his place in this world."

–Ian's mom

Children born prenatally alcohol-exposed come into the world with personal strengths, but also with biological vulnerabilities. Children who are affected by their prenatal alcohol exposure can show significant neurodevelopmental disabilities, even in the early years. These disabilities often go unidentified or misunderstood, but actually can be clinically diagnosed within a set of conditions collectively called Fetal Alcohol Spectrum Disorders (FASD). Early diagnosis, before age 6 years, has been identified as one of the most important 'protective' factors associated with greater odds of positive long-term outcomes for individuals with FASD [1]. Intervention provided in the early years has been shown to improve child and family outcome in the very few studies of children born prenatally alcohol-exposed carried out so far.

Early intervention has also been effective for other groups of children who experience similar life challenges, or have deficits like those who are affected by prenatal alcohol exposure. These include children who show developmental disabilities, polydrug exposure, traumatic brain injury, disruptive behavior disorders, and also children at high psychosocial risk or who have been maltreated. Early intervention is important, because it has the potential to take advantage of the newly understood plasticity of the developing brain to improve at least some of the neurological impairment resulting from alcohol's teratogenic effects.

There is a general lack of intervention research focused on children affected by prenatal alcohol exposure or known to have FASD, even though interest in this topic is rapidly growing [2-4]. This is especially true for intervention with very young children. Accordingly, this chapter reviews the small amount of available treatment outcome data for young children born prenatally alcohol-exposed, but focuses more on exploring some of the existing early intervention ideas and approaches that hold promise for this surprisingly large population of young children (birth to 8 years) and their families. The chapter emphasis is on treatments that improve children's early development or aim to improve care giving and family outcome. There is a special focus on treatments that improve children's behavioral regulation, given the importance of this early developmental achievement for overall life success.

Readers of this chapter will find information about how to look at the problem of FASD using a 'neurodevelopmental viewpoint' to better understand this disability. They will learn about the ins and outs of early identification, and explore treatment recommendations coming from experts (found in a clinical database) and from the wisdom of families (found in a review of personal exchanges over the internet). Readers of this chapter will also learn about a variety of promising approaches to early intervention for this population, and think about how they can use these ideas in their own area of practice to help children with FASD and the families that care for them.

A NEURODEVELOPMENTAL VIEWPOINT

In designing interventions for young children affected by prenatal alcohol exposure, or with FASD, an important first step is to change perspective. This means taking a 'neurodevelopmental viewpoint.' This viewpoint is based on research that explains the teratogenic effects of alcohol, the collective experience of families and researchers, and several important developmental theories. This viewpoint is also based on principles from 'developmental psychopathology'— a scientific field that explores the developmental influences on the life pathways children follow that lead to typical or atypical developmental outcomes. Taking this neurodevelopmental viewpoint can make it easier to see when certain types of intervention are not appropriate, or how to adapt treatment approaches (and change expectations) to increase effectiveness. This viewpoint is the foundation for a positive parenting intervention specialized for families raising children with neurodevelopmental disabilities (especially FASD) called the 'Families Moving Forward Program' [5(study #5)], discussed later in this chapter. The neurodevelopmental viewpoint and intervention basics have previously been discussed in depth as they apply to early intervention by Olson and her colleagues [6]. Many pioneering researchers and clinicians have led the way to developing this viewpoint and intervention ideas for this population [7-12].

Researcher Kodituwakku has recently presented his own neurodevelopmental framework, based on cognitive neuroscience principles, to guide development of skills-teaching interventions for children with FASD [13]. While there are differences from the viewpoint presented in this chapter, Kodituwakku's framework leads to some of the same conclusions about intervention in the field of FASD. Among these are the importance of paying attention to a child's cognitive-behavioral profile when designing interventions, and the central need to provide training on self-regulation as early as possible.

"Brain-Based" Difficulties

Alcohol is a neurobehavioral teratogen. A great deal of research shows that prenatal alcohol exposure is a risk factor that changes how the fetal brain and central nervous system develop, and that these changes result in functional difficulties that start early and persist lifelong. A central idea in thinking about individuals affected by prenatal alcohol exposure, including those with FASD, is that they have 'brain-based' difficulties in cognition, learning and memory, or what might be called a generalized deficit in processing complex information [14,15]. These difficulties may be misinterpreted (at least in part) as disruptive or dysfunctional behavior. In young children, brain-based difficulties can often be seen as problems or delays in behavior regulation. This can include negative affect and difficulties in arousal regulation, stress reactivity, impulse control, sensory integration, early attention skills, sleep and more. They may also show difficulties in fine and gross motor function, and in coordination and balance. These underlying neurodevelopmental problems may be called 'primary disabilities' [7]. Observed in the day-to-day life of young children, these disabilities also show up as markedly lowered adaptive function (children's ability to communicate, get along with other people socially, and do daily living skills). Further, these may show up as lifestyle problems for young children, including social skill deficits, difficulties in pre-academic and early academic achievement and, quite distressing to care givers, challenging and often disruptive behavior.

Intervention Basics

When working with those affected by prenatal alcohol exposure, or with FASD, it is vital for care givers and clinicians to go through a process of 'reframing' their understanding of the child's behavioral difficulties as, at least in part, 'brain-based.' This has been highlighted as a central intervention principle by Olson and her colleagues [5], and pioneering clinician Malbin [9]. The earlier the process of reframing can take place, the more likely it is thought that a good outcome will occur. Reframing helps parents gain a more positive view of their child, and of the parent-child relationship, which can help jumpstart the use of the most appropriate care giving methods, and move everyone down a more positive life path. The field of developmental disabilities refers to this process of reframing as gaining a more positive 'cognitive appraisal,' while the important framework of attachment theory calls this gaining a more positive 'relational schema.' Once the basic process of reframing has begun, it becomes clear to a care giver that many of a young child's learning and behavior problems are 'brain-based.' It is then easier for a care giver to have a more positive and realistic view of the affected individual, feel more effective, and be motivated and 'ready to change' their own ways of doing things. This can be true for parents, grandparents, school staff, and even daycare providers and coaches.

In addition to reframing, clinicians and researchers have come up with basic intervention processes that seem to be the 'heart' of what works with individuals affected by prenatal alcohol exposure, or with FASD, and their families. These intervention processes are part of the practical positive parenting intervention designed for families raising children with FASD, discussed later, called the "Families Moving Forward" program.

As a first line of treatment, it is logical for care givers to use methods that take into account these brain-based difficulties, and help improve how well the affected individual fits into his or her environment. Olson and her team use the term 'accommodations' for these care giving methods [5]. Accommodations include a wide variety of environmental modifications, many learned from research on 'cognitive rehabilitation' for individuals with traumatic brain injury. Some accommodations apply to most affected individuals, including young children, such as increasing structure and predictability in school or home routines, and making sure there is a high level of supervision [16]. These accommodations are geared to the child's 'developmental age' rather than chronological age. There are some accommodations that must be tailored to the needs of the particular individual with FASD. One example for young children might be a teacher who provides memory aids to a child who has problems remembering everyday information. Another example, used for a child who has trouble processing what they hear, might be parents trying to pause while speaking and using simple, concrete language. There are many, many creative ideas for accommodations, such as 'fidgets' to keep a child with high activity and restlessness appropriately focused, ear phones to help a child who cannot handle a noisy environment, or putting a 'picture schedule' on the wall to help a child stay organized during the daily routine. Accommodations largely focus on changing the environment or how the care giver behaves around the child.

There are other intervention processes that can help young children with 'primary disabilities' resulting from the effects of prenatal alcohol exposure. Parenting practices can be tailored to the needs of children in this population. Very early in life, 'relationship-focused' approaches to care giver training may be useful and have good scientific evidence to show improvements in child and family outcome. These include selected professional home visiting and/or infant mental health approaches. As children reach preschool age and beyond, 'positive parenting' interventions that use adapted behavioral principles and are useful for children with developmental disabilities (and/or high psychosocial risk), and their families, may be helpful.

One such behavioral approach is often called 'positive behavior support' (PBS) [17-19]. PBS (sometimes called functional behavioral assessment) has research data showing that it helps improve outcomes in individuals with developmental disabilities (and challenging behavior), and also improves the lives of their families. Learning a PBS approach helps parents (and teachers) understand how to 'shape' their own behavior and create careful behavior plans in order to help a child replace problem behavior with more desirable behavior. Care givers do this to help an affected individual meet needs and behave in ways that are adaptive and functional day-to-day (rather than showing challenging, often negative behavior). Helping care givers learn to use a 'user-friendly' PBS approach that has been adapted for children with FASD, and to do this on their own, is a promising parenting practice. Olson and her colleagues have called use of PBS by care givers a 'brainstorming' process [5].

There are many family needs when raising children affected by prenatal alcohol exposure, or with FASD [20]. Raising children with FASD is highly stressful for care givers [20,21]. Parents need support, both for emotional reasons and for help in figuring out the best parenting strategies, and when trying to reframe their understanding of a child's behavior. The need for parent support, either through parent groups or one-on-one relationships with other parents who have gone through the same situation, is another intervention basic. Research from the field of developmental disabilities suggests that parents and families with the right kind of support do better later on [22]. Parents also need education about FASD, advocacy, the importance of care giver self-care, and the need for respite services throughout the lifespan. Teachers (and coaches, therapists and, later on, employers) also need this kind of education.

Another intervention basic is the fact that a full continuum of care is needed for families raising individuals with FASD. Early intervention is important, because it may take advantage of plasticity of the young brain and help create a more positive life direction. But as affected individuals grow older, they need ongoing and ever-changing services. Early intervention is a time when families need to be prepared for the future, which often includes time for grieving and accepting what is to come. 'Anticipatory guidance,' or talking with families about what may come up and what will likely be needed to help, and how to advocate for services that can be hard to get, is an important part of early intervention. Early intervention providers must recognize that neurodevelopmental disabilities are lifelong. This means that services are needed at every phase in development, as clinical researchers Paley and O'Connor make quite clear in their recent intervention review [10].

There are evidence-based or scientifically-validated interventions, developed for other clinical populations, that are promising for use with young children affected by prenatal alcohol exposure, or with FASD. However, these interventions likely need to be adapted for use with this clinical population to improve effectiveness. FASD describes a clinical population that has complex cognitive and learning disabilities (which may sometimes be hard to measure or understand), who also often have experienced many psychosocial risks. Because of this, child behavior change and care giver understanding of brain-based difficulties will be slow to take place. Parents may feel unsuccessful and will be stressed and personally distressed. For these and other reasons, some necessary treatment adaptations for any early intervention approach used with this population are summarized in Table **1**.

Table 1: Suggested Adaptations for Evidenced Based Early Intervention Approaches Targeted to Children with FASD and/or Their Care givers

Adaptation	Examples
Offer services over a longer period of time	• Increase the prescribed number of treatment sessions, and repeat treatment modules, as needed • Divide up longer sessions or sessions with more content, as needed
Expect slower progress in intervention	• Repeat treatment modules, as needed • Review and practice concepts more often than prescribed • For care givers, help them understand children's brain-based difficulties and resulting slower progress • For children, repeat instructions as needed
Use examples, modalities and treatment goals that are appropriate for the population	• For care givers, if using videotaped materials for learning through observational methods, be sure examples show children with FASD • For children, add visual props to assist in learning and reduce verbal input • For children, aim first for improved adaptive behavior
Consider children's sensory sensitivities and behavior regulation problems in intervention	• For care givers, teach approaches that accommodate child problems, such as difficulty filtering out auditory input or issues with impulse control • For children, deliver services in small groups, quieter conditions, shorter sessions, etc. to reduce stimulation and allow children to stay calm
Build on care giver and child strengths and provide emotional support to care givers	• For many care givers, existing good basic parenting skills can be assets • For children, high social motivation and willingness to ask and receive help from care givers can be assets • For care givers, who may have many strengths, ongoing emotional support (or referral for therapy) will still be needed to tolerate slow progress, deal with high stress and personal distress, and improve feelings of effectiveness

Risk and Protective Factors

As all children develop, their life path and outcomes are negatively affected by the risks they face, and positively affected by life influences that protect them. Risks can include genetic factors (such as family history of major mental illness), medical factors (such as serious illness or head injury), as well as family and socioeconomic factors (such as abuse/neglect, poverty, unsafe neighborhoods, or poor access to social services). Protective factors can also be biological or environmental, and can help reduce risk and promote children's development. Examples of protective factors include a child's good innate intelligence, good nutrition, parental warmth and involvement, a supportive family or community, and many other influences that help a child's life move in a positive direction. Scientific research on development shows that a changing mix of risk and protective factors alters a child's developmental outcome over time. If the mix is tipped toward risk factors, the child's life path can lead to unwanted and undesirable outcomes. If the mix is tipped toward protective factors, the child's life path can be altered in a positive direction. Early intervention is often aimed toward tipping the mix in this positive direction. Risk and protective factors exist at the level of the individual, the levels of relationships and families, and at multiple levels in the wider world of systems and services surrounding the family. In developmental theory, this is called an 'ecological model' of developmental influences [23]. It is thought best to design treatments to decrease risks and promote protective factors (at all these levels) that are good for children in general, and those that are specific to the population.

Prenatal alcohol exposure is one crucial risk factor common to this population. Of course, children born alcohol-exposed often have other prenatal exposures that are also risk factors, such as to cigarettes or street drugs. In a clinical database, Olson and colleagues [6] found that 84.5% of 781 young children, birth to age 8 years, were prenatally exposed to cigarettes and/or licit or illicit drugs along with alcohol. These other prenatal exposures can lead to negative developmental outcomes. But a combination of prenatal exposures may have even greater negative consequences for development.

For children in general, as well as for those affected by prenatal alcohol exposure, individual child characteristics can act as postnatal risk or protective factors. Among young children, for example, developmental research generally shows that a 'difficult' temperament, high levels of negative effect, behavioral cues that are hard for care givers to read, disrupted sleep patterns, and problems in behavior regulation can all be notable risk factors that lead a child down a more difficult life path. Studies conducted to date suggest that all these difficulties commonly occur among young children born prenatally alcohol-exposed [7, 24-27]. Developmental research shows that areas of intact development (such as good basic language skills and individually variable areas of cognitive strength), an engaging manner, and high social motivation can all play a role in helping children travel a more positive life path. Clinical observations by Olson and others suggest these strengths commonly occur among young children with prenatal alcohol exposure [20]. Those who study developmental psychopathology point out that some children seem to be 'resilient,' which means they generally appear less affected by serious, negative influences on development than might typically be expected. The study of resilient individuals is an important area of research for the field of FASD that has not yet been accomplished— for very young children, or at any stage of life.

Developmental theories highlight many crucial environmental influences for young children at the level of their 'primary relationships.' These are their relationships with parents and those who care directly for them. Important influences in primary relationships are the quality of care giving (at home and in childcare), and the warmth and security of attachment and bonding between the child and primary care giver(s). For a young child, the 'goodness-of-fit' between the child and parent is vital. Also important are a child's success in learning affect and behavior regulation through 'attunement' with their parent as an infant, and learning social rules from their parents when they reach the toddlerhood and preschool years [28,29]. Serious problems, such as child maltreatment, can also be a pivotal influence in a child's primary relationships. Environmental influences for young children may also occur at the broader level of the family. These influences, such as strong social support for the family or the availability of services (such as respite care), are also very important for young children. Research on protective factors specific for FASD are discussed in the next section.

Discussing FASD, Streissguth [7] suggests that if those in the young child's world, at all these levels, respond inappropriately to the child's 'primary disabilities' (deficits caused by prenatal alcohol exposure combined with other risk factors), or do not provide adequate support, then the young child's path through life will not go well. Poor adaptive function will continue and problem behaviors will increase. Taken further, if there is an ongoing cycle of inappropriate responses, there may be what is called a negative developmental progression. Developmental psychologists see this as a line-up of 'chain reactions' that can lead to negative outcomes [30]. Over time, unless there is healthy natural change or some kind of effective intervention, secondary disabilities, such as disrupted school experiences or substance use, are likely to emerge from this negative developmental progression. Secondary disabilities bring lifelong negative consequences to the affected individual and their family.

Promising Directions for Early Intervention

Keeping a neurodevelopmental viewpoint in mind, the second half of this chapter has been organized into broad sections of important material about early intervention. These sections first cover descriptive research on the population. The following sections cover early intervention approaches the authors have selected as especially promising for use with young children affected by prenatal alcohol exposure, or with FASD, and (when applicable) their families. There are certainly other approaches, some that are considered evidence-based, which may also be useful in intervention with this population. Information about some of these approaches has been provided in the Appendices linked to this chapter. When there is research specifically with the population of children affected by prenatal alcohol exposure, this is highlighted. An important point to keep in mind is that multi-component interventions may be most effective with this clinical population. For instance, parenting interventions should likely be combined with linkage to parent support groups and to therapies that teach children specific important skills that are a problem because of prenatal alcohol exposure (such as better self-regulation).

RESEARCH ON CHARACTERISTICS OF YOUNG CHILDREN AFFECTED BY PRENATAL ALCOHOL EXPOSURE, THEIR FAMILIES AND PROTECTIVE FACTORS

What does research so far say about the characteristics of young children affected by prenatal alcohol exposure, and their families? What is known about protective factors? This body of research points the way to creating, choosing and adapting approaches to early intervention that will be most effective. There seem to be particular strengths that can be built upon in early intervention, and protective factors that can be put in place. There also are areas of difficulty for infants and young children and their families, and in the systems that serve them. These should be treatment targets for early intervention.

Strengths of Children and Families

The clinical literature and informal reports are filled with descriptions of how engaging, innocent, straightforward, amusing, curious, social and alert young children with an FASD can be, and the sometimes intriguing perspective they bring to understanding life. Many stories of families raising children with FASD are tales of courage, persistence, flexibility and the ability to stay optimistic in the face of challenge. Yet there are limited research data describing child and care giver strengths, especially for adoptive families [20]. Highlights of what is known about child and care giver strengths from data and clinical observations are briefly summarized in Table **2**.

Table 2: Positive Characteristics of Children with FASD and their Care givers

Child Strengths	Care giver Strengths
• Many positively engaged with their families • Many willing to seek/receive help from care givers • Often high social motivation and engaging manner, and interest in being connected emotionally to others • Often have good basic language skills (depending on overall IQ) • Individual children have their own unique profile of strengths	• *Birth parents:* Work to understand and cope with their child's neurodevelopmental problems • *Foster parents:* Often have positive motives for fostering and positive characteristics that enhance their parenting • *All parents (assuming in recovery/in stable households):* Often have good basic parenting practices • *All parents:* Experience both the 'special benefits' and 'common benefits' of parenting, and have their own unique profile of strengths

Data show that about half of a group of young children with FASD were reported by their parents to show positive characteristics, summarized as being engaged with their families and willing to receive (and even seek) help from their care givers [20]. Clinical observations reveal that young children with FASD often show aspects of good social relatedness and high motivation to be connected socially and emotionally, even with people they do not know well. This seems often to be the case despite higher environmental risks experienced by these children. These data all suggest that early intervention approaches where parents and teachers assist children in practicing new skills with their peers, should work well with this population because they build on children's high social motivation and willingness to receive help [20]. But sometimes children born prenatally exposed do show a diagnosed attachment disorder, or other significant psychological impact of maltreatment. When this occurs, early intervention must be adjusted to address this problem during treatment, and good social motivation cannot be counted upon. Promising intervention ideas for young children drawn from the field of child maltreatment are discussed later in this chapter.

Positive motives for successful fostering of children with FASD have been studied. Findings of positive motives included wanting to help children with disabilities and to help children stay connected with their families and communities [31]. Qualitative study of birth mothers raising children with FASD found these women worked independently to develop understanding and coping methods for their children's neurodevelopmental problems [32]. Very appropriate parenting attitudes have been reported by parents of all types raising preschool and school-aged children with FASD and very challenging behavior, even before treatment was applied [20]. As illustrated in the real-life 'scene' between Ian and his mother presented at the outset of this chapter, families raising children with FASD anecdotally report experiencing 'special benefits' as their parents, which are positives and benefits above and beyond the usual 'common benefits' of parenting. Care giver-focused interventions that emphasize the rewards of these 'special benefits' of parenting may keep adults involved, increase parenting satisfaction, and also promote care giver positive cognitive appraisal (or 'relational schema') and optimism [5,20]. Both relationship-building and 'positive parenting' interventions do this, to some extent, and are discussed later in the chapter.

Protective Factors for this Population

There is limited research identifying protective influences for the population of individuals with FASD or prenatal alcohol exposure. Available data are briefly summarized in Table **3** as applied to early intervention.

Table 3: Summary of Protective Factors for Individuals with FASD Based on Research

At the Level of Care giving
For foster parents: • Care giver ability to provide structure and a high level of organization • The right kind of personality and skills for raising children with FASD • A good diagnostic understanding of FASD
For all family types (birth, adoptive, foster): • Having an early diagnosis of a condition on the fetal alcohol spectrum (before age 6 years) • Descriptors of stable, nurturant, appropriately stimulating 'good quality' care giving (in early and middle childhood) • Child not living with parents involved with substance abuse or directly experiencing violence • Positive perceptions of the child and parent-child relationship by care givers, such as what may occur from 'reframing,' and other improvements in care giver attitudes • Improved care giver knowledge and parenting practices, such as: relationship-focused interventions; knowledge of FASD and advocacy; use of 'accommodations' and 'brainstorming;' or other positive parenting practices
At the Level of Systems and Supports
For all family types (birth, adoptive, foster): • Good parent support and self-help (see Appendix 1 for information on parent support) • Availability, positive nature and good quality of family and neighbor social support • Availability of social services funding • Availability of effective treatments for families raising young children with FASD, and adjunct treatments such as recovery support for parents

At the Level of Care Giving

Qualitative study of families raising children with FASD found what was needed for successful placements with foster parents were care giver protective factors. These included parental ability to provide structure and a high level of organization, and a good understanding of FASD. Also important was the right kind of personality and skills, such as having flexibility, dedication, love and endurance, though it was also considered important to match individual parent strengths with a particular child's needs [33].

For all family structures, descriptors of stable, nurturant, appropriately stimulating 'good quality' care giving (in early and middle childhood), and not living with parents involved with substance abuse or experiencing violence, were found to have a universally 'protective' influence on outcome. This meant lowered odds of secondary disabilities among affected individuals in natural history research on FASD [34]. Also, a more positive home environment (in terms of developmental stimulation) in elementary school was related to less severe alcohol effects on aspects of cognition at age 7½ years in longitudinal study of prenatal alcohol exposure [35]. Improved knowledge and altered care giver attitudes and behavior (relative to comparison groups) were found in several interventions applied to children with FASD and their families, coupled with findings of positive child outcome [5]. In the field of developmental disabilities, positive perceptions on the part of care givers have been found to serve as an adaptive coping mechanism [36]. These findings provide some guidance for early intervention. Needed are addiction treatment and recovery support (when necessary), knowledge about FASD, help with creating environmental structure and other 'accommodations,' encouragement of positive attitudes among care givers, and parenting programs specialized for this population.

At the Level of Systems and Supports

Protective influences at the wider level of the supports and services surrounding the family have been pinpointed by research in the field of FASD. Parent support and self-help were found to have positive effects on outcome for families raising children with FASD regardless of family type (birth, adoptive, foster) [20]. Availability of family and neighbor social support, and of social services funding, were recognized as important for successful foster placements [33]. Streissguth *et al.* [34] identified the availability of appropriate social services as an important factor associated with reduced odds of secondary disabilities in a diverse group of individuals with FASD across a wide age range. Studying disabilities in general, Bailey [22] stated that the nature and quality of social support available to families raising children with disabilities have repeatedly been demonstrated as vital to positive family adaptation. This means that parent support and linkage to appropriate social services are vital to early intervention. Parent support is discussed in supplementary material connected to this chapter (Appendix 1.)

Child Deficits

In a large clinical sample of children 8 years and younger born alcohol-exposed, Olson *et al.* [6] found that only just over half showed marked developmental delay in the first three years of life. This means that while some show global deficits, more than one-fourth of the sample had early developmental profiles well within normal limits using standard developmental tests. The same percentages applied to the smaller group of children later diagnosed with FAS or partial FAS. This suggests that deficits may not be obvious in standardized test results or many areas of function until middle childhood and beyond. But research so far does show that many infants and young children affected by prenatal alcohol exposure may show problems not often measured in developmental tests. These hard-to-measure problems are found in deficits in adaptive function, physiological processes and regulatory capacity, motor skills, and in certain precursor impairments of later-developing cognitive skills. It appears that special methods of early identification are necessary for this population, since the usual ways of finding children with problems may not work well. These are discussed in the next section of this chapter. Categories of difficulties for this population are briefly presented in Table **4**.

Adaptive Behavior Deficits

Among children with FASD aged 5 to 8 years, significantly greater problems in adaptive function were found compared to a group of typically developing peers [37]. Research has clearly identified adaptive behavior deficits among young children with prenatal alcohol exposure. These deficits were not attributable only to children's level of IQ, and did not seem related to postnatal disruption as measured by multiple home placements [38]. Children with FASD have been found to show delayed daily living skills even compared to those with ADHD, with socialization and communication increasing areas of difficulty as children with FASD grow older. Importantly, compared to healthy controls, young children with FASD much more frequently needed intensive levels of adaptive support from parents and teachers (presumably creating greater care giver burden) [37]. The extent of a child's need for adaptive support is a better predictor of service intensity than a child's level of adaptive behavior or maladaptive behavior alone. This suggests that early interventions for young children with FASD should be designed to improve child adaptive behavior (ability to function day-to-day), and help the family provide more intensive adaptive support. Most early intervention approaches discussed in this chapter have these dual aims.

Table 4: Difficulties for Young Children with FASD, Their Care givers and Families Based on Research

For Young Children
• Adaptive behavior deficits, with increased need for a higher level of care giver support to function well day-to-day
• Global or more subtle, wide-ranging developmental deficits (though subtle deficits may not become apparent until the child is older)
• Precursors of later deficits in higher-order cognitive skills, negative affectivity and problems in behavior regulation
• Disturbance of physiological processes and regulatory capacity, including deficits in early motor skills
• Social skills deficits and behavioral variability
• Potential for child psychopathology and child behavior problems
For Care givers/Families
For all family types (birth, adoptive, foster):
• High care giving stress related to the child
• High levels of unmet, important family needs
• Specific need for respite care and understanding of FASD by all service systems
• Often high psychosocial risk status for the family

Global or Wide-Ranging Developmental Deficits

Some individuals with FASD can show global developmental or intellectual delays. Broadly speaking, however, as many affected individuals grow older, deficits related to the teratogenic effects of alcohol can eventually emerge in many domains. These can include deficits in arousal and attention, behavior (or self) regulation, processing speed, cognition, learning and memory, executive functions, and higher-level integrative language abilities (especially social communication and pragmatics). Deficits can also occur in the ability to encode visual stimuli, visual-spatial abilities, neurological 'soft signs' indicating sensory-motor immaturities, and fine and gross motor skills (including difficulties in such areas as precision, dynamic balance, inefficient motor performance and handwriting). Further, deficits can occur in academic achievement, social skills, and behavior problems. No 'behavioral phenotype' (core set of characteristics) has been identified for FASD at this point in time, though it has been suggested that this population generally has difficulties with complex information-processing [14,15]. Because of the variable way in which alcohol exposure causes CNS damage and dysfunction, no two individuals with FASD are alike in specific clinical features, even if they share common areas of deficit.

The chapter in this book by Coles and her colleagues does a good job reviewing research on deficits found among children with FASD as these relate to educational interventions. However, research has documented these deficits primarily as of middle childhood and beyond. It is surprising how few studies look at the skills of very young children affected by prenatal alcohol exposure.

Precursors of Later Deficits in Higher-Order Cognitive Skills, Negative Affectivity, and Behavior Regulation

Developmental skills are highly interrelated in young children, so it is hard to identify subtle deficits or sort out deficits in specific domains. Developmental difficulties in these early years can show up as global delays, but may often be more subtle and found as impairments in the precursors of higher-level cognitive skills. Thought of most generally, problems among young children affected by prenatal alcohol exposure may have problems in emotional and behavioral regulation. This includes a general tendency toward 'negative affectivity' (internal feelings of distress and engagement with others that are not pleasurable; related to negative moods such as anger, fear, or worry) [39].

Problems in behavior regulation may be a central area of difficulty in young children affected by prenatal alcohol exposure. New research by the authors finds behavior regulation difficulties among young children (aged 4 to 8 years) diagnosed with FASD, compared to a matched group of peers from high-risk environments. Findings are presented in a short, interesting paper linked to this chapter (see Appendix 2). Developmental researchers who study behavior and self-regulation suggest that children with high physiological arousal and poor regulatory capacity fare worse in social situations [40,41]. Such children may have problems 'returning to baseline,' and 'settling down' to make good social decisions [42,43]. Unfortunately, this does not bode well for young children affected by prenatal alcohol exposure who show just these kinds of problems. For this group, interventions to help children improve behavior regulation are vital, and discussed later in this chapter.

Developmental systems research has traced the early life path of young children born prenatally alcohol-exposed, studying them within their primary care giving relationships. Programmatic studies indicate these children more often show individual characteristics that place them at risk for negative outcomes, including behavior problems. Biologically-based difficulties in their development negatively impact the quality of the early parent-child relationship, although parent characteristics certainly also affect this relationship. High psychosocial risk (such as poverty) worsens these negative effects on the parent-child relationship, and leads to even more difficulties in child outcome later on [24, 44-47]. Relationship-focused and positive parenting interventions that can help the early parent-child relationship go more smoothly are important for children born prenatally alcohol-exposed, and are discussed later in this chapter.

Disturbance of Physiological Processes and Regulatory Capacity, Including Deficits in Motor Skills

In young children affected by prenatal alcohol exposure or with FASD, 'brain-based' difficulties may first be seen in disturbances of physiological processes and regulatory capacity in daytime function, and even in disrupted sleep. Infants with prenatal alcohol exposure may have early motor problems, such as tone abnormalities, tremulousness, oral-motor difficulties, and delayed acquisition of motor milestones [48,49]. Infants born prenatally exposed to alcohol appear to have greater attention and arousal regulation problems, and greater stress reactivity. They may possibly encode environmental events differently at a neurophysiological level [27].

In a cutting-edge longitudinal study, Kable and Coles [27] examined early attentional regulation among 6-month-old infants. Using heart rate measures, infants more heavily exposed to alcohol responded more slowly to stimuli and were rated as significantly higher in arousal level when exposed to a series of auditory tones and picture stimuli. In a more recent study, Haley *et al.* [25] found that heavier exposure to alcohol before birth was associated with greater activation of infant stress response systems. Greater maternal drinking was related to faster heart rates, increased negative affect and other indicators of stress reactivity in infants of 5 to 7 months of age, when the babies were exposed to a mild social stressor. This was true even when controlling for other important confounding factors. There were differences in reactivity among girls and boys.

The study by Haley and his colleagues reflects a larger body of animal and human research on an interesting link between prenatal alcohol exposure and activation of a key component of the stress system (the limbic-hypothalamic-pituitary-adrenal [L-HPA] Axis). Abnormalities of what is generally called the HPA Axis can have negative effects for cognitive, affective and behavioral development. Interventions that improve function of the HPA Axis are of real interest for children born prenatally alcohol-exposed, with several such interventions discussed later in this chapter.

Social Skills Deficits and Behavioral Variability

Starting at about age 6 years, several studies reveal that social skills deficits are common among children diagnosed with FASD. Clinical observations have noted such problems as being overly friendly with strangers, socially immature, or being innocent, naïve and suggestible. Schonfeld *et al.* [50] found social skill deficits based on both parent and teacher report, with ratings of children's executive functioning predicting their level of social skills. Deficits can include problems in important areas of peer relations in children as young as 6 years, such as friendship skills [51]. A recent study has detected difficulties in social information processing in children as young as 7 years, suggesting there are problems with social cognitive processes underlying successful peer social interaction in children with heavy prenatal alcohol exposure [52]. Detailed classroom observation data show that young school-aged children also show higher rates of behavioral variability, compared to age- and gender-matched classroom peers [53]. Early intervention may be able to target some of the early impairment that lays the foundation for these later social skills deficits and behavioral variability.

Potential for Child Psychopathology and Challenging Behavior

Researchers O'Connor and Paley [39] emphasize that children born prenatally alcohol-exposed show "negative affectivity". However, they also note that eventual developmental outcomes depend on the responses and personal characteristics of the children's care givers. They conclude that prenatal alcohol exposure can act as a significant risk factor for early onset child psychopathology, along with other risks. O'Connor and Paley [39] have speculated that a developmental progression to conduct problems may occur in this population, given underlying problems in social information processing coupled with difficulties in self-regulation, and the presence of adverse environmental influences. O'Connor and Paley [47] also found an increased risk of childhood-onset depression in young children prenatally exposed to alcohol, with environmental influences playing an important role.

For young children in this population, behavior problems often discussed in the informal family literature include poor understanding of consequences, temper tantrums and angry outbursts, unpredictable behavior and changeable mood, noncompliance, impulsivity and difficulty inhibiting responses. A higher prevalence of behavioral difficulties and psychiatric conditions in this population not only occurs in childhood, but also in adolescence and adulthood. These difficulties can also be affected by both positive and negative environmental influences [39].

Care Giver/Family Difficulties

Recent studies consistently show very high child-related stress among care givers raising children with FASD (e.g., [20,21]. The source of this stress appears to lie more in children's problems with executive function than in their level of IQ or their diagnosis on the fetal alcohol spectrum [21]. Clinical wisdom suggests that stress and burden may occur in part because care givers may misunderstand the reasons for a child's dysfunctional behavior, and/or because home and school environments are not set up to accommodate the child's areas of deficit. Families raising children affected by prenatal alcohol exposure describe themes of family impact and family needs (e.g., care giver emotional and financial burden, impact on sibling function, lack of professional services) [20,32,33,54]. Town hall meetings emphasize the need for respite care and understanding of FASD by all service systems [55].

The Influence of Psychosocial Risk

Epidemiologic research reveals that environmental risk often characterizes the experience of families and young children born prenatally alcohol-exposed, and of those with FASD. Data from a large clinical database documents that the majority (82.6%) of young children (birth to 8 years) born prenatally alcohol-exposed, and those with FASD, whether they lived with birth, adoptive or foster parents, had clinical rankings of either "high" or "some" postnatal psychosocial risk [6]. Research also shows that prenatal alcohol exposure is highly associated with known postnatal environmental risk factors such as maternal drinking, care giver depression, and child maltreatment among birth parents at high psychosocial risk [56]. Developmental theory clearly states that children's outcomes are affected by an accumulation of risk from both biological and environmental factors. The problems experienced by children affected by prenatal alcohol exposure, or with an FASD, are the result of what has been called 'double jeopardy' coming from a mix of biological and environmental risks.

EARLY IDENTIFICATION OF CHILDREN BORN PRENATALLY ALCOHOL-EXPOSED

If intervention is to be provided as early as possible, there must be effective methods to identify young children with prenatal alcohol exposure. Preferably early identification would even pick out those who will later show effects of this exposure, and a diagnostic condition in the category of FASD. However, early identification is a challenge for many reasons. Unfortunately, passive identification systems such as birth defect registries do not include documentation of prenatal exposure. Providers in many settings where young children are seen (such as hospitals or early intervention programs) still miss infants and young children with characteristic facial features, and questions about prenatal alcohol exposure are not always asked. Innovative active identification systems are being tried, such as screening of digital facial photos for FAS features in young foster children in the U.S. [57] or experimental work on computerized 3-D modeling of facial features, but few children are screened at present. In countries such as Italy and South Africa, children are being screened in primary schools for possible effects of prenatal alcohol exposure [58,59], but this still misses very young children.

Research provides guidance on methods for detecting at-risk drinking. This is one way there can be very early identification of affected babies, or even detection before a child is born, although the practical value of these methods must be determined. Coles and her colleagues [60] examined the relative usefulness of several methods that could be used in neonatal healthcare settings to identify low birth weight children considered at-risk (because of prenatal substance exposure) to show developmental problems in the first year of life. While all methods were useful, the most sensitive and specific method was a 17-item maternal risk index of primarily substance use indicators, even though this method did lead to "false positives" (children identified as at risk even when they were not).

More recently, Chiodo *et al.* [61] set out to find detection methods useful during pregnancy that could predict learning problems presumably related to prenatal alcohol exposure in older preschoolers. The most useful method was a simple metric that defined a woman as 'at risk' if there was a 'yes' answer on any of several indices of self-reported maternal alcohol drinking during pregnancy (each considered a standard definition of 'at risk drinking'). The researchers recommended that clinical suspicions or positive screens be followed up with thorough assessment of drinking patterns and consequences. They also suggested their metric might improve how prenatal alcohol exposure is defined when children are examined in FASD diagnostic settings.

Early identification of young children affected by prenatal alcohol exposure needs to be folded into community practice. Although there has been progress, it is remarkable (and unfortunate) that questions about prenatal alcohol exposure are not routinely part of the standard of care for young children in settings where such questions could easily be asked, such as maternal-child health centers, parenting programs, or childcare centers. Providers caring for young children are not well-trained to recognize the physical or developmental indicators of alcohol effects. Changes are needed in professional practice.

Based on review of a large clinical database, Olson and her colleagues [6] pointed out that traditional indicators of problems in infancy, such as preterm birth, are not necessarily seen in children who are diagnosed with FASD up to age 8. The usual brief developmental screening methods used in early intervention, and even longer individually-administered developmental tests such as the Bayley Scales, may miss many children who later show the teratogenic effects of alcohol. When prenatal alcohol exposure is known, these researchers suggest that subtle facial features, microcephaly (small head size), mild growth impairment, subtle indicators of sensorimotor problems, and even behavior regulation problems may actually be more useful indicators for an FASD diagnostic referral than test scores. These indicators are not always recognized by those in early intervention settings.

Training is needed so early intervention providers can better carry out early identification of children affected by prenatal alcohol exposure. These providers also need clear guidance about what to do after questions are asked, and where to refer for FASD diagnosis. A list of training topics for early intervention providers is linked to this chapter (Appendix 3). Providers also need information about promising early interventions so they can do treatment planning. To that end, a variety of treatment recommendations and description of promising intervention approaches are discussed in the remainder of this chapter.

TREATMENT RECOMMENDATIONS FOR YOUNG CHILDREN DRAWN FROM AN FASD CLINICAL DATABASE

A statewide FASD diagnostic clinic network, called the Fetal Alcohol Syndrome Diagnostic Prevention Network (FAS DPN), has been operating since 1993 in Washington State. Over the years, a recommendations database based on expert opinion has been developed by the FAS DPN interdisciplinary professional teams. Delving into this database through record review, Jirikowic and her colleagues [62] described the most common referrals and recommendations received by 120 families of newly diagnosed children with FASD (age range: 0.2 to 16.5 years old).

Recommendations for social services were made for almost 90% of the families raising infants and toddlers (0-2 years). These services included family support programs/funding or advocacy for permanency placement. About 75% of these families received recommendations for family resources, such as parent support and education groups, advocacy training, care giver respite and self-care, and educational materials for self-help. Families with preschoolers (3-5 years) were more likely to receive recommendations for behavioral intervention than were families with younger children. It is important to note that behavioral intervention or learning accommodations were recommended for 50% of the overall sample of children birth to 16 years, showing the importance of these interventions. About 66% of families raising preschoolers received suggestions for anticipatory guidance (planning ahead for developmental and educational challenges) and developmental therapies (such as occupational therapy and speech-language therapy) [62].

FAMILY WISDOM ABOUT INTERVENTION FOR YOUNG CHILDREN AFFECTED BY PRENATAL ALCOHOL EXPOSURE

There is a growing body of observations by families and clinicians that provides crucial information about useful interventions for young children affected by prenatal alcohol exposure, or with FASD. However, these observations have not yet been validated through research. In town hall meetings held across the U.S. in 2002 and 2003, families and other participants identified two primary service needs across all family types (and across all ages of alcohol-affected individuals). Respite care was one basic need. Another was the need for all systems of care for children and families to understand FASD and provide appropriate services for this condition [55-63]. While the availability of respite care is still a problem, there is increasing availability of education on FASD for professionals in all systems of care. For instance, in the U.S. the Centers for Disease Control and Prevention have created a system of regional FASD training centers (**http://fasdcenter.samhsa.gov/documents/Flyerfasd_RTCs.pdf**) [64]. Around the world, there is a growing awareness of FASD through governmental education efforts, websites from parent organizations, and guidelines being developed by professional organizations.

A recent source of family wisdom on intervention comes from informal review of parenting forums, newsletters, and comments from support groups. This type of review was conducted over an 8-week period in 2009 for this chapter in order to find important trends in intervention for young children (*sources: FASlink [65]; Arctic FASPRTC [66]; NOFAS Parent Support Group [67]*). The review revealed that in these venues care givers often share experiences of parenting stress, and make efforts to find and partake of social support with other parents having similar problems with their young children. These trends fit well with data from the larger developmental disabilities literature indicating that informal social support, which often provides emotional support and practical childrearing input, is a form of intervention— and a powerful predictor of positive family and child outcome (Appendix 1).

In these parent support venues during the 2009 review, care givers shared ideas that are presented in italics below. They discussed *how to deal with the difficult behaviors* of their young alcohol-affected children and *how to manage care giver stress*. Frequently discussed interventions for the home centered around accommodations, or changing the environment so children's behavior is more functional (e.g., clear the child's room of everything but the essentials like a bed and blanket), and families seemed interested in these home adaptations. Parents offered advice to each other on *specific parenting techniques*, such as limiting verbal instructions when managing behavior and using repetition to help children learn, and hearing about strategies that work seemed to help families feel more confident and effective. Parents described trying to *help their young child identify their own feelings and how others feel*. Many parents posting on these listservs seemed to understand *how to deal with the sensory needs of young children* affected by prenatal alcohol exposure. Families appeared interested in finding *strategies to help their young child calm down*. Parents also seemed interested in *assistance with advocacy for their young child's educational rights*, and *help in explaining their child's special needs to those not informed about FASD*. There was strong *encouragement to stay hopeful and optimistic in parenting*.

This family wisdom informed the authors' selection of the scientifically validated early intervention approaches discussed next in this chapter.

RELATIONSHIP-FOCUSED EARLY INTERVENTION

Developmental research shows there can sometimes be significant problems in the early relationships between infants and toddlers affected by prenatal alcohol exposure and their primary care givers. This means that strategies to support and improve the early parent-child relationship are important interventions for them. The developmental literature offers several useful approaches.

First, because stable care giving environments lead to improved child outcome, a successful and efficient permanency planning process in the child welfare system is one important intervention. This process helps young children born prenatally alcohol-exposed move to stable adoptive homes. Alternatively, this process helps young children live in a more stable home because birth parents enter into recovery (perhaps because of motivating 'windows of opportunity' created by awareness of their child's exposure or diagnosis). Placement stability can create a more positive life trajectory for the child.

Second, relationship-focused interventions used early in life can help improve security of attachment—and also promote mutual regulation between parent and child, or the way in which parents and children interact together and stay in a calm and responsive state. For birth families, when needed, relationship-focused early intervention can be paired with parental depression and/or addiction treatment, to help birth parents become more sensitive and responsive care givers for their alcohol-affected young children. There are various types of relationship-focused interventions, including selected home visiting and infant mental health programs, discussed below and briefly presented in Table **5**.

Table 5: Relationship-Focused Approaches to Early Intervention

Selected Relationship-Focused Home Visiting and Infant Mental Health Programs
• *Nurse-Family Partnership*: Program of nurse home visitation that occurs prenatally and until the child's 2nd birthday. Aimed to improve women's prenatal health behavior and competent parenting during infancy and toddlerhood, and the life course development of the parent.
• *Promoting First Relationships*: Prevention program of parent education and support for care givers raising children with special needs, based on attachment theory. Includes videotaping parent-child interactions, discussing these with positive comments to build care giver competence with and commitment to their children, and focusing on emotional needs underlying children's challenging behaviors. Can be applied by early intervention service providers in multiple settings, or carried out in home visits.
• *Circle of Security*: Group infant mental health intervention, with additional individual visits focused on the unique parent-child relationship using analysis and clinician-parent dialogue about video vignettes of the parent and child together. Provides psychoeducation and psychotherapy for families at high-risk, based on attachment theory. Designed to help care givers provide a 'secure base' or safe haven for their children.
• *Child-Parent Psychotherapy*: Approach based on an integration of several theories for women at very high risk because of their own traumatic life experiences, often also including alcohol and drug abuse. Longer-term and more intensive therapy, with multiple components that focus on building a sense of trust and safe intimacy between parent and child. Includes helping parents understand their own viewpoint and their infant's distinct viewpoint, and build mutual understanding.

Relationship-Focused Home Visiting Programs

There is a great deal of literature on the impact of relationship-focused home visiting programs for parents raising infants and very young children. In these programs, a home visitor comes on a regular basis to the home of a parent with a new child, usually for at least a year. In 2000, Olds and colleagues [68] comprehensively reviewed these programs, which ranged widely from nurse visitors calling on pregnant and early parenting women at high risk (low income, unmarried, and/or first-time adolescent parents), to trained paraprofessional visitor programs. There were also programs in which home visits were made by professionals to families at risk for various reasons (such as high psychosocial risk, adoption, at risk for attachment disorders, or chemical dependency), and more. According to Olds *et al.* [68], not all home visiting programs are efficacious. They did find that home visiting services for parents with young children vulnerable because of low birth weight, illness or disability appear to be useful when programs are well-designed and well-conducted. They also found that home visiting programs carried out by professionals, guided by specific, carefully thought-out procedures grounded in theory on parent-child attachment, have shown beneficial effects on infant attachment. Olds and his colleagues have found long-term positive benefits of some home visiting programs for children and their parents. Specifically, they have found the *Nurse-Family Partnership* to be a useful and effective program [68,69].

Stern [59], a developmental researcher, has summarized information about home visiting programs. He noted that good quality home visiting programs seem to have a wide variety of positive effects. These include improvement in sensitive maternal behavior, richness of the parent's perception of the child, maternal mood, and healthy life choices. Stern noted that a more effective home visiting process seems to have several characteristics. This includes visits that occur at regular and frequent intervals, programs that start in the 1st month (or even before the baby is born), and careful pre-training and regular supervision for home visitors. Stern points out that home visitors are often mature women. Based on this and other observations, he notes that treatment effects may partly come from specific intervention techniques, but may actually arise mostly from therapeutic, 'non-specific' effects of the good quality relationship that is built between the home visitor and (usually) the mother. Stern theorizes that this visitor-mother relationship can actually be viewed as providing a secure attachment and 'holding environment' for the mother.

Lyons-Ruth and Easterbrooks [70] have tried to look at the effects of early home visiting over time. In their research, they looked at children's outcome at 18 months, 5 years and 7 years. They found there was no evidence of an "inoculation" effect of home visiting for an *individual* child. For *groups* of children (as a whole), however, they did find that good quality home visiting had positive effects later in life. The patterns of intervention-related effects over time were complicated. A pattern emerged showing that early home visiting services shift family dynamics of highly stressed families, and act to prevent a downward spiral. Their data suggested this was true only when services were intensive and lasting. Less intensive home visiting programs did not seem to have this result. These researchers also found a second pattern in their data. In this pattern, home visiting services in infancy and toddlerhood seemed to set in motion a better family process that evolved over time, continuing to have positive effects at each phase in development (even when there were episodes of difficulties with the child).

This research suggests that early home visiting programs may be useful for infants and toddlers affected by prenatal alcohol exposure, who are biologically vulnerable and may show disabilities. If home visiting programs are used, they should be well-conducted, carried out by well-trained, supervised home visitors, and (in these early years) likely grounded in attachment theory. Highly stressed families will probably benefit the most, but services to these families should be intensive and long-lasting. The effects may appear as a slowing of a downward spiral, and/or may have periodic positive effects at different developmental stages over time. Individual children and families may not always show the positive effects that are seen when looking at the group as a whole.

Infant Mental Health Interventions

Interventions taking an 'infant mental health' perspective are usually grounded in attachment theory. These interventions typically aim to improve attachment security between the young child and primary care givers, and improve the process of 'mutual regulation' between parent and child. Infant mental health interventions are typically applied in the first three years of life (and usually started in the child's first or second year). Some of these interventions are home visiting programs. All these programs are designed to lay the foundation for better mental health in childhood and beyond.

In infancy, these relationship-focused interventions help parents learn how to be sensitive and responsive to their baby. Parents are taught how to read their very young child's cues and appropriately soothe distress. In toddlerhood, these interventions help parents understand how to provide a 'supportive presence' and 'secure base' to their toddler, who is learning to be more independent and striving for mastery and competence. Parents are taught how to let their child try out things on their own (and make mistakes), but still assist, soothe and protect their child just enough to let them learn and be independent while staying safe and secure. Infant mental health interventions often also aim to help parents understand the viewpoint of their child, and develop positive perceptions ('relational schemas') about the parent-child relationship.

Infant mental health interventions have the goal of creating warmly engaged parent-child relationships and, as children grow older, the added goals of promoting proper limit-setting and monitoring provided by parents. If well supported, the underlying ideas are that, over time, the young child moves from care giver-imposed regulation to good ability to self-regulate and an improved ability to comply with parent instructions. Over time, if well supported, young children also learn and begin to follow social rules, both when guided by their parents and (eventually) on their own. Achieving all these developmental goals may be a harder process for children affected by prenatal exposure to alcohol. Because of this, they may need much more support. Infant mental health interventions can help care givers provide better support for their young alcohol-exposed children.

Infant mental health interventions can also help care givers understand how to use special environmental accommodations for young children who have biological vulnerabilities. One example is using less stimulating 'vertical rocking.' This is a technique in which a baby is held and rocked vertically, facing away from the parent (which can be calming), rather than in the usual rocking posture in which a child is cradled in a parent's arms and held face-to-face. In general, accommodations can be used to help children prone to arousal regulation problems, including those affected by prenatal alcohol exposure, avoid overstimulation and achieve better regulation of their 'state' (wake, sleep, distress, etc.).

A wide variety of infant mental health interventions exist, and books are available that discuss the broad scope of the field [71]. See Table **5** for a listing of a few of these intervention approaches that might be useful for families raising infants and toddlers with prenatal alcohol exposure, although there are other possibilities. Most likely, any of these interventions would need to be combined with care giver education on FASD and related topics. There are attachment-based infant mental health interventions such as *Promoting First Relationships* [72], *Circle of Security* [73-75], or others [76,77]. Some of these interventions are aimed at mothers at very high risk because of their own traumatic life experiences, often including substance abuse, such as *Child-Parent Psychotherapy* [78-80]. Some infant mental health approaches address various child mental health problems, such as attachment disorders [81] or depression [82], which may be co-morbid conditions experienced by young children with FASD. Many of these interventions take place through home visiting or bringing families into mental health clinics. But there are also approaches that integrate infant mental health interventions into settings already attended by young children with prenatal alcohol exposure. These settings range from Early Head Start, to substance abuse treatment programs for parents [83], to case management programs for very high-risk women with chemical dependency who are parenting young children who were born drug-exposed [84].

There are data to support the efficacy and utility of the various infant mental health interventions discussed above. However, while these interventions have been used for populations that undoubtedly include children born prenatally alcohol-exposed, no data are yet available showing efficacy for use specifically with children identified as prenatally alcohol-exposed, or with FASD. The wide range of infant mental health interventions are well-suited for matching to the diversity of families raising children affected by prenatal alcohol exposure. The particular technique(s) chosen should be matched to care giver needs (such as history of parental chemical dependency, or presence of maternal depression), severity of neurodevelopmental delay observed in the child, and co-morbid conditions (such as child attachment problems or evidence of childhood depression).

Tests of promising infant mental health interventions are an especially high priority for research on early intervention with infants affected by prenatal alcohol exposure. Research examining the efficacy of infant mental health interventions has begun, led by researcher Paley and her team. One good candidate for research is an intervention called *Promoting First Relationships* [72], which can be delivered in multiple settings, is easily adapted for children with special needs, and can be used with families at high risk. There are also interesting interventions developed for children with autism spectrum disorders that could be tried out with young children affected by prenatal alcohol exposure. Another research priority is to carry out "secondary data analysis' in more general studies of the effectiveness of infant mental health interventions. This could be done by identifying the children with prenatal alcohol exposure already being served, and comparing their outcome to non-exposed children receiving the intervention.

Interventions Designed for Children with Autism Spectrum Disorders

It is beyond the scope of this chapter to discuss all that has been learned from the study of intervention for children with Autism Spectrum Disorders (ASD), another important neurodevelopmental disability. However, several points drawn from a recent review of ASD interventions help in thinking about early intervention for FASD [85]. First, entry into treatment immediately after diagnosis (or when identified as high risk) has been nationally recommended for ASD. This also seems crucial for children born with heavy prenatal alcohol exposure or FASD. Second, an intervention recommendation for ASD is the creation of 'natural environments,' such as school and home, that build on strengths and compensate for deficits. From a neurodevelopmental viewpoint, this might be rephrased as working hard to provide 'accommodations' for children at home and at school, also thought to be vital for FASD. A third intervention recommendation is the strong need for education and support for care givers raising children with ASD. This is also important in FASD intervention.

In recent years, there has been a major effort to carry out research on intervention for ASD, using a variety of promising models. A surge of intervention research is also crucial for the field of FASD. As discussed in the recent review [85], the strongest evidence in early intervention for ASD (so far tested for children of preschool age and older) supports the effectiveness of behavioral techniques, such as intensive, individualized behavioral treatment to improve cognitive skills [e.g., 86]. Adapted behavioral techniques are likely very useful for children with FASD, at least from the preschool years on. There are also non-behavioral intervention models for ASD that focus on social-emotional growth and other areas of development that have some evidence of effectiveness, such as the Denver Early Start Model [87]. Several of these interventions focus on teaching parents general principles related to the factors that are thought to influence how children with ASD learn. These approaches then provide training to care givers on how to plan ways to help their young children with ASD improve in important deficit areas for this disability. In the same way, it seems vital to develop interventions that help care givers raising infants and young children with prenatal alcohol exposure or FASD to 'reframe' and take a 'neurodevelopmental viewpoint.' They can then plan ways for how to help their youngsters improve behavior regulation and other individual areas of difficulty, and decrease challenging behavior. All this means is that innovative infant mental health interventions, and the 'positive parenting interventions' discussed in the next section, may have special promise for FASD intervention.

POSITIVE PARENTING INTERVENTIONS

The present chapter focuses on a selected set of scientifically validated parenting interventions that seem especially promising for FASD intervention from a neurodevelopmental viewpoint. The current authors term these "positive parenting "interventions. These scientifically validated interventions teach positive parenting skills, and methods for dealing with the challenging behavior that is common in FASD. One program is designed especially for this clinical population. Table **6** provides a brief summary of these selected interventions.

There are a variety of parent training methods and treatment elements available, including those primarily developed for young children at risk for (or with) disruptive behavior disorders or ADHD, or focused on promoting school readiness. Appendix 4 has examples of evidence-based parenting interventions not covered in this chapter. With careful adaptation, these types of approaches might be useful for children affected by prenatal alcohol exposure. However, these approaches may not work well as stand-alone treatments, and it is important to note that the evidence base for these programs may not have included children with neurological impairment.

Table 6: Positive Parenting Interventions for Use with Families Raising Young Children

Selected Positive Parenting Interventions
• *Families Moving Forward Program:* Individualized behavioral consultation intervention designed for families raising preschool and school-aged children with prenatal alcohol exposure or FASD and behavior problems. Combines motivational interviewing techniques with care giver education, support and skills-teaching. Aims to have care givers take a neurodevelopmental viewpoint and use positive behavior support. Also provides targeted school and provider consultation, and linkages to community services. Delivered by specially trained clinicians in home or clinic visits.
• *Family Check-Up Model:* Prevention program designed for families at high psychosocial risk. Combines motivational interviewing techniques and promotes parent use of positive behavior support in visits at strategic developmental timepoints. Tested so far at the toddlerhood and preschool ages. Linked to an individually variable amount of customized parenting support services. Delivered by specially trained parent consultants in a variety of settings.
• *Triple P Stepping Stones Program:* Group parenting education program with some individual home observation sessions, used with families raising toddlers through young school-aged children with developmental disabilities. Based on behavioral family intervention and parent management training. Uses video vignettes of a variety of child management techniques, with discussion and some individual treatment planning. Delivered by specially trained clinicians in clinic settings and at home.

Positive parenting interventions are useful in the early years, starting in preschool, and across the years of childhood (principles from positive parenting interventions are even being adapted into interventions for adolescents and young adults with FASD) [88]. These interventions fit very well with the neurodevelopmental viewpoint. They take into account "brain-based difficulties" by focusing less on consequences for misbehavior, and more on how parents and teachers can set up home and school environments in which a child with special needs can be more functional. They teach useful parenting practices for children with developmental disabilities or high psychosocial risk. There are a few positive parenting intervention programs useful for families with young children. One was developed especially for parents raising children with FASD and behavior problems [5, see Study #5]. These positive parenting interventions were developed over about the past decade, and (in the time frame of treatment research) are relatively new.

The Families Moving Forward Program

The Families Moving Forward (FMF) Program is a positive parenting intervention, developed by Olson and colleagues [5, 89-92]. The FMF intervention model was designed specifically for the high priority group of families raising children with preschool and school-aged children with FASD, who also have clinically concerning behavior problems. This is a large segment of families who come into FASD diagnostic clinics or are seen in mental health settings. These children have low adaptive function and very high levels of behavior problems, and their care givers are nearly all highly stressed by the task of parenting children with FASD. These are children with very challenging problems.

The FMF model is a behavioral consultation intervention that combines a positive behavior support (PBS) approach with motivational interviewing and other scientifically-validated treatment techniques. The FMF intervention is specialized for families raising children with FASD, though it is likely useful for children with other neurodevelopmental disabilities. The FMF intervention is delivered individually to families by clinicians who have received specialized training on the model, and have access to supervision/consultation. There is a manual for the FMF intervention, but the intervention is also flexible enough to respond to the needs of the very diverse population of children with FASD and their families. The FMF intervention can be used for children aged as young as 4 years to as old as age 12 years (at the start of intervention). The efficacy of FMF services has been tested as home-based counseling delivered from a university setting and later by a community agency, with promising results so far. Delivery in clinic settings has also been tried and is quite feasible. The FMF Program has been designed to be affordable, and is now being disseminated to community agencies that have a special commitment to serving children with neurodevelopmental disabilities or FASD.

In the FMF intervention model, care givers are offered support and education, sustained behavioral consultation that includes coaching on skills, targeted school and provider consultation, advocacy assistance, and connection to community linkages. There is a strong emphasis on emotional support for care givers who must adjust to a disability that is often unrecognized by social systems, teachers and even health care providers. Other 'optional' treatment elements can be added, such as finding respite care or learning how to explain an FASD diagnosis to a child. Receiving FMF services does not preclude other services, and the FMF intervention model actually emphasizes links to other community resources.

The FMF Program is a care giver-focused intervention, designed to be used with families experiencing high care giving stress. Data on the FMF Program were gathered with the intervention offered in biweekly visits, usually each visit about 90 minutes long, occurring over a period of 9 to 11 months [5]. Recent experience suggests a somewhat shorter duration with more frequent visits is feasible, though no outcome data have been gathered. There is a highly collaborative and equal relationship between parent and professional (FMF Specialist).

The entire FMF intervention takes a neurodevelopmental viewpoint. A first aim of the FMF Program is to help parents "reframe" and understand their child's neurological impairment and ability to process emotions, changing attitudes in a more positive, realistic direction. A second aim is to help parents learn skills for how to come up with and use accommodations, such as modifications to the home or classroom. A third aim is to help parents learn how to set up practical behavior plans to reduce self-selected behavior problems. These plans rely less on setting up consequences for misbehavior. Instead, behavior plans rely more on parents thinking about the triggers and circumstances surrounding their children's problem behavior, and how to change them so the child's behavior problems decrease and the child acts in a more functional way. The idea is for parents to learn how to create behavior plans, so they have strategies to use in the future when new problem behaviors crop up. Parents receive a customized workbook, and do regular home activities to practice new skills and attitudes.

The FMF Program has been tested in a randomized control trial, and in a community-based efficacy trial just completed. More detailed results are presented in presentations and articles published or in preparation so far [5, 89-92]. The initial efficacy study compared two groups of families raising children with FASD and behavior problems randomized to receiving: (1) FMF services; and (2) the community standard of care. Families were very diverse in terms of ethnic background, social class, income level, and type of family structure (adoptive, birth, foster; grandparents, single parents, two-parent families). Immediately after treatment, relative to controls, findings showed the FMF group reported significantly greater family needs met, a greater sense of parenting efficacy, more parental self-care and decreased child disruptive behavior. While not all hypotheses were confirmed, parents reported high satisfaction with treatment, and both parents and clinicians reported good treatment acceptability. Treatment compliance was excellent, with 96% of families completing the basic intervention in this first efficacy trial.

More studies of the efficacy of the FMF Program are underway, with results in a community-based trial that are also promising and appear similar to the initial controlled trial. Treatment compliance in the community setting was about 86%. For more information, see the Families Moving Forward website: **http://depts.washington.edu/fmffasd** [81] and future publications.

The Family Check-Up

The Family Check-Up [93,94] is a positive parenting intervention that focuses on preventing problem behavior and negative interaction styles in families at high psychosocial risk. The goal of this intervention model is to support parents in a family-centered and 'ecologically-focused' manner. Like the FMF model, the Family Check-Up also uses motivational interviewing and strengthens parents' use of positive behavior support strategies. This model is delivered by specially trained parent consultants, and is linked to a variable amount of additional parenting support services customized for the family. The model was designed to be embedded into existing service systems, such as public school settings, and to be delivered at four transition time points in development. This model has so far been tested in the very early years, at the toddlerhood and preschool timepoints. There are promising results showing improvements in care giving skills and decreased child behavior problems [93].

The neurodevelopmental viewpoint suggests that the Family Check-Up model would likely not be intensive enough for most families raising children affected by prenatal alcohol exposure, even in the early years, unless sufficient follow-up parenting support sessions were provided. This type of follow-up appears to be possible in an extended version of the Family Check-Up model. This model would have to be adapted to offer specific information about FASD, work on acceptance of the task of raising a child with a disability and slower developmental progress, advocacy, and other topics important to families raising children with neurodevelopmental problems. Secondary data analysis would be useful to see if the Family Check-Up model holds promise for this clinical population. This analysis could identify children affected by prenatal alcohol exposure, and their families, who receive the Family Check-Up Model, and then examine their outcome compared to the larger group.

Stepping Stones Triple P Program

The Stepping Stones Triple P Program is also a positive parenting intervention, designed generally for young children with developmental disabilities and their families [95-97]. The age range tested so far is from 2 to 7 years (but has been extended up to children aged 9 who may be lower functioning). This intervention is based on principles of behavioral family intervention and parent management training. Parents learn to respond in a planned manner to their child's behavior and set up activities to minimize chances for disruptive behavior.

The Stepping Stones Triple P intervention was adapted from the evidence-based Triple P Positive Parenting Program. Adaptations included making content and materials more sensitive to families of children with disabilities, and covering additional issues relevant to this type of parenting (e.g., adjusting to having a child with a disability). Another adaptation was adding to the curriculum information about causes for behavior problems beyond those seen among children who are typically-developing, such as communication problems or disruptive efforts by the child to stop a disliked activity. Behavior change protocols for common problems associated with developmental disabilities (such as self-injurious behavior, or eating non-food substances) were included. Clinicians receive extensive specialized training and regular supervision.

The Stepping Stones Triple P Program is delivered in two-hour-long sessions. The 10-session curriculum includes examining causes of child behavior problems, and providing information on strategies for: developing positive relationships; encouraging desirable behavior; teaching new skills and behaviors; and managing misbehavior. Care givers receive a family workbook and watch videotaped demonstrations of positive parenting skills. Parents self-select goals and strategies to practice in clinic and several home observation sessions. In the original efficacy study, families with additional needs were offered additional sessions beyond the basic program to cover either Partner Support (marital communication and parenting teamwork) and/or Coping Skills (mood management and coping skills).

In a randomized control trial, an intervention group was compared with a waiting list control. Participants were preschoolers (up to age 7 years) with behavior problems and various developmental disabilities (none specifically identified as affected by prenatal alcohol exposure, or with FASD). When families had additional needs, the intervention included additional sessions offering training on partner support and/or coping skills for families with additional needs. Results were promising. The Stepping Stones Triple P intervention was associated with reduced child behavior problems as reported by mothers and independent observers, improved maternal and paternal parenting style, and decreased maternal stress. Some effects were maintained at 6-month follow-up. Families were well satisfied with treatment [95].

Further testing compared use of the Stepping Stones Triple P Program with and without the enhancements of parent coping skills, relative to waiting list controls. Participants were again families raising preschoolers (up to age 5 years) with developmental disabilities and behavior problems, who appeared to have milder adaptive behavior deficits than did participants in the earlier efficacy trial. Both the basic and enhanced interventions were equally effective, so there was no evidence that adding adjunctive treatment was superior to the standard behavioral training. After treatment, there were lower levels of observed negative child behavior, reduction in the number of care giving settings where children showed problem behavior, and improved parenting competence. No changes were seen in parent mood or couples adjustment. Families were again satisfied with treatment. Gains were maintained at one-year follow-up [96]. The Stepping Stones Triple P Program has also very recently been tested with families raising children aged 2 to 9 years with autism spectrum disorders, with significant improvements in parent-reported child behavior and parenting styles that were maintained over a 6-month follow-up [97].

INTERVENTIONS DRAWN FROM THE CHILD MALTREATMENT AND RESILIENCE LITERATURE

Young children affected by prenatal alcohol exposure, or with FASD, often experience psychosocial risk and sometimes actual maltreatment. Studies have shown that children with FASD and maltreatment have less positive outcomes than those who are not maltreated or victimized [1,98]. This means that appropriate maltreatment interventions are important for this population of young children. Federal laws passed in 2003 require infants and toddlers substantiated for maltreatment to be referred for early intervention under special education laws. Only a few children with maltreatment who were referred in this way showed a clear risk condition mandating services (3%). However, the most common 'established risk condition' making them eligible for early intervention services was FAS [99]. Interventions for maltreatment should be chosen carefully for young children with prenatal alcohol exposure and maltreatment, and Table **7** provides some useful intervention ideas.

In research on child maltreatment, there are various approaches including intensive family preservations services. For the children themselves, common interventions studied are consequence-based behavioral training methods that focus on reducing the occurrence of undesirable behaviors. Typically these are 'token economy' reinforcement systems (giving children chips or stickers for positive behavior so they can save up to earn rewards). While these strategies are useful for children of school age, they may not be developmentally appropriate for young children, or those with delays or neurological impairment such as children with FASD, who do not fully understand the idea of saving for a reward.

Trauma-Focused Cognitive Behavioral Therapy (TF-CBT), which is primarily aimed to children 10 years and older [100], is a well established, evidence-based intervention model. TF-CBT can be used with children as young as age 7 years, if developmentally modified, but may be hard to use with young children and/or those who have brain-based difficulties. This means that only certain treatment elements from TF-CBT may be useful, such as teaching children simple relaxation skills and ways to repeatedly practice becoming desensitized to trauma.

Table 7: Intervention Ideas Drawn from Child Maltreatment and Resilience Research

Useful Intervention Ideas
• Teach relaxation skills and other desensitization skills in a simple way.
• Use bibliotherapy (reading developmentally appropriate books on trauma topics and coping methods, and then talking with the child at their functional level in 'child-led' discussion).
• Teach children concrete skills, such as "the rules of touching" or appropriate friendship skills (this might include using the Social Stories method).
• Teach children important concepts related to maltreatment, such as the fact that the child is not alone in experiencing maltreatment, and that there are rules about people not hitting each other.
• Provide care giver education and consultation to schools related to child maltreatment.
• When appropriate, teach all care givers involved techniques to deal with reactive attachment disorder.

One recommended approach using these and other TF-CBT treatment elements starts with parent-assisted 'biblio therapy' where parents help children think about maltreatment, and teach children methods of child relaxation and coping, through examples in books. Reading these books can be followed by child-led discussion of trauma experiences, at times when the child spontaneously brings up the topic and during parent-child relationship-building activities. Importantly, child-led discussion can be paired with building a family 'narrative' that explains what happened. The parent can use this narrative to interpret the maltreatment experience to the child over a long period of time, gradually helping the child to create a new and healthier understanding of the experience. Parent involvement assumes that parents are not part of ongoing maltreatment and, if needed, are on their own path to addiction recovery and improved mental health.

Concrete skill-building may also be useful, directly teaching young children skills such as how to: start conversations; appropriately show affection; keep up personal space; ask for help appropriately and assertively; tell the difference between safe secrets and unsafe secrets; and so on. Another method is 'pre-teaching,' or using role-play with adults or coaching during peer interaction, to help young children learn important ideas such as the 'rules of touching.' The "Social Stories" method (discussed later) may also be helpful. To be effective with young children affected by prenatal alcohol exposure, these skill-building methods should be 'adult-assisted.' Care givers learn the methods, and then assist young children in using the skills over time and in real life. This brings learning as close as possible to the actual life situation and provides children with chances for repeated practice. Positive parenting interventions are also useful for children who have been maltreated.

No matter what therapeutic approach is used, there are important basic concepts to keep in mind when responding to child maltreatment. These ideas should be conveyed to the young child who has experienced maltreatment, and to their parents who can help the child understand these ideas over time. The first set of concepts is that the maltreatment experience does not mean the child is unique or alone, and that other children have experienced bad or frightening things and also may have reactions or problems because of this. The second set of concepts is that there are rules that "it is not OK for parents to hit", and "it is not OK for children to hit others". Consultation with the school or early intervention setting is important, and should focus on teaching providers about maltreatment, and on the importance of not isolating the child from their peers even if the child shows difficult behavior.

Some young children who have experienced maltreatment show diagnosed Reactive Attachment Disorder (RAD). When children show RAD, especially when they also have neurological impairment such as that seen in FASD, their intervention progress may be very slow. Care givers can still learn and use the skills discussed above and skills for how to respond when the child's behavior problems or anger escalate. Any approach to intervention with RAD should involve care giver consultation to go over the symptoms of RAD, the need for patience, coaching on how to prevent "indiscriminate" attachment behaviors (such as hugging everyone), and the probability that the child will only show slow change. It is vital to help care givers develop realistic expectations about what child symptoms and behavior problems are likely to change in response to treatment, and to sort out what issues may remain unchanged and so best be dealt with through accommodations.

SKILLS TEACHING WITH YOUNG CHILDREN TO IMPROVE BEHAVIORAL REGULATION AND RELATED SKILLS

Some early intervention methods improve later outcome by actively developing young children's self-regulation and related cognitive skills. This type of intervention is crucial. This is because young children affected by prenatal alcohol exposure often have difficulties with behavior regulation and stress reactivity, starting in early infancy. They also show lasting deficits in higher-order cognitive skills (executive functioning) that heighten the stress their care givers feel, and negatively affect other areas of their development.

For younger children with prenatal alcohol exposure, the most useful skills teaching programs are likely those in which children interact in groups. Treatment in groups allows young children to learn skills while involved in 'real life' social interaction with peers, typically accompanied by practice supported at school by their teachers and/or at home by their parents. In this child population, skills may best be learned through direct teaching [5]. For example, parent-assisted friendship skills training aims to help children learn concrete skills important to positive peer relations, and has been shown to have sustained effectiveness with children with FASD as young as age 6 years by O'Connor *et al.* [51]. (The chapter in this book by Coles and colleagues describes this and other child skills teaching programs useful for children with FASD who are somewhat older).

Two selected evidence-based group intervention models that use direct skills teaching, and one flexible intervention method, are discussed below. These are appropriate for younger children. While there are other programs, the authors consider those discussed here to be promising direct treatments for young children affected by prenatal alcohol exposure. However, each may need to be adapted to be most effective with this population. The two programs discussed below were designed for children at risk for or diagnosed with disruptive behavior disorders, but are also often useful for children with internalizing problems. These two programs aim for improvements in child social cognition, social competence, and 'executive functioning,' in an attempt to reduce child behavior problems or promote behavior regulation. Table **8** briefly lists these selected skills-teaching interventions.

Table 8: Skills-Teaching Interventions for Young Children to Improve Behavioral Regulation and Related Skills

Selected Interventions
• *Incredible Years-Child Training*: Videotape-based curriculum for children in preschool and early elementary school used in groups to teach problem-solving and social skills.
• *Promoting Alternative Thinking Strategies (PATHS) Program:* Classroom instruction in social-emotional skills used for groups of children in preschool and early elementary school.
• *Social Stories Method:* A direct skill-building method in which little customized books or cartoons are created for an individual child. These Social Stories are written at the child's developmental level and are individually created. The Social Stories visually show children steps for how to solve specific life skill problems, including particular social situations.

The Incredible Years Child Training Program (IY-CT)

The IY-CT Program is an 18-22 week videotape-based curriculum for 3 to 8-year olds who meet in small groups of 6-7 children with two therapists for two-hour weekly sessions [101]. Children view a wide variety of videotaped real-life vignettes filmed in home and school settings that model child problem-solving and social skills. After watching the vignettes, children are led by group leaders (sometimes using puppets) in discussion of feelings, generating ideas for more effective responses, and role-playing alternative scenarios. There are also group activities, reinforcers for participation, and workbooks to take home. The IY-CT treatment meets scientific criteria for a 'probably efficacious' treatment for children with disruptive behavior when delivered on its own (e.g., [101,102]. However, the IY-CT treatment it is usually delivered in association with the Incredible Years-Parent Training (IY-PT) Program. The IY-PT Program (see Appendix 4) is another interesting parenting intervention to examine, although as a group intervention it may be less feasible for FASD [103].

Aspects of the IY-CT program are well-suited to children with FASD or affected by prenatal alcohol exposure, including the use of observational learning, puppets to enhance child interest in discussion, adult assistance, small groups so that peer rejection is not a problem, and role-play with peers. The IY-CT program has not been tested with children with known FASD. Based on a neurodevelopmental viewpoint, it is possible that for this child population, the IY-CT Program might be less effective than expected. This is because of the issues of inattention and distractibility, difficulty generalizing information from one setting to another, and deficits in both integrative language abilities and working memory that characterize this population. Also, the increase in social cognitive skills targeted by the IY-CT Program might not lead to expected levels of decreased disruptive behavior because of the children's underlying neurodevelopmental disabilities. Adaptations may be necessary, such as viewing an increased number and variety of vignettes, more emphasis on role-play, or adding time to coach children through similar situations as they occur within the classroom or at home.

Promoting Alternative Thinking Strategies Program (PATHS)

The Promoting Alternative Thinking Strategies program (PATHS) involves theoretically–based classroom instruction in multiple social-emotional skill domains, such as emotion knowledge, self-control and calming, and problem-solving, delivered in a developmentally appropriate sequence. The curriculum is administered by trained teachers in 30 weekly sessions over the school year, in game, art, and reading formats. Goals are to increase social competence, reduce problem behavior, increase protective factors, and improve emotion awareness for the child and others [104]. Although developed for elementary-aged children, PATHS has been used with younger children. A randomized control trial of PATHS was recently completed for typically-developing children in 20 Head Start preschool classrooms [105]. In post-testing, children receiving PATHS increased their skills in emotion knowledge and emotion vocabulary more than controls. PATHS participants were more accurate in interpreting neutral emotions, rather than inaccurately seeing them as angry and attributing hostile intent. Teachers reported students involved in PATHS showed increased social skills and decreased internalizing problems and withdrawn behavior. Parents reported children receiving the intervention as more socially and emotionally competent, but did not report changes in externalizing or internalizing problems.

PATHS has also been tested in elementary school classrooms (1st to 3rd grades) for children with special needs. Kam and colleagues [106] evaluated the long-term effectiveness of PATHS used with a variety of children qualifying for special education services. They found substantial benefits from PATHS. Intervention was adapted to be delivered over a more intensive 60 lessons across a typical school year in nine classrooms (doubling the frequency of sessions), with a special education control group of nine classrooms. This likely meant increased practice and simpler delivery during lessons to teach component skills. Change over time was traced yearly for three years after intervention. Ratings of externalizing problems went down over time in the intervention group, while the same ratings went up over time for controls. In the intervention group, ratings of internalizing problems were slower to increase than were the same ratings for controls. For two years after treatment, this pattern of changes continued, with the intervention group improving and the control group showing increased problems.

Aspects of PATHS are well-suited to children with FASD or affected by prenatal alcohol exposure. PATHS is delivered in the school setting, which is a 'real life' natural environment for children. The intervention lasts the entire school year, follows a developmental sequence, and involves frequent 'teachable moments' in which teachers promote learning during structured social activities. This style of treatment delivery may foster initial learning and generalization of what has been learned for children with FASD. It may also capitalize on their apparently high social motivation. Also, PATHS outcomes of decreased anger and hostile attribution bias target an important deficit area recently identified among children with FASD [52].

However, PATHS has not been tested with this population. Children with FASD might show fewer intervention benefits, especially since it is known that children with better verbal abilities profit more from PATHS. Without adaptations to the curriculum, a neurodevelopmental viewpoint suggests that increased emotion knowledge may not result in expected levels of increased social competence and decreased problem behavior for children with FASD. Useful adaptations would likely include even more emphasis on role-play and teacher coaching, individualizing the curriculum when necessary, and employing those adaptations already discussed above that were used by Kam and his colleagues for children with special needs [106].

Social Stories

Social Stories are a direct skill-building method that may prove to be useful for younger children affected by prenatal alcohol exposure, perhaps especially when there has been child maltreatment. This method builds on the work being conducted with children diagnosed with autism (**http://www.thegraycenter.org/**) [107] and is used on an individual basis. Clinicians report Social Stories as very flexible and useful.

Social Stories are little customized books or cartoons for the child. Social Stories are written at the child's developmental level and are usually accompanied by pictures, drawings and/or words. Social Stories give children accurate information about situations they may find difficult or confusing. Using this method, a situation is described in child-friendly detail, such as what happens when other children refuse to play, what happens when inappropriate touching occurs, or even how to perform daily living skills. A Social Story focuses on a few key points: (1) important social cues; (2) events and reactions the child might expect to happen in the situation; (3) actions and reactions that might be expected of the child; and (4) why these might be expected. The goal of the story is to increase the child's understanding of the situation, increase the child's comfort level, and possibly suggest some appropriate responses to the situation in question.

Social Stories fit well with a neurodevelopmental viewpoint, as the stories provide visual, concrete stimuli to the child. Using Social Stories reduces demands on higher-level language abilities and working memory, and these stories can easily be geared to the child's developmental level. Examples can be found in the New Social Story Book [108].

EARLY INTERVENTION SETTINGS

Ramey and Ramey [109] have written about the characteristics of effective early intervention, primarily as these services relate to cognitive outcomes and school success. Intervention that begins earlier in children's development and lasts longer offers greater benefits to participants. Programs that are more intensive produce larger positive effects. Children receiving direct educational experiences show larger and more lasting effects than those that use intermediary routes, such as parent training, to impact children's competencies. More comprehensive and multimodal interventions generally have larger positive effects on children's development. Certain children show larger effects when given intervention, which seems to be related to their initial risk condition. Over time, initial positive effects of intervention will diminish, depending on whether or not there are adequate environmental supports available to maintain positive outcomes.

Table 9: Multi-Modal Early Intervention Programs

Selected Interventions
• *Math Interactive Learning Experience (MILE) Program:* Multimodal intervention program with a cognitive habilitation basis and aimed to improve child behavior and math function. Includes parent training in workshops and individualized educational intervention for children. Parent and child support also provided to improve learning readiness in children [See chapter in this book by Coles and colleagues for more complete description].
• *Early Intervention Foster Care (EIFC) Project:* Comprehensive, intensive multimodal early intervention with an attachment theory basis. Provides ongoing foster parent education and consultation, individual therapy and playgroups for children, and linkage to needed community resources.
• *Tools of the Mind Curriculum:* Preschool classroom curriculum designed to promote child self-regulation skills. Incorporates learning of self-regulation into pre-academic activities that promote complex play and self-talk, and offers supports through specialized teacher behavior and such prompts as visual cues in the classroom setting.

Three early intervention programs have been selected to be discussed here that appear promising for children affected by prenatal alcohol exposure. Each has been designed to provide developmental stimulation and environmental enrichment to combat social disadvantage and remediate developmental deficits. Each has a special focus on promoting child self-regulation. These are comprehensive and multi-modal interventions, and therefore may have larger positive effects on child development. But they may also cost more than interventions with fewer components. The first program was designed specifically for children known to be prenatally exposed to alcohol. The second was designed for children in foster care, who are at high psychosocial risk and where many are likely to be prenatally alcohol-exposed. The third was designed specifically as a preschool curriculum to promote child self-regulation, an important deficit among children affected by prenatal alcohol exposure. Table **9** briefly describes these programs.

Math Interactive Learning Experience Program

One research group that has systematically begun to test methods for intervention with children affected by prenatal alcohol exposure, including early intervention, carried out the Math Interactive Learning Experience Program (MILE) Program [5 (see Study #2)]. This multimodal intervention program served children with prenatal alcohol exposure, or FASD, aged 3 to 10 years, and their families. The program specifically focused on improving behavior and math functioning through parent training in workshops, individualized educational intervention that involved active learning, and multifaceted efforts to improve learning readiness and behavioral regulation in children. Gains were seen in decreased behavior problems and improved early math achievement after intervention [11], and these improvements were sustained over a 6-month follow-up and generalized to improved behavior in the school setting [110]. Direct skills-based intervention with the children was successful with families whose needs were met through additional parent education and family support services.

Multidimensional Treatment for Preschool Children in Foster Care

The Early Intervention Foster Care (EIFC) project (also known as Multidimensional Treatment Foster Care-Preschool) is a preventive intervention program, developed by Fisher and his colleagues. This program targets commonly co-occurring variables among preschoolers in foster care. These include behavior problems, physiological dysregulation within the neuroendocrine system (*i.e.*, HPA Axis activity), and developmental delays. This early intervention model is based primarily on animal research uncovering the negative effects of early stress on development. Theory behind the EIFC intervention emphasizes the importance of the care giver as an extension of the infant's regulatory system. The idea is that the care giver's actions protect the young child from the potential negative effects of outside stresses, promoting resilience. Without good quality care giving, the thought is that alterations in HPA Axis activity are likely to happen for the young child. The EIFC intervention is designed to support responsive and competent care giving for young children in foster care, trying to remediate the effects of early adversity.

In research on the EIFC intervention, outcomes studied have included placement stability, parent-child attachment quality, child behavioral regulation, and neuroendocrine and executive functioning. The EIFC intervention is delivered through a treatment team approach, and uses a developmental framework in which the issues of children in foster care are viewed as due to delayed maturation. Multiple layers of intervention are designed to create optimal environmental conditions to promote developmental progress. Foster parents receive pre-service training and ongoing consultation from program staff. Children have access to individual therapy and a therapeutic playgroup. The intervention emphasizes concrete encouragement for pro-social behavior, consistent and non-abusive limit-setting to deal with disruptive behavior, and careful, close supervision of the child. The aims are for foster parents to create a predictable daily routine, and to be responsive and consistent care givers.

In a randomized control trial, the EIFC intervention was compared to a regular foster care condition. Among other findings, after EIFC intervention, attachment behaviors were found to improve, with increased secure behaviors and decreased avoidant behaviors relative to the regular foster care condition [111]. For children with many foster placements (4 or more), a doubling in the rate of successful permanency attempts was found in the EIFC intervention group [112]. Findings from the EIFC intervention, and research on another attachment-based infant mental health intervention [76], show that care giver-focused interventions can help normalize HPA Axis activity. These physiological changes of improved stress reactivity co-occur with important positive changes in child behavior [113].

In research on the EIFC intervention, outcomes in the preschool years are expected to predict longer-term outcomes in early elementary school, including school behavior, long-term placement stability, and mental health status.

Childrearing practices of parents are expected to impact both the children's short-term and longer-term outcomes. Even though somewhat expensive in the short-term, the aim is that the EIFC intervention will be cost-effective long-term by reducing the length of time children spend in foster care, and reducing the need for later costly social, mental health and educational services.

Tools of the Mind Curriculum

The Tools of the Mind curriculum [114] was developed based on the principles of the Russian developmental theorist, Vygotsky, who suggested that children's cognitive development is built through play and learning-oriented social dialogue with adults [115]. The Tools of the Mind curriculum is designed to promote self-regulation skills for preschoolers by focusing on: (1) promoting child ability to regulate behavior and thoughts, attention, working memory, symbolic representation, and (2) increasing pre-academic skills, such as literacy and math abilities [116]. The curriculum is specifically designed to incorporate learning of self-regulation skills into pre-academic activities by promoting complex play and self-talk or private speech, and offers supports such as visual cues in the classroom setting. Teachers help children plan play themes and roles, remind children of rules, and help them make unique use of materials in imaginative play. When children learn to integrate others' plans and make a plan for themselves, they are practicing higher-order cognitive skills.

Vygotsky's theoretical framework suggests that children develop early self-regulation skills by practicing regulating the activity of others. They practice this by interacting with and directing their peers. Based on this concept, the Tools of the Mind curriculum also incorporates student-to-student activities such as turn-taking or checking the partner's work. Imaginative play also involves pre-play planning, development of imaginary roles, and explicit and implicit rules. Teachers and peers remind children if they do not follow these rules in order to promote self-monitoring of behavior during play. There is also an emphasis on using minimal props or using abstract play materials (such as a box with numbers drawn on it rather than a play cash register). This is done to increase creative and flexible thinking skills. Children also learn motor regulation by activities during games that require them to pose their body on command [117,118].

A multi-site test of efficacy of the Tools of the Mind curriculum was completed by Diamond and colleagues [119,120] with 147 preschoolers in low-income, urban preschools. This study compared the Tools of the Mind curriculum to a literacy curriculum that did not include material and activities focused on improvement of higher-order cognitive skills (executive functioning). Children who received the Tools of the Mind curriculum outperformed the literacy group on measures evaluating the following cognitive skills: inhibition; working memory; and attention switching. This study demonstrated that core components of 'executive functioning' can improve in a classroom setting for young children.

Because children with FASD have documented deficits in higher-order cognitive skills (executive functioning) and need to improve these if possible, Tools of the Mind may be a promising curriculum. The Tools of the Mind curriculum is woven into the natural environment of the preschool classroom, involves considerable teacher assistance, builds on social motivation, and uses sensory, motor and play activities for learning. These aspects of treatment delivery may make it especially applicable to children affected by prenatal alcohol exposure, or with FASD. However, with the attentional deficits, high activity level, and difficulties in social cognition and communication of this child population, the Tools of the Mind curriculum may not work as expected. Therefore, adaptations will probably be necessary, such as a higher teacher-child ratio with increased levels of adult support and structure for play activities, and perhaps less reliance on abstract play materials.

REALMS OF TREATMENT FOR YOUNG CHILDREN AFFECTED BY PRENATAL ALCOHOL EXPOSURE TO BE FURTHER EXPLORED

This chapter ends with a discussion of a variety of other promising treatment directions for young children affected by prenatal alcohol exposure that are in need of research investigation. Some are established interventions that should be enhanced to better target this child population. There are several new treatment directions for young children in this population based on intriguing animal research. Examining animal research for ideas, Hannigan *et al.* [121] found improved outcomes among alcohol-exposed animals using strategies such as: (1) neonatal handling;

(2) unstructured environmental enrichment that may increase social interaction and activity; and (3) rehabilitative (or 'therapeutic') motor training focused on specific behavioral targets with set learning criteria (not just simple exercise). In animals, these strategies can improve behavioral performance and reduce (or even eliminate) deficits in alcohol-exposed rats and mice. However, even though some animal studies report neuroanatomical changes associated with improvements in behavior, there still seems to be persistent impairment in the plasticity of neurons. Hannigan *et al.* suggest the exciting possibility that neonatal handling may alter changes in HPA Axis activity and, therefore, early response to stress. Mechanisms of change for most of these strategies are not yet determined, but it is important to reach an understanding of these mechanisms over time in order to build good treatments.

Table **10** briefly presents new realms for early intervention. These target areas of deficit commonly seen among young children affected by prenatal alcohol exposure, or with FASD.

Table 10: New Realms for Early Intervention

Intervention Categories
• *Developmental Therapies, including Motor Training*
• *Infant Massage, and Recreational Therapy/Exercise*
• *Sensory Integration-Based Treatments*
• *Occupational Therapy Consultation Model*
• *Alternative Approaches*
• *Monitoring for Emerging Problems in Language and Communication*
• *Treatment for Sleep Problems*
• *Other Treatment Realms: Nutritional Supplementation; Psychopharmacology*

Developmental Therapies, Including Motor Training

The large FAS DPN diagnostic clinic database discussed earlier shows that developmental therapies are often recommended for young children affected by prenatal alcohol exposure [62]. Occupational therapists (OTs), physical therapists (PTs) and speech-language pathologists (SLPs) can carry out individual therapy from infancy onward, training oral-motor, language, motor and life skills. This might be seen as 'rehabilitative training' moving toward learning criteria that are set ahead of time. In addition, very few pioneering research projects are underway to examine the effects of specific forms of motor training among young children in this population.

Infant Massage and Recreational Therapy/Exercise

Infant massage, with parents delivering the massage, may be a brief treatment worth trying with infants born prenatally alcohol-exposed. This idea assumes these very young infants can be identified. This method may be supported by the animal research discussed earlier. Infant massage has been shown to be efficacious for children who are biologically vulnerable because they are born preterm. While increased weight gain has been the outcome of interest in studies of infant massage, studies also show that moderate pressure massage for newborns also leads to more organized behavior in the child. Newborns receiving moderate pressure massage appeared more relaxed and less aroused than a light pressure massage group [122]. In another study, stress behavior and movement were decreased among newborns receiving massage, who also gained more weight [123]. Interestingly, mothers doing massage with their babies also experienced a decrease in depression and anxiety symptoms [124].

A wide variety of community-based recreational exercise programs are available for infants and young children. These activities such as music, dance or movement education, can be viewed as approaches to early education, and some may be promising targets for research [125]. Recreational exercise provides general developmental stimulation, skills training, and chances for socializing with peers. Benefits of this as an intervention may be supported by the animal research discussed earlier. Parents of children with FASD anecdotally report benefits from enrolling their children in these programs. Clinical wisdom suggests that recreational programs more likely to be successful with young children in this population are those that are individualized to child needs, rely less on verbal instruction, focus on individual rather than group performance, and emphasize effort over competition. Community programs include music programs, creative dance, tumbling and gymnastics programs, early sports (e.g., T-ball, swimming, martial arts). The Special Olympics Program (www.specialolympics.org) is especially likely to be successful with this child population. This organization offers a Young Athletes program in 21 countries for children with intellectual disabilities, aged 2 to 7 years [126].

Sensory Integration-Based Treatments

The ALERT Program for self-regulation was developed by Williams and Shellenberger [127,128]. This program of self-monitoring teaches children to monitor their physical and emotional level of upset feelings, such as frustration, anger, or sadness. Children learn to monitor their bodies and level of physiological arousal. They then learn strategies to help themselves tolerate distress and anticipate how to tolerate distress or focus attention when needed. This program was developed for children as young as preschool age [129] and has been adapted for children with FASD [130]. There are limited efficacy data on the ALERT Program or its use with children affected by prenatal alcohol exposure.

Principles from sensory integration-based programs such as the ALERT Program, and from literature on cognitive rehabilitation for pediatric traumatic brain injury, were incorporated into a group treatment used with foster or adopted children aged 6 to 11.9 years. Developed by Chasnoff and his colleagues, this is discussed in a paper on several FASD interventions with some efficacy data provided [5 (see Study #3)]. Briefly, their group included 12 weeks of intervention in small groups (approximately 5 children). Children were taught self-regulation skills using components of the ALERT program as well as additional skills targeting higher-order cognitive skills ('executive functioning' skills such as cause and effect, memory, sequencing, planning, and problem-solving).

Occupational Therapy Consultation Model

Jirikowic [131] described an occupational therapy (OT) consultation model focusing on sensory sensitivities and sensory integration issues of children with FASD. This short-term OT consultation model was used for intervention with families raising children with FASD, and may be especially useful for younger children, between the ages of 3 and 8. This model was first developed and used as part of a comprehensive positive parenting intervention known as the Families Moving Forward (FMF) Program (see [5] and earlier discussion in this chapter). It is possible that this OT consultation model could be used as a stand-alone treatment in mental health clinics and in schools.

In this model, an OT participates in developing parent education materials. The OT then trains behavior specialists working directly with families, and briefly consults with specialists on the issues of individual children, but does not have direct family contact. Parent education materials and clinician training focus on sensory-processing deficits and sensory-integration needs of children with FASD (especially those who are young), and how these may lead to behavior problems. Educational materials and consultation also cover sensory-based accommodations that can support positive child behavior. When consulting about individual children, the OT reviews clinical assessment data, and then assists behavior specialists in developing potential environmental or sensory accommodations that can help reduce problem behaviors. Examples include the use of sensory tools such as chair seats filled with water for a child who needs strong sensory input to reduce activity, calming methods such as "cool-off spots' in the classroom, or strategies such as reducing classroom noise. Through short-term OT consultation, behavioral specialists are 'cross-trained' and gain a working knowledge of possible antecedents for problem behaviors that could be sensory-based, and are also trained to collect sensory processing data.

Alternative Approaches

For young children, alternative treatment approaches to calming and self-regulation are of interest. For children of preschool age and older, alternative treatment approaches worth studying include applying the principles of "mindfulness" [132], and skills teaching of techniques for differential relaxation and yoga. Yoga might even be considered a type of motor training. Parents of children (including those with FASD or other special needs) anecdotally report trying these techniques with their children. (Interestingly, there are also approaches to 'mindful parenting,' such as the approach of *Listening Mothers* (www.listeningmothers.org) [133]).

These alternative approaches have not yet been studied systematically as treatments for children through well-designed research. For instance, the benefits of yoga for young children have not been fully clarified, although benefits are presumed to include more access to strategies for calming and improved overall child health [134]. To date, fewer than 20 randomized control trials on the use of yoga for children have been completed. In addition, research design for these studies has been criticized [135].

Monitoring for Emerging Problems in Language and Communication

Young children with FASD have been described as very "chatty," so language problems may not be evident in everyday life. Care givers may actually misconstrue young children's talkativeness as a strength and a sign of intellectual skill [136]. In the school years, however, Coggins *et al.* [137] found that 38% of 393 school-aged children in a clinic database showed severe impairments (>2SD below the mean) in at least one language domain. This percentage rose to 64% when assessments of complex discourse (e.g., narratives) were included.

Language delays have not been detected in recent careful longitudinal studies of the effects of prenatal alcohol exposure among two-year-old children [138]. In young children with heavy prenatal alcohol exposure, aged 3 to 5 years, in comparison to non-exposed controls, McGee *et al.* [139] found that receptive and expressive language abilities were impaired, but to no greater extent than was general intellectual functioning (Of course, many IQ tests are dependent on verbal abilities, so it is hard to separate these domains). McGee and her colleagues did conclude that existing language deficits would affect the behavioral function and social interactions of these young children. Certainly, when young children have problems in functional communication, and so have a hard time letting others know their wants and needs, they may then show challenging behavior. It also seems likely that young children's language deficits would affect success in socializing with peers because young children cannot do much to adjust to another child's language deficits.

As they grow older, language and communication deficits that emerge among children affected by prenatal alcohol exposure, or with FASD, may take the form of difficulties in the higher-level 'integrative' language abilities of middle childhood [140,141]. Higher-level language problems can be measured, such as difficulties in using language socially, or in constructing narratives (which are important at school and in social communication with peers) [142]. Research is very much needed to uncover how to measure the precursors of these problems when children are young.

In the early years, speech language therapy is clearly important to help with functional communication. But for all children affected by prenatal alcohol exposure, the most important intervention may be developmental monitoring of the child and anticipatory guidance for their parents and teachers. Care givers need to understand that early talkativeness, and mastery of vocabulary and basic grammar, may not be the best predictor of later linguistic skills. Parents and teachers especially need to know about the likelihood of subtle, yet compromising language and social communication deficits that may occur as children grow older.

Treatments for Sleep Problems

Recent research has highlighted a remarkably high rate of clinically significant sleep disturbances among children with FASD as young as age 4 years [143,144]. These sleep disturbances are seen both in care giver report and overnight sleep studies, and likely lead to fragmented sleep. Converging animal and human evidence strongly suggest an association between prenatal alcohol exposure and disrupted sleep that starts as early as infancy, and persists into adulthood [26, 145-148]. There are physiological reasons to believe that the teratogenic effects of alcohol may lead to sleep disturbance of various types. Studies of infant sleep are especially important to sort out what problems exist that can be linked more directly to the teratogenic effects of prenatal alcohol exposure.

Systematic clinical studies have not yet been carried out to understand the nature of sleep disturbances in children with FASD, how early they start, or their relationship to daytime function. It is interesting to realize that the neuropsychological and behavioral difficulties of children with FASD are quite similar to those seen among children with markedly disrupted sleep. Once sleep problems are better understood, diagnostic techniques, pharmacologic guidelines and targeted treatments can be developed.

Sleep treatments already used by parents and providers, including medication use, must be understood through research. There are scientifically-validated behavioral sleep treatments available to be tested for infants and children with FASD. Useful treatments focus on environmental accommodations. These include promoting good sleep hygiene (such as a consistent, soothing bedtime routine and predictable bedtime), and providing self-soothing methods for the child who has frequent night wakings. Accommodations for sensory issues (such as using a weighted blanket) may be useful to help reduce the length and frequency of sleep problems. Treatment of disturbances in 'circadian rhythm' (the day-night cycle) may require detailed rearranging of family activities and the child's sleep schedule, and perhaps treatments such as melatonin. For persistent sleep problems, including sleep movement disorders such as periodic limb movements, evaluation and treatment by a sleep medicine specialist is important.

Other Treatment Realms that Should be Explored

There are other early intervention methods now being explored or in need of further research. Some are so early in the process of development that most research has so far been reported only with animal models. Nutritional supplementation is one such approach. Innovative researchers have proposed the use of choline, a nutritional supplement, as a method for increasing learning and memory [149]. Documented improvement has been shown in animal models [149-151] through increasing cholinergic neurotransmission and cell function (such as repair and connectivity). Caution should be exercised in applying these findings, as details regarding dose and timing are still under scrutiny. Human studies are a next step.

Psychopharmacology for young children is mostly 'off-label,' because there is a limited database for medication use in the early years. There are many developmental considerations. Among these are the unknown impact of psychoactive medications on a young child's developing brain and body. Safety and efficacy data on psychoactive medication use for children with FASD is almost completely lacking [3]. Diagnosis and assessment is often challenging for very young children, making it hard to guide medication choice. Yet many individuals with FASD receive diagnoses of other psychiatric conditions [39], including younger children with FASD and behavior problems [89]. Psychoactive medications are often prescribed. Frankel and colleagues [152] report varied medications being used for school-aged children with FASD, including neuroleptics, antidepressants, mood stabilizers, adjunctive treatments for sleep, and others. Limited studies do exist on the use of stimulant medication for children with FASD and co-morbid ADHD/ADD symptoms. But the overlap of ADHD and FASD is problematic. In general, children with FASD are more sensitive to medication dosing and may experience paradoxical reactions [153]. Further, there are complex factors involved in the use of psychopharmacology in preschoolers. As Gleason [154] notes, for nearly all disorders, psychosocial interventions have a stronger evidence based than pharmacological treatment and may offer sustained effects not seen with psychopharmacology. There is no single answer for every family. If medications are used, collaborative, multidisciplinary care models are important, along with frequent peer and specialty consultation for prescribing physicians.

SUPPORTIVE MATERIALS

1. Appendix 1: The importance of parent support for families raising children affected by prenatal alcohol exposure.

2. Appendix 2: Preliminary results suggesting that behavior regulation deficits may be an area of central difficulty for children with prenatal alcohol exposure.

3. Appendix 3 (Single Powerpoint Slide): Suggested training topics for early intervention providers working with children affected by parental substance abuse.

4. Appendix 4 (Two Powerpoint Slides): Selected additional evidence based parenting interventions for young children birth to age eight.

ACKNOWLEDGEMENTS

We wish to acknowledge the following valuable research team members and colleagues, without whom this chapter, the behavior regulation study, and the Families Moving Forward research program would not have been possible:

Stephanie King, Kayla Pippitt, Joe Picciano, Beverly Wilson, Kyle Dehnert, and Tracy Jirikowic. Also helpful to manuscript preparation were Andrea Maikovich-Fong and Sue Kerns.

We deeply appreciate the contributions of Ian and his mother, Sheri Maxwell, who sent us the wonderful scene and quotation that leads off this chapter. We are very grateful to all the families who participated in our FASD intervention research. Their grace and courage are an inspiration to us all.

Most important to our FASD intervention research effort was funding from the Centers on Disease Control and Prevention, Grant No. U01-12DD000038, awarded to Heather Carmichael Olson, Ph.D. The contributions of faculty and students of Seattle Pacific University (SPU) were most helpful in our behavior regulation research; research for the comparison sample was supported by funding from the SPU Brain Center awarded to Beverly Wilson, Ph.D. and Karin Frey, Ph.D. The support of the Seattle Children's Hospital Research Institute and University of Washington School of Medicine, sites of research and manuscript preparation, are also gratefully acknowledged.

REFERENCES

[1]   Streissguth AP, Bookstein FL, Barr HM, Sampson PD, O'Malley K, Young JK. Risk factors for adverse life outcomes in fetal alcohol syndrome and fetal alcohol effects. J Dev Behav Pediatr 2004; 25(4): 228-38.

[2]   Chandrasena AN, Mukherjee RAS, Turk J. Fetal alcohol spectrum disorders: An overview of interventions for affected individuals. Child Adolesc Ment Health 2009; 14(4):162-7.

[3]   Peadon E, Rhys-Jones B, Bower C, Elliott EJ. Systematic review of interventions for children with Fetal Alcohol Spectrum Disorders. BMC Pediatr 2009; 9: 35-43.

[4]   Premji S, Benzies K, Serrett K, Hayden KA. Research-based interventions for children and youth with a Fetal Alcohol Spectrum Disorder: revealing the gap. Child Care Health Dev 2007; 33: 389-97.

[5]   Bertrand J. Interventions for children with fetal alcohol spectrum disorders (FASDs): Overview of findings for five innovative research projects. Res Dev Disabil 2009; 30: 986-1006.

[6]   Olson HC, Jirikowic T, Kartin D, Astley S. Responding to the challenge of early intervention for fetal alcohol spectrum disorders. Infants Young Child 2007; 20(2): 172-89.

[7]   Streissguth AP. Fetal alcohol syndrome: A guide to families and communities. Baltimore: Paul H. Brookes Publishing Company 1997.

[8]   Weiner L, Morse BA. Intervention and the child with FAS. Alcohol Health Res World 1994; 18(1): 67-72.

[9]   Malbin D. Fetal alcohol spectrum disorders: Trying differently rather than harder, 2nd Ed. Portland, OR: Fetal Alcohol Spectrum Consultation,Education and Training Services, Inc. 2002.

[10]   Paley B, O'Connor MJ. Intervention for individuals with fetal alcohol spectrum disorders: Treatment approaches and case management. Dev Disabil Res Rev 2009; 15(3): 258-67.

[11]   Coles CD, Kable JA, Taddeo E. Math performance and behavior problems in children affected by prenatal alcohol exposure: Intervention and follow-up. J Dev Behav Pediatr 2009; 30(1):7-15.

[12]   Kleinfeld J, Wescott S. Fantastic Antone Succeeds: Experiences in Educating Children with Fetal Alcohol Syndrome. Fairbanks, AK: University of Alaska Press 1993.

[13]   Kodituwakku PW. Neurocognitive profile in children with fetal alcohol spectrum disorders. Dev Disabil Res Rev 2009; 15(3): 218-24.

[14]   Kodituwakku PW. Defining the behavioral phenotype in children with fetal alcohol spectrum disorders: A review. Neurosci Biobehav Rev 2007; 31: 192-201.

[15]   Kodituwakku PW. Neurocognitive profile in children with fetal alcohol spectrum disorders. Dev Disabil Res Rev 2009; 15(3): 218-24.

[16]   Kalberg WO, Buckley D. FASD: What types of intervention and rehabilitation are useful? Neurosci Biobehav Rev 2007; 31: 278-85.

[17]   Koegel LK, Koegel RL, Dunlap G. Positive behavioral support: Including people with difficult behavior in the community. Baltimore, MD: Brookes Publishing 1996.

[18]   Lucyshyn JM, Dunlap G, Albin RW. Families and positive behavior support: Addressing problems behaviors in family contexts. Baltimore, MD: Brookes Publishing 2002.

[19]   Hieneman M, Childs K, Sergay J. Parenting with positive behavior support: A practical guide to resolving your child's difficult behavior. Baltimore, MD: Brookes Publishing 2006.

[20]   Olson HC, Oti R, Gelo J, Beck S. "Family matters:" Fetal alcohol spectrum disorders and the family. Dev Disabil Res Rev 2009; 15: 235-49. *(Also referenced in electronic databases under Carmichael Olson H)*

[21]   Paley B, O'Connor MJ, Frankel F, Marquardt R. Predictors of stress in parents of children with fetal alcohol spectrum disorders. J Dev Behav Pediatr 2006; 27: 396-404.

[22]   Bailey DB. Introduction: Family adaptation to intellectual and developmental disabilities. Ment Retard Dev Disabil Res Rev 2007; 13: 291-2.

[23]   Bronfrenbrenner U. The ecology of human development: Experiments by nature and design. Cambridge, MA: Harvard University Press 1979.

[24]   O'Connor MJ. Prenatal alcohol exposure and infant negative affect as precursors of depressive features in children. Infant Ment Health J 2001; 22(3): 291-9.

[25]   Haley DW, Handmaker NS, Lowe J. Infant stress reactivity and prenatal alcohol exposure. Alcohol Clin Exp Res 2006; 30(12):2055-64.

[26]   Troese M, Fukumizu M, Sallinen BJ, *et al.* Sleep fragmentation and evidence for sleep debt in alcohol-exposed infants. Early Hum Dev 2008; 84(9): 577-85.

[27]   Kable JA, Coles, CD. The impact of prenatal alcohol exposure on neurophysiological encoding of environmental events at six months. Alcohol Clin Exp Res 2004; 28(3): 489-96.

[28]   Schore A. The experience-dependent maturation of a regulatory system in the orbital prefrontal cortex and the origin of developmental psychopathology. Dev Psychopathol 1996; 8: 59-87.

[29]   Maccoby E. Social development: Psychological growth and the parent-child relationship. New York: Harcourt Brace Jovanovich, Inc 1980.

[30]   Patterson GR, DeBaryshe BD, Ramsey E. A developmental perspective on antisocial behavior. Am Psychol 1989; 44:329-35.

[31]   Brown JD, Sigvaldason N, Bednar LM. Motives for fostering children with alcohol-related disabilities. J Child Fam Stud 2007; 16: 197-208.

[32]   Salmon J. Fetal alcohol spectrum disorder: New Zealand birth mothers' experiences. Can J Clin Pharmacol 2008; 15(2): e191-e213.

[33]   Brown JD, Sigvaldason N, Bednar LM. Foster parent perceptions of placement needs for children with a fetal alcohol spectrum disorder. Child Youth Serv Rev 2005; 27: 309-27.

[34]   Streissguth AP, Bookstein FL, Barr HM, Sampson PD, O'Malley K, Young JK. Risk factors for adverse life outcomes in fetal alcohol syndrome and fetal alcohol effects. J Dev Behav Pediatr 2004; 25(4): 228-38.

[35]   Jacobson SW, Jacobson JL, Sokol RJ, Chiodo LM, Corobana R. (2004). Maternal age, alcohol abuse history, and quality of parenting as moderators of the effects of prenatal alcohol exposure on 7.5-year intellectual function. Alcohol Clin Exp Res 2004; 28(11):1732-45.

[36]   Blacher J, Baker BL. Positive impact of intellectual disability on families. Am J Ment Retard 2007; 112(5): 330-48.

[37]   Jirikowic T, Kartin D, Olson HC (2008). Children with fetal alcohol spectrum disorders: A descriptive profile of adaptive function. Can J Occup Ther 2008; 75(4): 238-48.

[38]   Whaley SE, O'Connor MJ, Gunderson B. Comparison of the adaptive functioning of children prenatally exposed to alcohol to a nonexposed clinical sample. Alcohol Clin Exp Res 2001; 25(7): 1018-24.

[39]   O'Connor MJ, Paley B. Psychiatric conditions associated with prenatal alcohol exposure. Dev Disabil Res Rev 2009; 15(3): 225-34.

[40]   Calkins S. Cardiac vagal tone indices of temperamental reactivity and behavioral regulation. Dev Psychobiol 1997; 31: 125-35.

[41]   Fox NA, Stifter CA. Biological and behavioral differences in infant reactivity and regulation. In: Kohnstamm GA, Bates J, Rothbart MK, Eds. Temperament in childhood. Sussex, England: Wiley 1989. pp. 169-83.

[42]   Eisenberg N, Guthrie IK, Fabes RA, *et al.* Prediction of elementary school children's externalizing problem behaviors and behavioral regulation and negative emotionality. Child Dev 2000; 71: 1367-82.

[43]   Eisenberg N, Sadovsky A, Spinrad TL, *et al.* The relations of problem behavior status to children's negative emotionality, effortful control, and impulsivity: Concurrent relations and prediction of change. Dev Psychol 2005; 41: 193-211.

[44]   O'Connor MJ, Sigman M, Kasari C. Interactional model for the association among maternal alcohol use, mother-infant interaction and infant cognitive development. Infant Behav Dev 1993; 16: 177-92.

[45]   O'Connor MJ, Kasari C. Prenatal alcohol and depressive features in children. Alcohol Clin Exp Res 2000; 24(7): 1084-92.

[46]   O'Connor MJ, Kogan N, Findlay R. Prenatal alcohol exposure and attachment behavior in children. Alcohol Clin Exp Res 2001; 26(10): 1592-1602.

[47]   O'Connor MJ, Paley B. The relationship of prenatal alcohol exposure and the postnatal environment to child depressive symptoms. J Pediatr Psychol 2006; 31(1): 50-64.

[48]   Harris SR, Osborn JA, Weinberg J, Loock C, Junaid K. Effects of prenatal alcohol exposure on neuromotor and cognitive development during early childhood; A series of case reports. Phys Ther 1993; 73: 608-17.

[49]   Riley EP, McGee CL. Fetal alcohol spectrum disorders: an overview with emphasis on changes in brain and behavior. Exp Biol Med 2005; 230(6): 357-65.

[50]   Schonfeld AM, Paley B, Frankel F, O'Connor MJ. Executive functioning predicts social skills following prenatal alcohol exposure. Child Neuropsychol 2006; 12(6): 439-52.

[51]   O'Connor MJ, Frankel F, Paley B, *et al.* A controlled social skills training for children with fetal alcohol spectrum disorders. Alcohol Clin Exp Res 2006: 24(4): 639-48.

[52]   McGee CL, Bjorkquist OA, Price JM, Mattson SN, Riley EP. Social information processing skills in children with histories of heavy prenatal alcohol exposure. J Abnorm Child Psychol 2009; 37(6): 817-30.

[53]   Olswang L, Svensson L, Astley S. Observation of classroom social communication: Do children with fetal alcohol syndrome disorders spend their time differently than their typical peers? J Speech Lang Hear Res 2010; 53:1687-1703.

[54]   Brown JD, Bednar LM, Sivaldason N. Causes of placement breakdown for foster children affected by alcohol. Child Adolesc Social Work J 2007a; 24(4): 313-31.

[55]   Ryan DM, Bonnett DM, Cass CB. Sobering thoughts: Town Hall meetings on fetal alcohol spectrum disorders. Am J Public Health 2006; 96(12): 2098-101.

[56]   Sood B, Delaney-Black V, Covington C, *et al.* Prenatal alcohol exposure and childhood behavior at age 6 to 7 years: I. Dose-response effect. Pediatrics 2001: 108(2): E34.

[57]   Astley SJ, Stachowiak J, Clarren SK, Clausen C. Application of the fetal alcohol syndrome facial photographic screening tool in a foster care population. J Pediatr 2002; 141(5): 712-7.

[58]   May PA, Fiorentino D, Gossage JP, *et al.* Epidemiology of FASD in a province in Italy: Prevalence and characteristics of children in a random sample of schools. Alcohol Clin Exp Res 2006; 30(9): 1562-75.

[59]   May PA, Gossage JP, Marais AS, *et al.* The epidemiology of fetal alcohol syndrome and partial FAS in a South African community. Drug Alcohol Depend 2007; 88(2-3): 259-71.

[60]   Coles CD, Kable JA, Drwes-Botsch C, Falek A. Early identification of risk for effects of prenatal alcohol exposure. J Stud Alcohol 2000; 61: 607-16.

[61]   Chiodo LM, Janisse J, Delaney-Black V, Sokol RJ, Hannigan JH.A metric of maternal prenatal risk drinking predicts neurobehavioral outcomes in preschool children. Alcohol Clinic Exp Res 2009; 33(4): 634-44.

[62]   Jirikowic T, Gelo J. Children and youth with fetal alcohol spectrum disorders: A summary of services, supports, and resources following clinical diagnosis. Intellect Dev Disabil 2010; 48(5): 330-344.

[63]   Substance Abuse and Mental Health Services Administration (SAMHSA) Fetal Alcohol Spectrum Disorders Center for Excellence [homepage on the Internet]. Rockville, MD: SAMHSA FASD Center for Excellence; [updated 2010 February 4; cited 2010 February 9]; Available from: http://www.fasdcenter.samhsa.gov/

[64]   Substance Abuse and Mental Health Services Administration (SAMHSA) Fetal Alcohol Spectrum Disorders Regional Training Centers. [accessed 2010 April 18]; Available from: http://www.fasdcenter.samhsa.gov/documents/FlyerFASD_RTCs.pdf

[65]   Fetal Alcohol Disorders Society FASlink Discussion Forum Internet Mail List [homepage on the Internet]. Bright's Grove, Ontario, Canada; [accessed 2009 August through November] Available from: http://www.faslink.org/faslink.htm.

[66]   Arctic Fetal Alcohol Spectrum Disorders Regional Training Center (FASPRTC). FASt Facts - The Arctic FASD RTC Monthly Email Newsletter [accessed 2009 August through November]; Available from: http://www.uaa.alaska.edu/arcticfasdrtc/fastfacts/.

[67]   National Organization for Fetal Alcohol Syndrome (NOFAS). Washington Chapter. Parent Support Group. Everett, WA. [accessed 2009 August through November]; Available from: http://www.nofaswa.org.

[68]   Olds D, Hill P, Robinson J, Song N, Little C. Update on home visiting for pregnant women and parents of young children. Curr Probl Pediat 2000; 30:109-41.

[69]   Kitzman HJ, Olds DL, Cole RE, *et al.* Enduring effects of prenatal and infancy home visiting by nurses on children. Arch Pediatr Adolesc Med 2010; 164(5): 412-18.

[70]   Lyons-Ruth K, Easterbrooks MA. Assessing mediated models of family change in response to infant home visiting: A two-phase longitudinal analysis. Infant Ment Health J 2006, 27(1): 55-69.

[71]   Zeanah CH, Ed. Handbook of infant mental health, 3rd Edition. New York, New York: The Guilford Press 2009.

[72]   Kelly JF, Zuckerman T, Rosenblatt S. Promoting first relationships: A relationship-focused early intervention approach. Infants Young Child 2008; 21(4): 285-95.

[73]   Hoffman KT, Marvin RS, Cooper G, Powell B. Changing toddlers' and preschoolers' attachment classifications: The circle of security intervention. J Consult Clin Psychol 2006; 74: 1017-26.

[74]   Marvin RS, Cooper G, Hoffman KT, Powell B. The Circle of Security project: Attachment-based intervention with caregiver-pre-school child dyads. Attach Hum Dev 2002; 4: 107-24.

[75]   Powell B, Cooper G, Hoffman K, Marvin R. The Circle of Security. In: Zeanah CH, editor. Handbook of infant mental health, Third Edition. New York: The Guilford Press 2009; pp. 450-67.

[76]   Dozier M, Peloso E, Lindhiem O, Gordon MK, Manni M, Sepulveda S. Developing evidence-based interventions for foster children: An example of a randomized clinical trial with infants and toddlers. J Soc Issues 2006; 62: 767-85.

[77]   Smyke AT, Breidenstine AS. Foster care in early childhood. In: Zeanah CH, Ed. Handbook of infant mental health, 3rd Ed. New York: The Guilford Press 2009; pp. 500-15.

[78]   Lieberman A, Ippen C, Van Horn P. Child-Parent Psychotherapy: 6-Month Follow-up of a Randomized Controlled Trial. J Am Acad Child Adoles Psychiatry 2006; 45: 913-18.

[79]   Lieberman A. Ghosts and angels: Intergenerational patterns in the transmission and treatment of the traumatic sequelae of domestic violence. Infant Ment Health J 2007; 28(4): 422-39.

[80]   Lieberman A, Van Horn P. Giving voice to the unsayable: Repairing the effects of trauma in infancy and early childhood. Child Adoles Psychiatr Clin N Am 2009; 18: 707-20.

[81]   Zeanah CH, Smyke AT. Attachment Disorders. In: Zeanah CH, Ed. Handbook of infant mental health, 3rd Edition. New York: The Guilford Press 2009; pp. 421-34.

[82]   Luby JL. Depression. In: Zeanah CH, Ed. Handbook of infant mental health, 3rd Edition. New York: The Guilford Press 2009; pp. 409-20.

[83]   Suchman N, DeCoste C, Mayes L, The Mother and Toddlers Program: An attachment-based intervention for mothers in substance abuse treatment. In: Zeanah CH, editor. Handbook of infant mental health, Third Edition. New York: The Guilford Press 2009; pp. 485-99.

[84]   Grant TM, Weston DW, Huggins JE. A pilot intervention with mothers who used methamphetamine prenatally and their children, 12th Annual NCAST-AVENUW Institute, Bellevue, WA 2007.

[85]   Carr T, Lord C. Autism spectrum disorders. In: Zeanah CH, ed. Handbook of infant mental health, Third Edition. New York: The Guilford Press 2009; pp. 301-17.

[86]   Harris SL, Weiss MJ. Right From the Start: Behavioral Intervention for Young Children With Autism, Second Edition. Bethesda, MD: Woodbine House, Inc. 2007.

[87]   Rogers S, Hall T, Osaki D, Reaven J, Herbison J. The Denver model: A comprehensive, integrated educational approach to young children with autism and their families. In: Handleman JS, Harris SL, eds. Preschool Education Programs for Children with Autism, Second Edition. Austin, TX: Pro-Ed 2000; pp. 95-113.

[88]   Bertrand J, Dang E, O'Connor MJ, Tenkku L, Olson HC, Grant T. CDC-funded interventions for youth and young adults with fetal alcohol spectrum disorders. Poster presented at: The Fourth National Biennial Conference on Adolescents and Adults with Fetal Alcohol Spectrum Disorder; 2010 April 14-17; University of British Columbia; British Columbia, Canada.

[89]   Carmichael Olson H, Brooks A, Davis C, Astley SJ. Creating and testing a new model of behavioral consulation for families raising school-aged children with FAS/ARND and behavior problems. Alcohol Clin Exp Res 2004; 28 (Suppl.)

[90]   Carmichael Olson H, Quamma J, Brooks A, Lehman K, Ranna M, Astley S. Efficacy of a new model of behavioral consultation for families raising school-aged children with FASD and behavior problems. Alcohol Clin Exp Res 2005; 28(Suppl. 5): 718.

[91]   Carmichael Olson H, Brooks A, Quamma J, *et al.* Efficacy of a novel model of behavioral consultation for families raising children with FASD and behavior problems. Manuscript in preparation.

[92]   Families Moving Forward. [home page on the Internet]. Seattle, WA: Families Moving Forward Program; [updated 2007 June; cited 2010 Jan 3]. Available from: http://depts.washington.edu/fmffasd/.

[93]   Dishion TJ, Shaw D, Connel A, Gardner F, Weaver C, Wilson M. The family check-up with high-risk indigent families: Prevention problem behavior by increasing parents' positive behavior support in early childhood. Child Dev 2008; 79(5): 1395-1414.

[94]   Gill AM, Hyde LW, Shaw DS, Dishion TJ, Wilson MN. The family check-up in early childhood: A case study of intervention process and change. J Clin Child Adolesc Psychol 2008; 37(4): 893-904.

[95]   Roberts C, Mazzucchelli T, Studman L, Sanders MR. Behavioral family intervention for children with developmental disabilities and behavioral problems. J Clin Child Adolesc Psychol 2006; 35: 180-93.

[96]   Plant KM, Sanders MR. Reducing problem behavior during care-giving in families of preschool-aged children with developmental disabilities. Res Dev Disabil 2007; 28: 362-85.

[97]   Whittingham K, Sofronoff K, Sheffield J, Sanders, MR. Stepping Stones Triple P: An RCT of a parenting program with parents of a child diagnosed with an autism spectrum disorder. J Abnorm Child Psych 2009; 37: 469-80.

[98]   Henry J, Sloane M, Black-Pond C. Neurobiology and neurodevelopmental impact of childhood traumatic stress and prenatal alcohol exposure. Lang Speech Hear Serv Sch 2007; 38:99-108.

[99]   Barth RP, Scarborough A, Lloyd EC, Losby J, Casanueva C, Mann T. Developmental status and early intervention services needs of maltreated children. Washington, D.C.: U.S. Department of Health and Human Services, Office of the Assistant Secretary for Planning and Evaluation 2007.

[100] Cohen JA, Mannarino AP, Murray LK, Ingelman R. Psychosocial interventions for maltreated and violence- exposed children. J Soc Issues 2006; 62: 737-66.

[101] Webster-Stratton C. The Incredible Years training series. Office of juvenile justice and delinquency prevention, Office of Justice Programs, U.S. Department of Justice. Juvenile justice bulletin 2000: 1-24.

[102] Webster-Stratton C, Reid MJ, Hammond M. Treating children with early-conduct problems: Intervention outcomes for parent, child, and teacher training. J Clin Child Adolesc Psychol 2004; 33: 105-24.

[103] McIntyre L. Parent training for young children with developmental disabilities: A randomized control trial. Am J Ment Retard 2008, 113(5): 356-68.

[104] Greenberg MT, Kusche CA. Building social and emotional competence: the PATHS curriculum. In: Jimerson SR, editor. Handbook of school violence and school safety. Mahwah, New Jersey: Lawrence Erlbaum Associates 2006. pp. 395-412.

[105] [Domitrovich CE, Cortes RC, Greenberg MT. Improving young children's social and emotional competence: A randomized trial of the preschool 'PATHS' curriculum, J Prim Prev 2007; 28(2):67-91.

[106] Kam C-M, Greenberg MT, Kusche CA. Sustained effects of the PATHS curriculum on the social and psychological adjustment of children in Special Education. J Emot Behav Disord 2004; 12: 66-78.

[107] The Gray Center for social learning and understanding [homepage on the internet]. Zeeland, MI: The Gray Center [accessed 2010 March 17]. Available from: http://www.thegraycenter.org/.

[108] Gray C. The new social story book: Illustrated Edition. Arlington, Texas: Future Horizons 2000.

[109] Ramey CT, Ramey SL. Early intervention and early experience. Am Psychol 1998; 53(2): 109-20.

[110] Coles CD, Kable JA, Taddeo E. Math performance and behavior problems in children affected by prenatal alcohol exposure: Intervention and follow-up. J Dev Behav Pediatr 2009; 30(1): 7-15.

[111] Fisher PA, Kim HK. Intervention effects on foster preschoolers' attachment-related behaviors from a randomized trial. Prev Sci 2007; 8: 161-70.

[112] Fisher PA, Kim HK, Pears KC. Effects of multidimensional treatment foster care for preschoolers (MTFC-P) on reducing permanent placement failures among children with placement instability. Child Youth Serv Rev 2009; 31: 541-46.

[113] Fisher PA, Gunnar MR, Dozier M, Bruce J, Pears KC. Effects of therapeutic interventions for foster children on behavioral problems, caregiver attachment, and stress regulatory neural systems. Ann N Y Acad Sci 2007; 1094: 215-25.

[114] Bedrova E, Leong DJ. Tools of the mind: A Vygotskian-based early childhood curriculum. Early Child Serv 2009; 3: 245-62.

[115] Vygotsky LS. Mind in society: The development of higher psychological processes. Cambridge, MA:Harvard Press 1978.

[116] Bedrova E, Leong DJ. Vygotskian perspectives on teaching and learning early literacy. In: Dickenson D, Neuman S, Eds. Handbook of research in early literacy development, 2nd Ed. New York: Guilford Press 2006; pp. 243-56.

[117] Bedrova E, Leong DJ. Tools of the Mind: The Vygotskian approach to early childhood education, 2nd Edition. Upper Saddle River, NJ: Prentice Hall 2007.

[118] Bedrova E, Leong DJ. Tools of the mind: A case study of implementing the Vygotskian approach in American early childhood and primary classrooms. Geneva, Switzerland: International Bureau of Education 2001.

[119] Diamond A, Barnett WS, Thomas J, Munro S. Preschool program improves cognitive control. Science 2007a; 317: 1387-8.

[120] Diamond A, Barnett WS, Thomas J, Munro S. Supporting online material for 'Preschool program improves cognitive control.' Science 2007b; 317: 1-24. [accessed 2009 January 29]; Available from: www.sciencemag.org/cgi/content/full/318/5855/1387/DC1.

[121] Hannigan JH, O'Leary-Moore SK, Berman RF. Postnatal environmental or experiential amelioration of neurobehavioral effects of perinatal alcohol exposure in rats. Neurosci Biobehav Rev 2007; 31: 202-11.

[122] Field T, Diego MA, Hernandez-Reif M, Deeds O, Figuereido B. Moderate versus light pressure massage therapy leads to greater weight gain in preterm infants. Infant Behav Dev 2006; 29: 574-78.

[123] Hernandez-Reif M, Diego M, Field T. Preterm infants show reduced stress behaviors and activity after 5 days of massage therapy. Infant Behav Dev 2007; 30: 557-61.

[124] Feijo L, Hernandez-Reif M, Field T, Burns W, Valley-Gray S, Simco E. Mother's depressed mood and anxiety levels are reduced after massaging their preterm infants. Infant Behav Dev 2006; 29: 476-80.

[125] Spodek B, Saracho ON, editors. Handbook of research on the education of young children. Second Edition. Mahwah, NJ: Lawrence Erlbaum Associates 2006.

[126] Special Olympics [homepage on the Internet]. Washington, DC: Special Olympics; c2010 [cited 2010 May 2 Available from: http://www.specialolympics.org/young_athletes.aspx.

[127] Williams MS, Shellenberger S. The Alert Program™ for self-regulation. American Occupational Therapy Association Sensory Integration Special Interest Section Newsletter 1994; 17; 1-3.

[128] Williams MS, Shellenberger S. How Does Your Engine Run? A Leader's Guide to the Alert Program® for Self-Regulation. Albuquerque, New Mexico: TherapyWorks 1996.

[129]   Pliscofsky G, Cashriel C. Playing together. ADVANCE for Occupational Therapists 2006; October: 22-23.

[130]   Schwab D. Reframing Perceptions: How Children with FAS/E Sense the World. In: Mayer L, editor. Living and working with fetal alcohol syndrome/effects. Winnipeg: Interagency FAS/E Program 1999; pp. 97-100.

[131]   Jirikowic T. Home-based behavioral intervention for children with fetal alcohol spectrum disorders: The role of occupational therapy consultation. Poster session presented at: 88th Annual Conference of the American Occupational Therapy Association 2008 April 10-13; Long Beach, CA.

[132]   Semple RJ, Reid EFG, Miller L. Treating anxiety with mindfulness: An open trial of mindfulness training for anxious children. J Cogn Psychother 2005; 19:379-92.

[133]   Community of Mindful Parents: Listening Mothers [homepage on the Internet]. Community of Mindful Parents [cited 2010 Mar 17]. Available from: http://www.listeningmothers.org/.

[134]   White LS. Yoga for children. Pediatr Nurs 2009; 35(5): 277-95.

[135]   Birdee GS, Yeh GY, Wayne PM, Phillips RS, Davis RB, Gardiner P. Clinical applications of yoga for the pediatric population: A systematic review. Acad Pediatr 2009; 9(4): 212-20.

[136]   Olson HC. The effects of prenatal alcohol exposure on child development. Infants Young Child 1994; 6(3):10-25.

[137]   Coggins TE, Timler GR, Olswang, LB. A state of double jeopardy: Impact of prenatal alcohol exposure and adverse environments on the social communicative abilities of school-age children with fetal alcohol spectrum disorder. Lang Speech Hear Serv Sch 2007; 38(2), 117-27.

[138]   O'Leary CM, Zubrick SR, Taylor CL, Dixon G, Bower C. Prenatal alcohol exposure and language delay in 2-year-old children: The importance of dose and timing on risk. Pediatrics 2009; 123(2): 547-54.

[139]   McGee CL, Bjorkquist OA, Riley EP, Mattson SN. Impaired language performance in young children with heavy prenatal alcohol exposure. Neurotoxicol Teratol 2009; 31(2): 71-5.

[140]   Thorne JC, Jirikowic T, Brooks A, Davies J. Fetal alcohol spectrum disorders. In: Nass R and Frank Y, Eds. Cognitive and behavioral abnormalities of pediatric diseases. Oxford, UK: Oxford University Press 2010; pp. 577-86.

[141]   Coggins TE, Olswang LB, Carmichael Olson H, Timler GR. On becoming socially competent communicators: The challenge for children with fetal alcohol exposure. In: Abbeduto L, Ed. Language & Communication in Mental Retardation. International Review in Research on Mental Retardation, Vol. 27. New York: Academic Press 2003; pp. 121-50.

[142]   Thorne JC, Coggins TE. A diagnostically promising technique for tallying nominal reference errors in the narratives of school-aged children with Fetal Alcohol Spectrum Disorders (FASD). Int J Lang Commun Disord 2008; 43(5): 570-94.

[143]   Chen ML, Olson HC, Astley SJ. Sleepless in Seattle: preliminary data suggesting sleep disorders in those with FASD. Research Society for Alcoholism, Fetal Alcohol Spectrum Disorders Study Group 2006.

[144]   Chen ML, Carmichael Olson H. Caregiver report of sleep problems in children with fetal alcohol spectrum disorders. Am J Respir Crit Care Medicine 2008; 177: A707.

[145]   Allen GC, West JR, Chen WJ, Earnest DJ. Neonatal alcohol exposure permanently disrupts the circadian properties and photic entrainment of the activity rhythm in adult rats. Alcohol Clin Exp Res 2005; 29(10): 1845-52.

[146]   Green CR, Mihic AM, Nikkel SM, Stade BC, Rasmussen C, Munoz DP. Executive function deficits in children with fetal alcohol spectrum disorders (FASD) measured using the Cambridge Neuropsychological Tests Automated Battery (CANTAB). J Child Psychol Psychiatry 2009; 50(6): 688-97.

[147]   Pesonen AK, Raikkonen K, Matthews K, *et al.* Prenatal origins of poor sleep in children. Sleep 2009; 32(8): 1086-92.

[148]   Steinhausen HC, Spohr HL. Long-term outcome of children with fetal alcohol syndrome: psychopathology, behavior, and intelligence. Alcohol Clin Exp Res 1998; 22(2): 334-8.

[149]   Thomas JD, La Fiette MH, Quinn VR, Riley EP. Neonatal choline supplementation ameliorates the effects of prenatal alcohol exposure on a discrimination learning task in rats. Neurotoxicol Teratol 2000; 22: 703-11.

[150]   Thomas JD, GarrisonM, O'Neill TM. Perinatal choline supplementation attenuates behavioral alterations associated with neonatal alcohol exposure in rats. Neurotoxicol Teratol 2004; 26: 35-45.

[151]   Thomas JD, Biane JS, O'Bryan KA, O'Neill TM, Dominguez HD. Choline supplementation following third-trimester-equivalent alcohol exposure attenuates behavioural alterations in rats. Behav Neurosci 2007; 121: 120-30.

[152]   Frankel F, Paley B, Marquardt R, O'Connor M. Stimulants, neuroleptics, and children's friendship training for children with fetal alcohol spectrum disorders. J Child Adolesc Psychopharmacol 2006; 16(6): 777-89.

[153]   O'Malley DK, Nanson J. Clinical implications of a link between fetal alcohol spectrum disorder and attention-deficit hyperactivity disorder. Can J Psychiatry 2002; 47: 349-54.

[154]   Gleason MM. Psychopharmacology in early childhood: Does it have a role? In: Zeanah CH, Ed. Handbook of infant mental health, 3rd Edition. New York: The Guilford Press 2009; pp. 516-30.

APPENDIX I

Parent Support

Research in the general field of developmental disabilities repeatedly shows that the nature and quality of social support that is available to families is vital to positive family adaptation [1]. Social support comes from many sources, but a number of studies show that strong 'informal' (parent-to-parent) support systems are more likely to lead to positive outcomes. In the field of FASD, families with young children affected by prenatal exposure to alcohol often seek parent support and use methods of self-help. Experts agree this is a good idea. In fact, analysis of recommendations from the FAS DPN clinical database show that family resources, such as parent support, are often suggested for families with young children.

Support of good quality is always important. But population characteristics are likely to determine what the most appropriate type of parent support is. For example, for families raising children with FASD, support needs undoubtedly vary by type of family placement (non-relative adoptive, non-relative foster, kinship, birth parent) [2]. The importance of different types of support for different types of family placement can be seen in the spontaneous evolution of parent support mechanisms in the field of FASD. For example, special, separate 'birth mother support networks' and peer mentoring programs have been created which can deal with the unique stresses and concerns of birth parents [3]. Summarized testimony from birth parents indicates their special concerns that; for them, childrearing is associated with feelings of guilt and shame, financial strain, frustration with the lack of knowledgeable professionals, stress related to the child's involvement in the judicial system, and multiple time demands [4]. The concerns of foster and adoptive parents are somewhat different (e.g. Brown *et al.*) [5].

In recent years, and especially with the advent of web-based communication, 'informal' parent support has grown in many ways to become more sustainable and organized. There are statewide networks of general parent-to-parent support, fathers' networks, and parent support models such as the Program for Early Parenting Support (**PEPS; http://www.pepsgroup.org/**) [6]. There are also parent-to-parent support programs specialized for different disabilities. With an internet presence in the form of websites, and *via* list servs, email, and other types of web-based communication, parent support groups provide a rapid and flexible means of dialogue and support from other parents. These groups also provide access to parent-led community education and self-help. Beyond web-based connections, parent support networks can also be the platform for other parent-led services.

Parent support has grown quickly in the field of FASD, suggesting families find it useful. Support groups began to appear in the 1980's with growing momentum by the early 1990's and this momentum has been sustained to the present day. There is now a lively national FASD parent support organization in the U.S. (with multiple affiliates at the state level) called NOFAS (www.nofas.org) [7]. Other countries, such as United Kingdom (www.nofas-uk.org) [8], Canada (**http://www.faslink.org/faslink.htm**) [9], and others, also have very active FASD parent support organizations. These organizations have grown and matured, especially in countries with national leadership efforts, and are beginning to link internationally.

There are also many community-level FASD parent support groups (for listings by state and country see: **http://depts.washington.edu/fadu/Support.Groups.OI.html**) [10]. These groups may simply be a platform for peer support between parents. But they may also sponsor a diversity of services, such as summer camps, social skills groups, teen groups, respite care, parent education efforts, and personal advocacy. Some of these groups even act as publication outlets, carry out public policy activities, or provide platforms for FASD diagnostic services.

Parent support and self-help mechanisms in the field of FASD appear not to have been formally evaluated in the scientific literature. Because of the importance of parent support to child and family outcome, evaluation research is very much needed. Both internet-based support mechanisms, and more traditional means of parent support and self-help, should be investigated.

REFERENCES

[1]   Bailey DB. Introduction: Family adaptation to intellectual and developmental disabilities. Ment Retard Dev Disabil Res Rev 2007; 13: 291-2.

[2]   Olson HC, Oti R, Gelo J, Beck S. "Family matters:" Fetal alcohol spectrum disorders and the family. Dev Disabil Res Rev 2009; 15: 235-49.*(Also referenced in electronic databases under Carmichael Olson H)*

[3]   Salmon J. Fetal alcohol spectrum disorder: New Zealand birth mothers' experiences. Can J Clin Pharmacol 2008; 15(2): e191-e213.

[4]   Substance Abuse and Mental Health Services Administration (SAMHSA) Fetal Alcohol Spectrum Disorders Center for Excellence. Hope for Women in Recovery Summit. Understanding and Addressing the Impact of Prenatal Alcohol Exposure;   2005.   [cited   2009   February   28];   [about   2   screens].   Available   from: http://fascenter.samhsa.gov/initiatives/summitsForWomen.cfm.

[5]   Brown JD, Sigvaldason N, Bednar LM. Motives for fostering children with alcohol-related disabilities. J Child Fam Stud 2007; 16: 197-208.

[6]   Program for Early Parenting Support. [homepage on the Internet] 2007; [cited 2009 February 9]; Available from: http://www.pepsgroup.org/.children and families affected by fetal alcohol spectrum disorders. Pediatr Nurs 2006; 32(4): 299-306.

[7]   National Organization for Fetal Alcohol Syndrome (NOFAS). Washington Chapter. [homepage on the Internet] 2008; [cited 2010 February 10]; Available from: http://www.nofaswa.org.

[8]   National Organisation on Fetal Alcohol Syndrome (NOFAS) – UK [homepage on the Internet]. London, England: NOFAS-UK c2007-2010; [cited 2010 February 10]; Available from: http://www.nofas-uk.org/

[9]   Fetal Alcohol Disorders Society FASlink Discussion Forum Internet Mail List [homepage on the Internet]. Bright's Grove, Ontario, Canada; [accessed 2009 August through November] Available from: http://www.faslink.org/faslink.htm FASWORLD

[10]   Parent Support Groups [homepage on the Internet] Fetal Alcohol and Drug Unit, University of Washington; [updated 2008 April 16; cited 2010 February 10]; Available from: http://depts.washington.edu/fadu/Support.Groups.US.html

APPENDIX II

A Central Difficulty: Behavioral Regulation Problems Among Young Children Affected by Prenatal Alcohol Exposure

In the usual course of development from infancy into toddlerhood and the preschool years, children achieve self-awareness and learn to regulate their behavior. For children affected by prenatal alcohol exposure, the usual developmental process may not go well. Problems in behavior regulation, which can negatively affect their early social relationships, seem to be common among these young children. Therefore, interventions to improve behavioral regulation should be a central focus for young children affected by prenatal alcohol exposure.

Behavior regulation is one aspect of a broader construct known as self-regulation. The term "self-regulation," rather than behavioral regulation, is often used by developmentalists when talking about children who have reached the preschool years and beyond.

Self-regulation is a complex construct with many related abilities involving the regulation of behavior, emotion and cognition including a group of cognitive abilities collectively termed executive functions. Self-regulation skills develop rapidly during the preschool and early elementary years [1]. At the same time, the emergence of executive functions is associated with the ongoing development of part of the brain called the prefrontal cortex, which matures quickly during early childhood with ongoing maturation through adolescence [2-3]. Children's early executive function skills predict later social competence [4-5]. The early years of life are an important period of brain development, and there is potential during this time for intervention to improve deficits in self-regulation skills.

One important aspect of self-regulation is 'inhibitory control,' or children's ability to inhibit their internal and external reactions to environmental stimuli. Inhibitory control involves the inhibition of a well-learned or automatic response, or what are called 'pre-potent' responses in the face of temptation [6]. In children who are typically developing, inhibitory control develops during the preschool years, especially between ages 3 and 5 [7]. Inhibitory control predicts later academic and social competence, and even what has been called development of the "conscience" during childhood [8-9]. Children with disabilities, such as those with ADHD, typically show problems in inhibitory control when they are older [10-11]. Parent ratings of young children diagnosed with an FASD suggest these children have significant problems in behaviors reflecting executive functioning. Specifically, Rasmussen and colleagues found all scales on the Behavior Rating Inventory of Executive Function (BRIEF) were clinically elevated, indicating problems, but that for young children (5 to 8 years) the 'Inhibit' scale showed the highest elevation [12]. If direct testing data confirms the existence of these deficits in young children, interventions to remediate problems in inhibitory control (or teach care givers how to accommodate these difficulties) may help improve children's adaptive function.

Inhibitory control among children with FASD has primarily been examined using parent report, and data on young children are scarce. The authors and their colleagues, Wilson and Picciano, recently completed a pilot study involving observations of the inhibitory control of children with FASD and the findings are currently in preparation. The researchers plan to report the results of this study more fully in a subsequent publication, along with data on the related construct of attention regulation. But because findings are of interest when thinking about interventions for young children with FASD, preliminary results are included here.

A group of young children with FASD were compared to a group of high-risk, typically-developing peers on measures of inhibitory control. Using a high-risk comparison group was considered important because the children diagnosed with FASD also typically experienced high levels of cumulative psychosocial risk, which itself can impact inhibitory control [13]. The research hypothesis was that the group of children with FASD would perform more poorly on measures of inhibitory control than comparison peers.

A sample of 13 children with a clear diagnosis of FASD, with chronological age ranging from 5.2 to 8.3 years old, was matched to a group of 13 high-risk, typically-developing peers. Matching was based on mental age calculated from direct testing of verbal reasoning skills. Inhibitory control was assessed with two tasks carried out in the laboratory that are often used with young children. Task performance was coded live during the task, or afterwards from videotapes, by trained examiners who achieved acceptable inter-rater reliability. The battery included: (1) the well-known Simon Says task [8], which resembles the childhood game of the same name; and (2) the Delay of Gratification task [14], in which children must wait alone in a room for seven minutes before eating a snack, with the snack sitting on the table before them. Children's comprehension of task instructions was checked before the actual inhibition tasks were given. This presumably minimized demands on working memory, a consistent problem for children with FASD [15] and raised the likelihood that inhibitory control (and not simply task understanding or recall of instructions) was evaluated, which has been a problem in earlier direct testing of inhibitory control in preschoolers [16].

Preliminary findings revealed significant group differences on the Simon Says task, a measure of suppression of movement in the face of changing instructions that is especially sensitive to deficits across the developmental age period of ages 4 to 6 [7], and likely through age 10 years [17]. Children with FASD had significantly more difficulty inhibiting their behavior during this task. Group differences were quite clear, even in this relatively small sample. Differences in motor skill were not seen as the sole reason for group differences, because both groups of children could adequately perform the movements in the Simon Says task. In contrast, the two groups of children did not perform differently on the Delay of Gratification task, a measure of suppression of an impulse to eat a preferred treat. The Simon Says task was considered more complex because it required the child to repeatedly inhibit responses and follow a generalized rule across different situations and in changing form. For example, some trials required inhibition of touching their nose and other trials involved making large movements like clapping or waving hands. The Delay of Gratification task only required the child to adhere to a simple rule (resist the temptation to eat). Results so far suggest that some aspects of inhibitory control may be affected in children with an FASD, especially when children are required to exercise inhibitory control in the face of more complexity. For these young children with FASD, initial findings suggest that deficits in inhibitory control are explained by disability status rather than intellectual level or psychosocial risk. If these findings hold true in future replication studies, interventions to improve deficits in inhibitory control and, more broadly, in behavioral and self-regulation, are indicated for young children with FASD.

REFERENCES

[1]   Espy KA. Using developmental, cognitive, and neuroscience approaches to understand executive control in young children. Dev Neuropsychol 2004; 26: 379-84.

[2]   Lowel S, Singer W. Experience dependent plasticity of intercortical connections. In: Fahle M, Tomaso P, Eds. Perceptual learning. Cambridge, Massachusetts: MIT Press 2002. pp. 1-18.

[3]   Segalowitz S, Davies P. Charting the maturation of the frontal lobe: an electrophysiological strategy. Brain Cog 2004; 55(1): 116-33.

[4]   Carlson SM, Wang TS. Inhibitory control and emotion regulation in preschool children. Cogn Dev 2007; 22: 489-510.

[5]   Hughes C, White A, Sharpen J, Dunn J. Antisocial, angry and unsympathetic: 'Hard to manage' preschoolers' peer problems, and possible social and cognitive influences. J Child Psychol Psychiatry 2000; 41: 169-79.

[6]   McCabe LA, Cunnington M, Brooks-Gunn J. The development of self-regulation in youg children: Individual characteristics and environmental contexts. In: Baumeister RF, Vohs KD, editors. Handbook of self-regulation: Research, theory, and applications. New York, New York: Guilford Press 2004. pp. 340-356.

[7]   Carlson SM. Developmentally sensitive measures of executive function in preschool children. Dev Neuropsychol 2005; 28(2): 595-616.

[8]   Kochanska G, Murray K, Coy KC. Inhibitory control as a contributor to conscience in childhood: From toddler to early school age. Child Dev 1997; 68: 263–77.

[9]   Kochanska G, Murray KT, Jacques TY, Koenig AL, Vandegeest KA. Inhibitory control in young children and its role in emerging internalization. Child Dev 1996; 67: 490-507

[10]   Mahone EM, Powell SK, Loftis CW, Goldberg MC, Denckla MB, Mostofsky SH. Motor persistence and inhibition in autism and ADHD. J Int Neuropsychol Soc 2006; 12: 622-31.

[11]   Quay HC. Inhibition and attention deficit hyperactivity disorder. J Abnorm Child Psychol 1997; 25:7-13.

[12]   Rasmussen C, McAuley R, Andrew G. Parental ratings of children with fetal alcohol spectrum disorder on the behavior rating inventory of executive function (BRIEF). J FAS Int 2007; 5(e2): 1-8.

[13]   Raikes HA, Robinson JL, Bradley RH, Raikes HH, Ayoub CC. Developmental trends in self-regulation among low-income toddlers. Soc Dev 2007; 16(1): 128-49.

[14] Mischel W, Shoda Y, Rodriguez ML. Delay of gratification in children. Science 1989; 244:933–8.

[15] Rasmussen C. Executive functioning and working memory in fetal alcohol spectrum disorder. Alcohol Clin Exp Res 2005; 29(8): 1359-67.

[16] Noland JS, Singer LT, Arendt RE, Minnes S, Short EJ, Bearer CF. Executive functioning in preschool-age children prenatally exposed to alcohol, cocaine and marijuana. Alcohol Clin Exp Res 2003; 27: 647-56.

[17] Lengua L. Associations among emotionality, self-regulation, adjustment problems, and positive adjustment in middle childhood. Appl Dev Psychol 2003; 24: 595-618.

APPENDIX III

Suggested training topics for early intervention providers working with children by parental substance abused (Adapted from Olson *et al.*, 2007, p. 184)
How to ask questions about prenatal exposure.
The process of addiction and recovery; harm reduction and relapse prevention.
How to provide FASD prevention information.
How to recognize and screen for the characteristic facial features of FAS, small head size, and mild or greater growth impairment.
Key behavioral symptoms signaling need for diagnostic referral when in the presence of alcohol exposure.
Advocacy skills to help children at risk continue to be monitored or qualify for services even with subtle deficits, and to promote services in the next intervention setting.
Neurodevelopmental disabilities, and specifics about FASD; how brain development and function are affected by prenatal alcohol exposure.
How to provide appropriate early intervention given current data on FASD, with a focus on environmental modification and antecedent-based positive behavior support planning.
The family experience of raising children with FASD, and differences between different family structures.
How parental substance abuse affects children's lives.
CAPTA and IDEA regulations, and interagency efforts to improve services for children affected by parental substance abuse.
Systems of care for chemical dependency treatment, FASD diagnosis, child welfare, crisis placement, foster care, adoption, adult corrections, and adult developmental disabilities services.

APPENDIX IV

Key References	Key References
Incredible Years: www.incredible years.com **Webster-Stratton C. The Incredible Years: Parents, teachers and children training series. Res Treatment Children Youth 2001;18(3)31-46.** **Webster-Stratton C, Reid MJ, Hammond M. Treating children with early-onset conduct problems: Intervention outcomes for parent, child, and teacher training. J Clin Child Adolesc Psychol 2004;33:105-24.**	**Parent-Child Interaction Therapy (PCIT):** **Eyberg SM, Nelson MM, Boggs SR. Evidence-based psychosocial treatments for children and adolescents with disruptive behavior. J Clin Child Adolesc Psychol 2008;37(1):215-37.** **Eyberg SM. Parent-child interaction therapy: Integrity checklists and session materials. Unpublished manuscript, University of Florida at Gainesville 1999. [Updated 2010 February; accessed 2010 March 10];** http://pcit.phhp.ufl.edu/measures/indiv%20pcit%20manual%2 0feb%202010.pdf. **Data on use with children with FASD:** **Bertrand J. Interventions for children with fetal alcohol spectrum disorders (FASDs): Overview of findings for five innovative research projects. Res Dev Disabil 2009;30:986-1006.**

Parent Management Training: Patterson GR, Chamberlain P, Reid JB. A comparative evaluation of parent training procedures. Behav Ther 1982;13:638-50 Kazdin A. Parent Management Training: Treatment for Oppositional, Aggressive, and Antisocial Behavior in Children and Adolescents. New York: Oxford University Press; 2005.	***Parent-Child Home Program*** *(one example of a program focused on parenting and school readiness)* www.parent-child.org Kamerman SB, Kahn AJ. Starting Right. New York: Oxford
Helping the Noncompliant Child: Peed S, Roberts M, Forehand RL. Evaluation of the effectiveness of a standardized parent training program in altering the interaction of mothers and their noncompliant children. Behav Mod 1977;1(3):323-50. McMahon RJ, Forehand RL. Helping the noncompliant child: Family based treatment for oppositional behavior, Second Edition. New York: Guilford Press; 2005.	***Treatment for ADHD: Barkley Model*** Barkley RA. Attention-Deficit Hyperactivity Disorder, Third Edition: A Handbook for Diagnosis and Treatment. New York: The Guilford Press

Selected Additional Evidence Based on Parenting Interventions for Young Children Birth to Adulthood
Incredible Years - Parent Training
Parent Management Training
Helping the Noncompliant Child
Parent-Child Interaction Therapy (PCIT)
Parent-Child Home Program
(One example of a program focused on both parenting & school
Treatment for ADHD: Barkley Model

Innovative Educational Interventions with School-Aged Children Affected by Fetal Alcohol Spectrum Disorders (FASD)

Claire D. Coles[*], Elles Taddeo and Molly Millians

FASD Center at the Marcus Autism Center, 1920 Briarcliff Road, Atlanta, Georgia, 30329, USA and Departments of Psychiatry and Behavioral Sciences and Pediatrics, Emory University School of Medicine, 1256 Briarcliff Road, Atlanta, Georgia, 30306

> ***Every student can learn, just not on the same day, or the same way***
>
> George Evans

Abstract: Fetal Alcohol Spectrum Disorders (FASD) has been estimated to affect as many as one in 100 children. Children with prenatal alcohol exposure may exhibit physical alterations and compromised cognitive functioning. The neurodevelopmental deficits associated with FASD range from global intellectual impairments to specific processing deficits, and learning disabilities that can hinder academic performance and adaptive functioning. The purpose of this chapter is to provide an overview of the impact of FASD on children's education, and to present a brief summary of the evidence-based programs and other interventions that may support better educational and behavioral outcomes for alcohol-affected children.

INTRODUCTION

Fetal Alcohol Syndrome (FAS) and the spectrum of associated conditions that result from maternal alcohol use during gestation (*i.e.*, Fetal Alcohol Spectrum Disorders, FASD) are among the most common developmental disorders and may affect as many as one in 100 children [1,2]. The prevalence of FASD is higher than, or similar to, the prevalence of other common developmental disabilities, such as Down syndrome, Spina Bifida, Autism Spectrum Disorder (ASD), and Fragile X [3]. Thus, it is a concern that, although the prevalence of FASD is similar to other developmental disabilities, there has been much less attention paid to investigating educational functioning and interventions for alcohol- affected children [3].

Children most severely affected by alcohol receive a clinical diagnosis of FAS, and display physical characteristics such as dysmorphic facial features and growth deficits, as well as evidence of the neurocognitive impact of their prenatal exposure. Cognitive impairments also are associated with Fetal Alcohol Spectrum Disorders (FASD) although the physical features may not be apparent. These cognitive impairments can range from global intellectual deficits to specific processing and academic deficits that interfere with children's success in school [4]. Often children diagnosed with alcohol-related disabilities have behavior and emotional problems as well. Such problems may be the result of the effects of their prenatal exposure or of non-optimal postnatal environments; or, as is most likely, of the interaction of these factors. Thus, the alcohol-affected child comes to the learning environment with a number of challenges. Given the spectrum of outcomes associated with an alcohol-related diagnosis, it is important for teachers, professionals, and caregivers working with children with FASD to understand the range of these effects and their impact on learning.

This chapter presents an overview of the educational needs of, and interventions for, children with alcohol-related diagnoses. In addition to the research on the cognitive and behavioral effects of prenatal alcohol exposure, the information for this chapter is compiled from the limited available research that has investigated educational interventions for children with FASD and clinical observations from professionals working with children with an alcohol- related diagnosis. We have also taken into account insights from the extensive body of research into the efficacy of interventions for children with other developmental disabilities which may have overlapping characteristics [5,6]. The first goal of this chapter is to provide information about the impact of the consequences of the neuro developmental

---

*Address correspondence to Claire D. Coles: Departments of Psychiatry and Behavioral Sciences and Pediatrics, Emory University School of Medicine, 1256 Briarcliff Road, Atlanta, Georgia 3030, USA; E-mail: Claire.Coles@choa.org

Susan A. Adubato and Deborah E. Cohen (Eds)

effects of alcohol and of environmental experiences on the learning and achievement of children with FASD. To do so, the authors will first outline specific cognitive and academic problems observed in children with FASD, and then provide a discussion of interventions. This discussion will include a review of several studies that have investigated interventions to improve academic, social, and adaptive skills in children with FASD. Additionally, the authors will provide suggestions for interventions found to be useful in clinical settings for children with FASDs and with other developmental disabilities that share similar cognitive profiles as children with an alcohol- related diagnosis.

NEURODEVELOPMENTAL DELAYS ASSOCIATED WITH PRENATAL ALCOHOL EXPOSURE AND ENVIRONMENTAL CONDITIONS THAT IMPACT LEARNING

In 1973, Kenneth Lyon Jones' and David Smith's article "Recognition of Fetal Alcohol Syndrome in Early Infancy" was published in the journal, Lancet [7]. The article described the impact of gestational alcohol exposure on offspring. Since the publication of the Jones and Smith article, many studies have taken place confirming the effects that were reported and expanding the understanding of these disorders in children. Over time, it has been recognized that prenatal alcohol exposure may lead to a spectrum of effects including the clinical diagnoses of Fetal Alcohol Syndrome (FAS) and Partial Fetal Alcohol Syndrome (pFAS) [8] as well as a number of outcomes that are summarized by the term FASD. Although it is not a diagnostic term, the phrase Fetal Alcohol Spectrum Disorders (FASD) is currently used in most literature.

Until recently, FASD research focused almost exclusively on the prevention of the consequences of maternal alcohol abuse by encouraging abstinence in pregnancy and, when observing children, on the neurodevelopmental and physiological deficits in offspring. Some of these effects and their educational implications are summarized in Table 1. It is evident that deficits are widespread and have the potential to affect children's academic achievement. In the last decade, neuroimaging research has confirmed in human samples what was obvious from animal models: that alcohol affects the structure of the brain and these alterations probably account for many later learning problems [9]. The size and function of the frontal cortex are affected [9-11] and this difference may be associated with problems observed in working memory, complex problem solving, and abstract thinking [2,12-15]. Several researchers have found abnormalities in gray and white matters in the brain, and in some individuals with FAS, the corpus callosum was greatly diminished or missing [16-19]. Even when the corpus callosum is intact, there is evidence that white matter is diminished, a condition that could affect the efficiency of information processing [20-22]. Other studies report that the hippocampus, which is known to be associated with learning and memory, is smaller in alcohol-affected individuals [23, 24].

Behavioral effects of prenatal alcohol exposure have been documented both clinically and through a number of research studies [25,26]. Children with FASD may exhibit IQ scores ranging from 45 to 110 (with averages of 65 to 67) [27,28]. Children who are affected by prenatal alcohol exposure but do not meet the criteria for a diagnosis of FAS may have higher general intellectual functioning, yet have a variety of learning deficiencies.

White matter damage to the brain may impair encoding of verbal and visual information and affect processing speed [20]. Additionally, deficits in visuo-spatial skills and problems with executive functioning are associated with gestational alcohol exposure [21,29-32]. Executive functioning encompasses the abilities to plan, to execute, to shift problem solving techniques, and to monitor and adjust the thinking processes. Additionally, executive functioning incorporates the process of cognitive flexibility and efficiency [33-35]. Impairments such as those associated with the effects from prenatal alcohol exposure often lead to secondary learning difficulties [36].

Although it is shown that prenatal exposure to alcohol can affect neurodevelopment, this is not the only risk faced by children whose mothers drink during pregnancy. Frequently, women who use alcohol also use other substances, most often tobacco, and in some cases have other social problems and/or mental health issues. They may also associate with other individuals with substance abuse problems. Thus, the environment provided by caregivers who have problems with chronic substance abuse can also be a source of risk to alcohol-affected children. Though many studies have investigated the impact of environmental neglect on children, only a few have focused specifically on the impact of the environment on children with FASD [37-39]. However, children with FASD have neurodevelopmental vulnerabilities that may be confounded by environmental deprivation. Risks include neglect, abuse, continued parental substance use, and multiple home placements that can negatively impact children's intellectual development as well as acquisition of language, early learning skills, and behavior [38, 40-43]. It may be due to such risk factors that a recent study conducted in Canada found that children with FASD reported a significantly lower quality of life in comparison to a control group of children with various types of cancers [44].

Table 1: Processing Impairments Associated with FASD and the Potential Impact on Learning

Impairment	Impact on Functioning	Displayed at School
Speed of Processing [20]	• Slow rate of intake of information • Slow rate of output of information	• Inconsistent grasp of information presented in the classroom • Misses relevant information due to poor grasp of intake • Slow production of work
Encoding of Visual Stimuli [4,45,46]	• Poor registration of visual information into the memory system - hinders visual recall • Difficulties with integration of information	• Difficulties interpreting information and forming conclusions due to their retention of partial intake • Inconsistent learning; requires extended exposure
Visuo-spatial Abilities [32,47,48]	• Problems with organizing visually presented information • Poor judgment of distance • Difficulties scanning a page from left-to-right, top-to bottom • Difficulties orientating an object and/or themselves in a mental or physical space • Difficulties reconstructing an image or object from a given model • Difficulties with reconstructing an image or pattern from memory • Difficulties remembering sequences of visually presented objects • Poor mental manipulation of object to solve a problems • Inefficient use of visual imagery to support problem solving	• Frequently misplaces objects or forgets to turn in assignments; appears disorganized • Stands too close to classmates in line; difficulties judging personal boundaries • Difficulties with finding a position when playing a team sport in Physical Education • Problems remembering the locations of the classrooms when changing classes • Struggles to remember the class schedule, the order of routines, or the steps to tasks • Difficulties copying information from the board due to visual distractions from extraneous material or decorations • Difficulties planning the layout of work on a page. For example, starts writing in the center of page instead of on the upper, left-hand line. • Misses relevant information presented near the edges of a page in a text. Poor scanning abilities.
Gross and/or Fine Motor Skills [28,49]	• Poor hand-eye coordination • Appear clumsy • Difficulties with visual-motor integration • Poor graphomotor skills (handwriting) • Poor fine motor skills	• Difficulties with skills such as cutting with scissors, coloring, or sewing • Difficulties tying shoes • Poor letter formation and slow rate of writing speed • Difficulties completing tasks that require the hand to be guided by visual stimuli such as artwork and/or crafts • Difficulties with hitting and/or catching a ball
Self-regulation [50-52]	• Difficulties adjusting responses to the environment or setting • Inconsistent ability to attend to stimuli on cue • Inability to control or shift physical and/or emotional responses as the setting changes • Poor energy modulation, such as having difficulties with calming when needed to prepare to complete a quiet task • Poor internal sense of time • Unaware of their actions on others	• Cannot sit still in class • Easily startled • Runs in the hall and/or into the classroom when entering from an outside activity or recess • Difficulties controlling vocal intonations, may talk too loud for indoors • Problems stopping an action when asked by an instructor or a peer • Appears defiant when asked to shift to a calm state • Works in spurts and requires frequent adult assistance to complete task

Impairment	Impact on Functioning	Displayed at School
Executive Functioning Skills [15,31,35]	• Difficulties with planning and predicting outcomes • Poor concept formation • Poor cognitive flexibility • Poor selection and application of problem solving strategies • Unaware of the effectiveness of the strategy • Difficulties shifting a strategy • Poor interpretation and understanding of cause and effect	• Difficulties selecting the relevant information and organizing the information to make a plan • Problems predicting outcomes or goals • Frequently asks what comes next or checks to see if they are finished with an activity • Unaware that an assignment or task is being completed inaccurately • Over-reliance on a strategy that works for a specific type of problem • Difficulties shifting strategy use and frequently makes the same errors on a task • Frustrated and/or resistant to shifting to a new task or activity • Difficulties synthesizing the information to form a conclusion or generalization
Language Pragmatics [42,53,54]	• Problems with social communication • Use of ambiguous language to convey an event or a story • Difficulties accessing succinct words to refer and/or name objects during narratives and/or conversations • Problems with determining and/or interpreting another's state of mind to support interactions • Difficulties interpreting the subtle nuances that occur during interpersonal exchanges, e.g. intent, nonverbal cues, mood. • Predicting and interpreting responses in order to respond appropriately	• Able to understand the conventions of social communication, such as taking turns • Difficulties following the topic or conversation • Provides remarks that are off topic or unrelated to the discussion • Retells an event or story that is hard to follow, contains extraneous information, and lacks a conclusion or a point • Difficulties interpreting the implied intent conveyed in language • Misuse of figurative language, jokes, and sarcasm. At times, the misuse of language angers or annoys peers • Poor social timing, for example, attempting to joke around after a peer has shifted focus to a learning task • Difficulties interpreting nonverbal cues and body language

CHILDREN WITH FASD AND LEARNING

Because of the neurodevelopmental problems caused by prenatal alcohol exposure, and in some cases, by environmental deprivation and neglect, many children with FASD have problems in their educational setting. Children with FASD perform poorly on academic achievement tests and in their classroom settings [36,55]. Problems are noted in behavior and self-regulation, and impairments in processing numerical information, as well as weaknesses with visuo-spatial skills, have been documented. These impairments contribute to the deficits in mathematics associated with the effects from prenatal alcohol exposure [32,56,57]. In the next section, we review research that identifies and describes specific learning and behavioral deficits in children with FASD.

FASD, SELF-REGULATION AND BEHAVIOR

Sometimes the initial concern about alcohol-affected children is their behavior in the classroom. In addition to problems with processing and organizing information, which is required for appropriate adjustment to the school setting, children with FASD have difficulties modulating their physical and/or emotional reactions to their environment as it changes [4]. The functions associated with self-regulation have a biological basis. The ability to activate the functions required for self-regulation which includes coping and self-soothing, can be disrupted by biological and/or environmental factors [50]. In school-aged children, difficulties with self-regulation may interfere with the ability to transition smoothly to new activities and to maintain a consistent state of mental alertness, especially in a classroom or group setting. Often the behaviors demonstrated by children with difficulties with self-regulation are similar to the behaviors observed in children with behavioral disorders. However, there are often differences in the goals and purposes of these behaviors.

There have been inconclusive results regarding a direct correlation between the effects from prenatal alcohol exposure and challenging behaviors [43]. Some researchers have found that children with FASD have elevated scores on externalizing behaviors, such as tantrums and impulsivity, on behavior checklists. However, many of the studies investigating behavior difficulties in children with FASD did not account for the impact of neglectful environments and/or intellectual impairments on behaviors. Also, most of the studies investigating a direct connection between FASD and behavior difficulties, recruited participants who were referred for clinical services [58] thus ensuring that challenging behaviors would be present. The challenging behaviors of children with FASD need to be viewed on an individual basis in relation to their cognitive functioning and the adequacy of their care giving environment. Although "clinical lore" has suggested that the behavioral problems seen in FASD are resistant to standard behavioral interventions, some of the recent studies reported below have identified effective methods for moderating behavior problems [59]. However, these methods have not yet been evaluated in the classroom.

FASD AND ACADEMICS

School problems and academic failure are commonly reported in clinically-referred individuals with FASD [60]. While some of these problems are attributable to environmental and behavior problems, mathematics has been identified by a number of studies as a specific weakness in children affected by prenatal alcohol exposure [4,36,61]. Aspects of language functioning also have been identified as problematic [54]. There is less evidence regarding other academic areas and there is little specificity about the age of the child when problems occur or methods for remediation [62-63]. Parents and teachers often report that children with FASD appear to struggle in academic subjects that require higher order thinking skills, cognitive organization, and the effective use of problem solving techniques [5,6,45,64]. Additional research is needed to investigate the impact of FASD on learning across academic subjects.

FASD AND LANGUAGE SKILLS NECESSARY FOR SCHOOL SUCCESS

Many children with FASD show relative strengths in their naming vocabulary and surface language skills, such as describing personal events and responding to concrete questions [54]. However, studies have suggested that children with FASD exhibit difficulties with language pragmatics, which is the ability to use language effectively across contexts and often includes social language [53,65]. In these studies, children with FASD were able to use the conventions of social discourse, such as turn-taking, yet struggled to maintain a conversational topic especially when the conversation or topic became more complex. In addition to difficulties with language pragmatics, children with FASD may have weaknesses encoding verbal information which can hinder their acquisition of linguistic concepts [54,66]. Difficulties with social discourse along with deficits in self-regulation and/or in processing may interfere with the ability to conduct successful social interactions in a school environment [67,68] and contribute to the problems often observed in this group of children.

FASD AND MATHEMATICS

Relative deficits in mathematics achievement have been identified in both longitudinal and clinical studies [36,56]. Specifically, research has noted that many children and adolescents with FASD demonstrate difficulties processing numerical information [56]. In addition, children with FASD show difficulties with estimation, interpreting mathematic symbols, representing mathematical information in different forms, and solving word problems [29,32,36,56]. It is speculated that these problems in mathematics exhibited by children with FASD may be related to weaknesses in maintaining information in the working memory system [57]. It is also possible that problems in the areas of interhemispheric integration of verbal and visual information and the self-monitoring functions moderated by the executive functioning system may impact mathematics performance in some children with FASD [69-72].

However, some children with FASD do acquire basic arithmetic skills, such as recognizing written numbers, comparing the value of two numbers, reciting numbers in order, and computing single addition, subtraction, multiplication, and division problems [56,57]. Clinical observation suggests that difficulties in mathematics appear when children are required to combine skills to compute problems within a designated amount of time, to shift between mathematic procedures such as adding and subtracting, or to transform information into abstract representations [29, 56,73]. Research continues to investigate the specific mathematic domains impacted by FASD as well as instructional interventions to support learning.

UNDERLYING ACADEMIC SKILLS AND CHILDREN WITH FASD

In order to achieve in a school setting, children must have available certain prerequisite skills. Such skills may be referred to as "preliminary learning skills" and include, for instance, the ability to attend to relevant information, take in all the available information, and the ability to scan for information in a systematic manner. Generally, a child learns these skills prior to entering school through early interactions with caregivers. If there is no adequate interaction, or if the child is not able to benefit from the interaction, the preliminary learning skills may not be acquired sufficiently, which may result in difficulties with learning later on [74].

It appears that some children with FASD exhibit difficulties with these preliminary learning skills. Taddeo [75] conducted an observational study of the underlying "thinking skills" in a clinical sample of 56 children with FASD. Underlying thinking skills, termed cognitive functions by Feuerstein [74] are the rudimentary skills children need in order to learn. These skills include the ability to search systematically for information on a page, the ability to put information in a time/space perspective, the ability to take into account all the available information, and the ability to attend to relevant information [74]. These preliminary thinking skills can be assessed on three levels, first, the intake of information, secondly, the processing of information, and finally, the output or communication of the processed information. According to the study's findings, more than 60% of the alcohol-affected children exhibited difficulties with the basic thinking skills required to take in the necessary information to solve problems. For instance, many of the children had difficulty attending to more than one piece of information at one time, or they did not search a page from left to right and from top to bottom, skipping all over a page to find the information [76].

Often children with FASD exhibit problems selecting and assimilating the relevant information needed to approach and solve a problem. When a child does not attend to relevant information, he or she will assign equal importance to each word in a sentence. For instance, in a math word-problem where the learner is required to compute the total amount of 3 plastic cars and 7 wooden cars, all the words in the math sentence will be read accurately and with equal emphasis. However, the words "total amount" and the numbers "3" and "7" will not be recognized as the only facts needed to solve the problem, resulting in either an inability to start solving it, or a haphazard attempt to solve it with an incorrect outcome. In a classroom situation it is important to recognize the inability of the child to identify relevant information, so that he or she is not misjudged as being stubborn, defiant or inattentive when the assigned task is not started immediately, or appears to be avoided.

Additionally, when a child has not acquired the skill to search systematically for information, a page will not be scanned from left to right and from top to bottom. With this type of unsystematic and probably incomplete data gathering, important information needed to solve a problem may be missed. For instance, when presented with a sheet of simple addition and subtraction problems, children with FASD often overlooked the mathematical signs that indicated the correct operation as they tried to complete the math problems. Many times, when they began with addition, children continued to add all the problems even though the operation sign changed to indicate that subtraction was required. Problems attending to the changes in mathematical signs impact children's accuracy when completing mathematic problems. Thus, children with FASD may require specific instruction to learn how to scan and detect the changes in mathematic procedures, as well as how to take into account all the information that is available to them on the math page. Because the underlying thinking skills in which they show deficits are considered to be teachable skills [77-79], it is important to recognize that children with FASD may not have acquired these skills, and to identify areas of deficit. Specifically teaching these skills may help them increase their cognitive flexibility and their ability to shift attention to different aspects of presented information. Teachers who consider these thinking processes and provide the necessary interventions to address identified weaknesses can support more effective learning.

EVIDENCE-BASED PROGRAMS FOR ALCOHOL-AFFECTED CHILDREN

Given the known environmental risks as well as the neurocognitive, behavioral and educational problems documented in FASD, caregivers, researchers and advocates have called for an increase in medical, social, and educational services for children with FASD [1,8] as well as for research on effective, evidenced-based treatments that can be used in school and communities. However, such services are rare and only a few studies have addressed specifically educational interventions for alcohol-affected individuals [63,80,81]. Despite 30 years of research into the effects of prenatal alcohol exposure, it is not until very recently that interventions were developed targeting the problems associated with these conditions [82]. As there are only a limited number of studies, it is possible to describe briefly the evidence- based interventions that have been developed, or more usually, adapted for alcohol-affected children [63, 80-82]. Of these few studies, the majority of the interventions have focused on preschool and school-aged children. There is no published information on adolescents at this time.

SCHOOL-BASED LANGUAGE AND LITERACY TRAINING (LLT) [62]

In this South African study, they addressed the well known effects on cognition, academic achievement, and behavior among children with FASD. Forty, third grade children diagnosed with FASD were randomly assigned to a Language and Literacy Training (LLT) group or a non-treated control group and compared to non-exposed controls from the same school systems. At pretest, children with FASD in both groups were significantly weaker than controls in reading, spelling, and phonological awareness as well as arithmetic skills. The intervention was administered in the children's classroom in a group format for 30 minutes, twice a week by a speech and language therapist. Half of the time was spent on phonological awareness and half on language therapy. At follow-up, the group receiving LLT demonstrated improved outcomes on language and literacy measures relative to the non-treated FASD group, whereas the non-treated group did not improve. Both FASD groups continued to perform more poorly than the non-exposed controls on these outcome measures. However, improvement was specific to language and literacy with no effects seen on overall scholastic achievement (e.g., math outcomes) indicating that specific and explicit instruction is important in remediating the effects of prenatal exposure. The authors suggest that methods developed for remediation with other groups of learning disabled children can be applied effectively to those with FASD. Attempts to involve parents in this intervention were not as effective as anticipated, probably due to poverty and limited family resources.

MATH INTERACTIVE LEARNING EXPERIENCE (MILE) [59, 69]

While prenatal alcohol exposure affects cognitive and academic functioning in many areas, cognitive skills that contribute to the development of mathematics are particularly vulnerable. These problems may be attributed to the effects of alcohol exposure on the brain as well as lack of adequate environmental support. The MILE program addressed this problem through parent training, individualized educational intervention, and modifying arousal regulation to improve behavior and math functioning in clinically-referred children ages 3 to 10. In a study carried out at the Marcus Institute in Atlanta, Georgia, 61 children were randomly assigned to either a math tutoring program or a standard psychoeducational contrast group. Parents in both groups were provided information about the neurodevelopmental impact of FASD on learning and behavior, methods for interacting with educational and social systems, and behavioral management techniques. The Math group received six sessions of individual tutoring while parents were provided with "home work" to support math development. An active learning approach adapted from the methodology developed by the High-Scope Perry Preschool Project [83] was used. At follow-up, children in both groups showed fewer behavior problems and those in the math group had significantly more gains in math achievement. At a 6-month follow-up, improvements in both areas were maintained and teachers reported significant declines in behavior problems at school.

PROJECT BRUIN BUDDIES: A SOCIAL SKILLS TRAINING PROGRAM [68, 84]

Alcohol-affected children, from early school age through young adulthood, have difficulties making friends and developing and using appropriate social skills [85]. Researchers at the University of California at Los Angeles adapted a social skills program based on social learning theory [86] for use with alcohol-exposed children, ages 6 to 12. They modified Frankel's well-researched protocol to accommodate the neurodevelopmental deficits associated with FASD by changing how the treatment was delivered rather than by altering content. Significant skills, including social network formation, goal-directed information exchange, group entry ("slipping in"), play dates and conflict avoidance, were taught in a group format. In addition, parents were taught how to "coach" children to support skill development. Half of the 96 children were randomly assigned to parent-assisted Children's Friendship Training (CFT) and half to a Delayed Treatment Control (DTC). The intervention included 12 sessions and was evaluated immediately after completion and 3 months later. Children showed significantly improved knowledge of appropriate social behavior and parents reported improved social skills and decreased problem behavior at home. Teachers, however, did not report significant improvements at school. Observed gains were maintained over the 3-month follow-up period. Parents reported increased understanding of FASD and satisfaction with treatment. In a follow-up, this program was successfully replicated in a community setting [84].

"GAMES THAT WORK": USING COMPUTER GAMES TO TEACH ALCOHOL-AFFECTED CHILDREN ABOUT SAFETY [87, 88]

Adaptive skills are frequently a concern in clinically-referred children with FASD and cognitive limitations and behavior problems in such children place them at high risk for unintentional injuries that are a leading cause of death and disability in this age group. Teaching safety skills can prevent such injuries but this may be a difficult task for parents and teachers because of the need to tailor the instruction to the specific needs of the child and to persist until the skill is mastered. In this project, 32 children, ages 4-10, diagnosed with FAS or FASD, learned fire and street safety through computer games that used "virtual worlds" to teach recommended safety skills. These skills sets were chosen because of the significance of street and fire safety issues for young children. The game format addressed children's skill learning deficits by allowing repeated, consistent practice, clear on-screen guidance (provided by a cartoon dog named, "Buddy"), safe learning situations, control of input stimuli and complexity to help with appropriate task focus, and strong engagement value in the teaching format. Methods first developed for use with autistic children were adapted for the different characteristics of alcohol-affected children. Changes included more emphasis on language and language-based instruction and simplification of visual/motor and visual/spatial aspects to accommodate to the problems experienced by alcohol-affected children. Children were randomly assigned to either the fire or street safety condition and each group acted as a control to the other group. Following play, children showed significant improvement in knowledge of safety skills. This verbal knowledge also generalized to actions in the real-world environment and was retained over a week's time at follow-up. These outcomes suggest that this may be an effective and convenient method for teaching alcohol-affected children.

This brief review of educational methods demonstrates that, in the right circumstances, prenatally exposed children respond well and demonstrate significant improvements in development and behavior. These findings point out both the importance of early identification of affected children as well as the need for resources in this area. In addition, it is evident that certain factors greatly increase the likelihood that interventions will be successful. First, particularly with young children, involvement in and commitment to the treatment process by caregivers are important to successful outcomes. Second, is the answer to the frequently asked question about whether there is a need for interventions specifically designed for alcohol and drug-exposed children. Is it not possible that their needs can be met through the "usual and customary" methods used to treat other neurodevelopmentally based disorders? The answer to these questions is "yes and no". Clearly, prenatally exposed children respond in most ways as others do. However, prenatal exposure does lead to particular patterns of neurodevelopment and is associated more often with certain kinds of life experiences. Understanding these patterns allows greater efficiency in designing effective interventions for this group.

It has been demonstrated previously with other disability groups, that to be effective, intervention strategies must target disability-specific strengths and weakness and adapt techniques to accommodate to these characteristics [89]. All of the studies reviewed used methods that were developed for other groups of children, including those with learning disabilities, psychiatric disorders and behavior problems. When these methods were adapted to accommodate the neurodevelopmental characteristics associated with prenatal exposure as well as the impact of postnatal environment, children were able to benefit significantly from the interventions. In the past, it has been suggested that alcohol and drug-exposed children are particularly resistant to treatment, perhaps because "brain-damage" resulting from their exposure makes them unable to learn or change or react in ways that other children can. This suggestion is often made either to deny children services or to excuse a lack of effort to improve outcomes. Happily, the studies mentioned in this article directly refute this idea and may help avoid such negative thinking in the future.

DESIGNING EDUCATIONAL INTERVENTIONS FOR ALCOHOL-AFFECTED CHILDREN

The preceding reviews of deficits in individuals with FASD and existing interventions, suggest that the educator will find it necessary to identify appropriate methods to support educational success in alcohol-affected children. There is a wide spectrum of effects caused by prenatal alcohol exposure, so children with an alcohol -related diagnosis may have a variety of learning needs. Given the range of deficits associated with FASD, a single behavioral phenotype is not likely to describe children effectively or provide adequate guidance to the instructor. As with any child, the individual's learning strengths and challenges need to be considered when devising educational programs for children with FASD. This process will include assessing children's overall intellectual functioning, processing patterns, and academic skills. Subsequent formal and informal assessments need to be completed to determine the educational needs and to guide educational planning [90,91].

Often aspects of the deficits associated with FASD are similar to those found in other developmental disabilities or learning disorders, such as Nonverbal Learning Disabilities and Mathematics Disorders. Some children affected by prenatal alcohol exposure exhibit average cognition but problems with processing skills may require accommodations to support their performance in the learning environment. However, other children with FASD who have significant cognitive impairments may require specialized educational interventions. Educational interventions need to be designed according to the needs of the individual with FASD. Because of the overlapping learning difficulties with other developmental disabilities and learning disorders, educational interventions devised for learning disabilities may be used to teach children with an alcohol related diagnosis. The website www.ldonline.org provides articles and access to online discussions for parents and professionals to inquire about learning disabilities. Also, the Learning Disabilities Association (LDA) is a valuable resource for parents, teachers, and other professionals working with children with learning disorders (www.ldanatl.org).

PUBLIC EDUCATION IN THE UNITED STATES AND CHILDREN WITH FASD

In planning for the education of alcohol-affected children, it is important to consider the context of that education. This context will include not only the individual school and school system but the laws and regulations that govern them. Since the late 1990's, educational policy has moved toward educating children with disabilities with their non-disabled peers [92,93]. This practice is termed "inclusion". The movement toward inclusive education is embedded in the revised Individuals with Disabilities Education Improvement Act of 2004 (IDEA; PL 108-446). According to IDEA, children with disabilities need to be educated in the least restrictive environment and often within a general classroom setting. The recent revision of IDEA aligned their requirements with those of the No Child Left Behind Act (NCLB; PL 107-110 115 Stat.1425). According to NCLB all children need to be instructed using evidenced-based curriculum regardless of their disability. The US Department of Education has published the website "IDEA, Building the Legacy" that explains the rules and regulation of IDEA. The website is http://idea.ed/gov.

Many parents and professionals assume that having a medical diagnosis will qualify a child for special education services. However, children with a medical related disability, including those with Fetal Alcohol Syndrome (FAS), need to show that they have academic deficits in their classroom setting to be considered for special education services. According to IDEA, a multi-level assessment and intervention process must be conducted before children are determined to need special education services. A process called Response to Intervention (RTI) is implemented in order to increase the accuracy of identifying children who require special education instruction [94]. Many school districts have adopted a multi-tiered system to address children's learning difficulties in the classroom setting. Fig **1** shows an example of the RTI framework.

According to the RTI framework, Tier 1 refers to adjustments to the curriculum or instructional methods on a school-wide basis. School-wide means that changes are made in all classrooms to ensure that students, regardless of academic struggles, are receiving quality instruction. Tier 2 of RTI provides adjustments to the instructional methods for a struggling student. Such adjustments may include providing extra time or providing further explanation of the directions. Tier 3 increases the intensity of the interventions and may include providing small group instruction. Children's progress through each tier is monitored [94,95]. Children are referred for consideration for special education services if they are "resistant" to these different levels of interventions. That is, if they do not demonstrate appropriate educational gains under these conditions. The premise of the RTI framework is consistent across school districts. However, some districts use a different number of tiers and different types of strategies for intervention. This includes receiving related educational services such as speech and language therapy, physical therapy, and/or occupational therapy. Often children with an alcohol related diagnosis require therapies to address weaknesses in language, fine motor skills, grapho-motor skills as well as in other areas to ensure their success in a classroom setting.

The implementation of the RTI process varies according to the educational guidelines for each state. It is important to confer with the state's department of education and/or the specific school district to inquire about the implementation of the RTI.. The Response to Intervention Action Network supported by the National Center for Learning Disabilities provides extensive information about RTI. Their website is **www.rtinetwork.org**

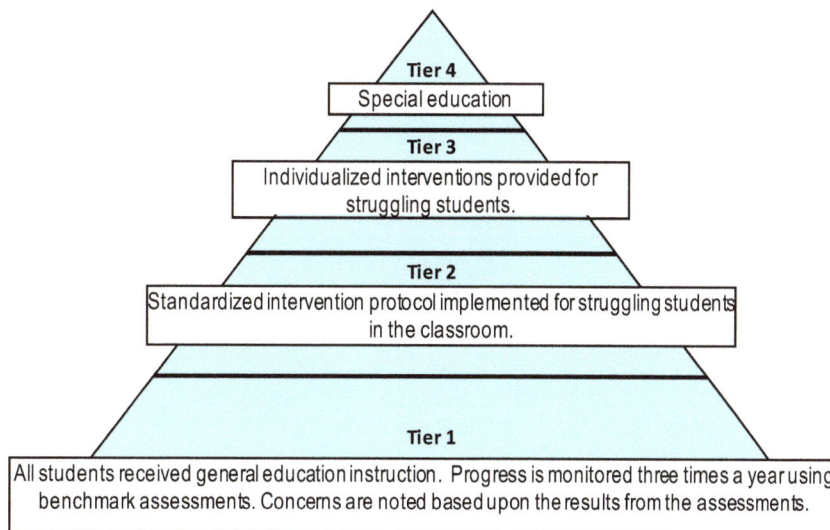

Tier 4
Special education

Tier 3
Individualized interventions provided for struggling students.

Tier 2
Standardized intervention protocol implemented for struggling students in the classroom.

Tier 1
All students received general education instruction. Progress is monitored three times a year using benchmark assessments. Concerns are noted based upon the results from the assessments.

Figure 1: Response to Intervention (RTI).

SUPPORTING CHILDREN WITH FASD IN THEIR EDUCATIONAL ENVIRONMENT: PRACTICAL ADVICE FOR EDUCATORS

Children with FASD require specific strategies to support their interactions in the classroom and their academic progress. Specifically, the supports must address the deficits that have been identified as affecting their neurodevelopment and behavior. These may include encoding new information (learning), visuo-spatial processing, and speed of processing, as well as their difficulties with self-regulation [96-97]. This section will discuss the types of educational supports children with FASD need in order to maneuver within their classroom setting and achieve academic progress.

Maneuvering the Classroom

Problems with visuo-spatial processing and motor skills associated with FASD often hinder a child's ability to negotiate the classroom setting, including following the daily schedule, managing transitions in the schedule and/or adapting to classroom routines. Children with FASD frequently require structure to support daily expectations in the classroom such as remembering their schedule, adjusting to schedule changes, shifting to new activities, recalling the steps to complete tasks, and maneuvering the physical space of a classroom. There are a number of supports that can be instituted by the teacher to support success in these areas. These include using visual schedules and picture cues to provide children with consistent exposure to the information to which they can refer at need without relying on memory. Such picture cues have been found to be successful for individuals with severe developmental disabilities and have helped to improve their skills to self-manage tasks [53,91,98].

Children with FASD also may benefit from a classroom layout that is easy to navigate. Changes that can be implemented to improve the classroom layout include designating consistent locations for books, papers, and supplies, and having regular classroom routines. The website **www.do2learn.com** provides ways to adjust the classroom environment to meet children's needs.

Behavior in the Classroom

Due to a variety of factors, some children with FASD exhibit difficulties with behavior in the classroom. As noted earlier in this chapter, behavior problems are commonly found although it is not clear whether there is a direct connection between behavior and the effects of prenatal alcohol or whether these difficulties occur due to environmental factors associated with prenatal alcohol exposure [43,58].

Regardless of the underlying causes of the behavior problems, a positive and consistent approach is needed to address behavioral issues. For some children, appropriate interventions may require contact with the school counselor to request that the school behavioral specialist conduct a Functional Behavioral Analysis (FBA) to assess the triggers, the setting, the frequency, duration, and intensity of problem behaviors. In addition, a reward and punishment survey should be done to outline the consequences that reward positive and negative behaviors. Once the FBA is completed, a behavior intervention plan (BIP) is devised. The purpose of the BIP is to teach children how to use appropriate actions across settings. The BIP needs to include hypotheses concerning the factors that maintain behaviors: a clear behavioral definition of the targeted behaviors, an explicit method for providing replacement behaviors, and it should indicate methods for providing feedback [99]. The website Positive Behavioral Interventions and Supports (www.pbis.org) provides information on devising effective behavior intervention plans.

Children with FASD may need instruction and strategies on how to modulate their interactions across settings. Difficulties with self-regulation may impact children's ability to attend to the cues in the environment, adjust and shift their perspective to solve problems, and to modulate their pacing in the classroom or group setting. Students with FASD need support as well as instruction to teach self-awareness and strategies to regulate their behavior [100]. Strategies to teach self regulation may include giving the children advance warning before shifting or ending an activity; giving frequent breaks and using sand timers or time-timers to measure the time before the break; if different tasks need to be done, giving the child the choice as to which task will be done first; assigning a quiet place where the task can be completed.

Additionally, in understanding children's behavior and learning, it is important to be aware of the effects of the expectations and demands placed on children with FASD. Children with FASD who have processing impairments may misunderstand directions or situations in which they find themselves. Communication can be improved by using short, concise statements. Verbal messages should coincide with nonverbal signals to help children with FASD understand directions and expectations [4, 101]. Instructions should outline preferred actions rather than emphasizing negative behaviors. An example of a statement that outlines the preferred behavior would be, "keep your hands by the side of your body when walking down the hall." This is in contrast to the instruction, "Don't touch other people", which may be more difficult for the child to follow. Finally, when a child exhibits the correct behavior, provide praise using statements that identify the appropriate behavior. "Thank you for keeping your hands to yourself as we walked down the hall. Because of that, we were able to get into the lunch line and get our food first." This practice tells children why the behavior was successful and identifies what needs to be repeated.

Presentation of Information During Classroom Instruction

Understanding the cognitive deficits associated with FASD and their impact on academic functioning will help the teacher present information in a way that is accessible to the child with special needs. Children with FASD may have difficulties retaining information due to the deficits in encoding (learning) and retrieving information. Therefore, many children with FASD demonstrate inconsistent recall. They may remember factual information presented one day but cannot recall the information the next day when asked a similar question. They require frequent practice and review of information to help them encode and process information presented through class lectures, discussion, and/or direct instruction. It is also the case that many children learn differently, with one modality more efficient than another. Therefore presenting information in as many modalities as possible, such as verbal and/or pictorial will be beneficial. This can be accomplished by pairing orally presented information with a visual cue [102]. Monitoring the rate of speech when presenting verbal directions will accommodate to the slow speed of processing associated with FASD [45]. To assure that children understand, information needs to be repeated frequently while requesting that the students paraphrase the directions in their own words in order to check for understanding and to help them to process the information further.

Children with FASD may need additional time to generate a response because they require more time to process information [102]. Therefore, if a child is asked to respond to a question, the teacher needs to wait 10 seconds before moving to another student or providing the answer. While waiting, the teacher can look at the student in an expectant manner after the question has been asked in order to circumvent any learned avoidance behavior. This practice gives the student the opportunity to interact with the teacher in a positive manner, even if the right answer may not be forthcoming.

Given the processing difficulties associated with FASD, an older student may require a study guide during classroom presentations. Using a study guide enables the student to focus on the information presented verbally and lessen the cognitive demands of note-taking. According to Roth [103] lessening the demands of note-taking enables students to process and retain the information more efficiently. Additionally, this practice helps to support children with grapho-motor difficulties, another common disability associated with FASD.

INSTRUCTION: SPECIFIC METHODS FOR IMPROVING OUTCOMES

As was discussed earlier in this chapter, there are a limited number of studies that have evaluated interventions for children with FASD. For this reason, teachers often use strategies and intervention methods found successful for children with other disabilities in working with these students. For example, often children with FASD exhibit relative strengths in surface language skills and in academic skills, such as naming vocabulary and reading individual words. At the same time, they may demonstrate weaknesses in abstract reasoning, applied mathematics, and maintaining appropriate social interactions. This profile reflects attributes that are similar to those of children diagnosed with a Nonverbal Learning Disability (NVLD) [104-106]. Clinical observations suggest that the strategies used to support children with NVLD may be successful for children with FASD as well.

Strategies cannot be applied uncritically. Selected strategies for children with FASD need to be based upon the results of a comprehensive educational assessment and consistent monitoring of progress [90]. As noted above, children with FASD require thoughtful instructional methods to support information processing, and strategy use to complete academic tasks [75]. Instruction in these areas may help children with FASD develop the skills to learn efficiently in the classroom. Lessons need to be scaffolded so they build upon previously learned skills. Also, skills that are lacking need to be explicitly taught. This provides children with FASD the review and the framework to recognize the connections among ideas. Unlike typical children, they will not spontaneously bring effective learning skills to a new situation, so it is important to establish the purpose and to provide instructional questions to children with FASD in order to support their deficits in selecting relevant information and to support encoding of new material [107].

Mediated Learning

A mediated, metacognitive learning approach has proved effective in instruction with this group [69]. To use this approach, the instructor uses statements and/or questions to help the student to figure out presented problems and to draw conclusions that lead to the desired outcome without directly providing the children with the answer. This approach supports the development of more effective learning habits. Once a student learns to figure out learning challenges, less emphasis needs to be placed upon the memory function, which is often weak in children with FASD. This learning approach encourages teachers to "question" or discuss both right and wrong answers in order to provide the opportunity for the student to reflect on the process that he/she used to derive at the answer. For example, if the child makes an error in calculating a simple arithmetic problem, the teacher may say, "I see that your answer to 7+4=3." "How did you get that answer?" After asking the question, the teacher has the child, usingcounters or small objects, demonstrate the process by which they came to their original answer. If the child combines a pile of 7 with a pile of 4, the teacher makes a statement such as "it seems that you put them together." This observation directs them to attend to the outcome. Then ask "what happened to the piles?" Many times, children will respond that the piles were put together and became higher. After this occurs, direct the children to compare the process to the problem, 7+4=11. Have the children compare the results from using the objects, to their initial answer, which was possibly the result of misreading the operation sign and subtracting, rather than adding. Finally, have the children correct their answer and restate why the answer needed adjusting. Using this kind of procedure allows the child to come to an understanding of the meaning of addition as well as identifying the correct answer to the problem.

Self-Talk and Task Sequencing

Children with FASD often have difficulties in the processes related to executive functioning, specifically with selecting problem solving strategies and shifting their attention effectively from one aspect of a task to another [35,108]. While such deficits are observed regularly in individuals with FASD, it is possible to teach methods for improving functioning in this area. In a math study for children with FASD, Kable, *et al.* [69] found that the use of a mediated learning approach, the FAR method (Focus and plan – Act – Reflect), was beneficial in guiding the students to plan their actions before beginning a task, to think about how they were going to complete it, and to reflect upon the task to improve cognitive organization, shifting, and generalization of information. In other words, this method explicitly provided the "executive functioning" skills that the children were not applying spontaneously.

A Saturday Tutoring Program carried out from 2007-2008 used a process based upon the FAR method [69], and clinical observations of the effectiveness of this and other methods were recorded [109]. Children were required to use a series of self-questions during the completion of tasks. The sessions were conducted on an individual basis. Three index cards were presented to the children. The beginning card contained the question "what do I need to do?" The second card contained the question "what am I doing?" The final card contained the question "what do I need to remember?" The children pointed to the question that corresponded to the sequence of the task completion in which they currently were engaged and verbalized the answer. The children's progress was monitored through their spontaneous use of the method, the accuracy of their answers while completing tasks, and their ability to self-correct items. Over the semester, these children showed an increase in their problem solving accuracy leading to the conclusion that this process helps in learning to select relevant information, organize thought processes, and helps to support generalization to other areas [110].

Mapping Techniques

Another method that has proved helpful with this group of children is the use of visual mapping. Mapping techniques help students learn by transforming information into a visual format that depicts the connections among topics. From the visual layout students are able to select pertinent information and organize the information into categories. The categories enable students to shift the information into an outline form. This strategy can be helpful to students when organizing notes to study for a test or information to write an essay [111].

Direct Instruction

In many cases, children with FASD exhibit academic deficits that require direct, educational interventions. The need for direct instruction or remediation needs to be based upon the findings from a comprehensive educational evaluation which will identify the specific areas that require intervention. Direct instruction may be provided in school through special education services. However, some children with FASD may not qualify for special education instruction services and may seek services from other professionals. Programs such as Orton-Gillingham Reading (www.orton-gillingham.com) may be beneficial to address specific problems in reading. For grapho-motor difficulties that interfere with handwriting, the program Handwriting without Tears (www.hwtears.com) is available and has been found to be very effective in remediating the deficits associated with FASD [59,69]. Instructors may use Number Worlds (www.sra.com) to provide remedial mathematic instruction

In addition to what can be provided in the school setting, private tutors may provide remedial instruction. When selecting a tutoring program, determining the qualifications of the tutor (trained remedial instructor and/or volunteer), the administration of the program (small group and/or individual), the program outline (established curriculum and/or individualized), and the expectations of the program (remediation and/or improving standardized test scores) must be considered. The book, **A Parents Guide to Tutors and Tutoring: How to Support the Unique Needs of Your Child**, by **James Mendelson** provides information on selecting appropriate tutors and programs for children.

Use of Technology

There are a number of ways in which technology and/or software programs can support learning for children with FASD. Programs such as word processing, organizational programs, and those providing keyboarding instruction will lessen the demand on handwriting and provide an alternative method to produce work for students with FASD. Software programs also can be used as supplements to review, practice, and to help maintain previously learned skills. Also, software programs can provide reinforcement to help the child develop information that needs to be automatically known, such as math facts and certain adaptive skills. For example, www.do2learn.com has developed games to teach safety skills using computer games that train the children through game play on how to respond in dangerous situations. These games have been found to be effective in teaching children such skills both in the virtual world and in a real world context [87].

Home-School Communication

Home-School communication is important for all students, but even more so for children with FASD. Having teachers and parents "on the same page" benefits everyone concerned in the educational process- the child, the parent and school personnel. In addition to providing a clear and well integrated support for learning, good communication also lessens the possibility of the child triangulating or manipulating the system. To streamline the communication between teachers and caregivers, all parties need to agree upon the type of information that must be conveyed home to support academic progress. Also, everyone needs to agree upon the frequency and method of communication between home and school. For example, some teachers and caregivers prefer to discuss the issues over the telephone or by e-mail. Many find that it is necessary to establish a home-school communication notebook to support bringing papers back and forth from home to school [6]. If a child has multiple instructors, it is important to select a specific contact person at school, for instance the school counselor or the student's special education instructor, to facilitate the communication between home and school. Finally, it is essential to set up the communication system so that it is used to support the student, and is not used as a punishment or as a prelude to punishment.

CONCLUDING THOUGHTS

Research has shown that prenatal alcohol exposure can cause global intellectual impairments as well as deficits in processing, encoding, interhemispheric integration of verbal and visual information, working memory, and executive functioning [4,15,29,35,45,57]. In addition, many children experience negative caregiving environments and disruptions in custody. All of these factors have an impact on learning and educational achievement and many children with FASD demonstrate significant problems in this area. Nevertheless, caregivers, clinicians, and educators report that often children with FASD are successful in their learning environment. Research and clinical acumen suggest that alcohol-affected children succeed in their educational setting when provided with instructional supports that begin early and continue through high school and into adulthood. At the present time, research has begun to add to the knowledge about the cognitive impairments associated with FASD and the ways in which these problems can be addressed in educational settings. This increase in knowledge and experience can provide the support necessary to allow successful outcomes to become the norm rather than the exception for this population.

However, because there are still few resources for individuals with FASD and those working to help them, it is important to continue and expand investigations into educational interventions and treatment [90,112]. Certainly more research is needed at all ages but particularly for infants and toddlers and for adolescents since there are currently no such studies. Early intervention should be a primary focus since prevention of secondary disabilities in behavior and cognition is of vital importance. A second goal should be to increase the resources available to educators to support children's learning, by ensuring that more research on evidenced based interventions are carried out in the educational settings where most learning will take place. At this point in time, most of the evidenced-based interventions available were carried out in a clinical context. It is important to expand research on these to determine if such methods can be implemented successfully in the classroom and in other contexts where children are cared for. Therefore, in addition to continuing to develop novel and innovative methods, future research should focus on the application of existing methods in a naturalistic environment (e.g. classroom or small group setting).

In addition, support for these investigations must be found to allow continued development of innovative methods or adaptation of existing methods tailored to the needs of alcohol-affected individuals. Such support might be through an increase in research funding by agencies like the Centers for Disease Control and Prevention and the National Institutes of Health or by encouraging attention to this issue in the wider context that is impacted by FASD, for instance, by the Department of Education or the Department of Juvenile Justice. Public policy decisions must be made that include FASD as a condition worthy of attention and services similar to those decision made about autism spectrum disorder in recent years. In many cases, children with FASD are able to become productive adults when they are provided access to defined, successful interventions and receive the necessary educational supports.

Meeting the educational needs of children with FASD will contribute to changing to the long-term implications of the condition and help affected individuals become productive, well adjusted members of their community.

REFERENCES

[1]   Olson HC, Ohlemiller MM, O'Connor MJ, Brown CW, Morris CA, Damus K. A call to action: Advancing Essential Services and Research on Fetal Alcohol Spectrum Disorder – A report of the National Task Force on Fetal Alcohol Syndrome and Fetal Alcohol Effects 2009. http://www.cdc.gov/ncbddd/fasd/documents/08_121973CallActionBk+Cov.pdf

[2]   Sampson PD. Kerr B, Carmichael-Olsen H, *et al*. The effects of prenatal alcohol exposure on adolescent cognitive processing: A speed-accuracy tradeoff. Intelligence 1997; 24(2): 329-53.

[3]   National Center on Birth Defects and Developmental Disabilities, Centers for Disease Control and Prevention, Department of Health and Human Services, & National Task Force on Fetal Alcohol Syndrome and Fetal Alcohol Effects. Fetal alcohol syndrome: Guidelines for referral and diagnosis. Atlanta: CDC; 2004.

[4]   Kable JA, Coles CD. Teratology of alcohol: Implications for school settings. In Brown R, editor. Handbook of pediatric psychology in school settings.. Mahwah, New Jersey: Lawrence Erlbaum Associates, Inc. 2004; pp.379-404.

[5]   Miller D. Students with fetal alcohol syndrome: updating our knowledge, improving their programs, Teach Except Child 2006; 38(40): 12-8.

[6]   Duquette, C, Stodel E, Fullarton S, Hagglund K. Teaching students with developmental disabilities: Tips from teens and young adults with fetal alcohol spectrum disorder. Teach Except Child 2006; 39(2): 28-31.

[7]   Jones KL, Smith DW. Recognition of fetal alcohol syndrome in early infancy. Lancet 1973; 2: 999-1001.

[8]   Stratton L, Howe C, Battaglia F, editors. Fetal alcohol syndrome: Diagnosis, epidemiology, prevention, and treatment. Washington, DC: National Academy Press; 1996.

[9]   Sowell ER, Thompson PM, Mattson SN, *et al*. Regional brain shape abnormalities persist into adolescence after heavy prenatal alcohol exposure. Cereb Cortex 2002; 12: 56-65.

[10]   Wass TS, Persutte WH, Hobbins JC The impact of prenatal alcohol exposure on frontal cortex development in utero. Am J Obstet Gynecol 2001; 185: 737-42.

[11]   Fryer SL, Frank LR, Spandoni AD, *et al*. Microstructural integrity of the corpus callosum linked with neuropsychological performance in adolescents. Brain Cogn 2008; 67: 225-33.

[12]   Connor PD, Streissguth AP. Effects of prenatal exposure to alcohol across the life span. Alcohol Health Res World 1996; 20(3): 170-4.

[13]   Kerns KA, Don A, Mateer CA, Streissguth AP. Cognitive deficits in non-retarded adults with fetal alcohol syndrome. J Learn Disabil 1997; 30(6); 685-93.

[14]   Kable JA, Coles CD, Drews-Botsch C, Falek A. The effects of maternal drinking prenatally on patterns of pre-academic mathematical concept development. Symposium conducted at the meeting of the 22nd Annual Scientific Meeting of the Research Society on Alcoholism; Santa Barbara, CA. 1999

[15]   Kodituwakku PW, Kalberg W, May PA. The effects of prenatal alcohol exposure on executive functioning. Alcohol Res Health 2001; 25(3): 192-8.

[16]   Riikonen R, Salonen I, Partanen K, Verbo S. Brain perfusion SPECT and MRI in foetal alcohol syndrome. Dev Med Child Neurol 1999; 41: 652-9.

[17]   Johnson VP, Swayze VW II, Sato Y, Andreasen NC. Fetal alcohol syndrome; Craniofacial and central nervous system manifestations. Am J Med Genet 1996; 61(4): 329-39.

[18]   Mattson SN, Riley EP, Jernigan TL, *et al*. Fetal alcohol syndrome: A case report of neuropsychological, MRI and EEG assessment of two children. Alcohol Clin Exp Res 1992; 16 (5):1001-3.

[19]   Swayze VW II, Johnson VP. Magnetic resonance imaging of brain anomalies in fetal alcohol syndrome. Pediatrics 1997; 98(2): 232-40.

[20]   Ma X, Coles CD, Lynch ME, *et al*. Evaluation of corpus callosum anisotropy in young adults with fetal alcohol syndrome according to diffusion tensor imaging. Alcohol Clin Exp Res 2005; 29: 1214-22.

[21]   Li L, Coles CD, Lynch ME, Hu X. Voxelwise and skeleton-based region of interest analysis of fetal alcohol spectrum disorders in young adults. Hum Brain Mapp 2009; 30(10); PMID 19278010.

[22]   Wozniak R, Muetzel RL, Mueller BA, *et al*. Microstructural corpus callosum anomalies in children with prenatal alcohol exposure: An extension of previous diffusion tensor imaging findings. Alcohol Clin Exp Res 2009; 33(10): 1825-35.

[23]   Chen X, Coles CD, Lynch ME, Hu X. Understanding specific effects of prenatal alcohol exposure on brain structure in young adults. Hum Brain Mapp 2011; v 32. (in press).

[24]   Willoughby KA, Sheard ED, Nash K, Rovet J. Effects of prenatal alcohol exposure on hippocampal volume, verbal learning, and verbal and spatial recall in late childhood. J Int Neuropsychol Soc 2008; 14: 1022-33.

[25]   Coles CD. Prenatal Alcohol Exposure and Human Development. In M. W. Miller, (Ed), Brain development: Normal processes and the effects of alcohol and nicotine. New York, Oxford University Press 2006; pp. 123-42.

[26]   Kodituwakku PW. Defining the behavioral phenotype in children with fetal alcohol spectrum disorders: A review. Neurosci Biobehav Rev 2007; 31: 192-201.

[27]   Weiner L, Morse BA. Intervention and the child with FASD. Alcohol Health Res World 1994; 18(1): 67-72.

[28]   Adnams C, Kodituwakku P, Hay A, Molteno C, Viljoen D, May P. Patterns of cognitive-motor development in children with fetal alcohol syndrome from a community in South Africa. Alcohol Clin Exp Res 2001; 25(4): 557-62.

[29]   Burden J, Jacobson S, Jacobson J. Relation of prenatal alcohol exposure to cognitive processing speed and efficiency in childhood. Alcohol Clin Exp Res 2005; 29(8): 1473-83.

[30]   Coles CD, Platzman K, Raskind-Hood C, Brown R, Falek A, Smith I. A comparison of children affected by prenatal alcohol exposure and attention deficit hyperactivity disorder. Alcohol Clin Exp Res 1997; 21(1): 150-61.

[31]   McGee C, Schonfeld A, Roebuck-Spencer T, Riley E, Mattson S. Children with heavy prenatal alcohol exposure demonstrate deficits on multiple measures of concept formation. Alcohol Clin Exp Res 2008; 32: 1388-97.

[32]   Uecker A, Nadel L. Spatial locations gone awry: Object and spatial memory deficits in children with fetal alcohol syndrome. Neuropsychologia 1996; 34 (3): 209-23.

[33]   Rasmussen C, Bisanz J. Executive functioning in children with fetal alcohol spectrum disorders: Profiles and age-related differences. Child Neuropsychol 2008; 15: 201-15.

[34]   Morris R. Relationships and distinctions among the concepts of attention, memory, and executive function: A developmental perspective. In Lyon GR, Krasnegor N, editors. Attention, Memory, and Executive Function. Baltimore, MD, Brookes 1996; pp.11-6.

[35]   Mattson S, Calarco K, Lang A. Focused and shifting attention in children with heavy prenatal alcohol exposure. Neuropsychology 2006; 20(3): 361-9.

[36]   Howell K, Lynch ME, Platzman K, Smith H, Coles CD. Prenatal alcohol exposure and ability, academic achievement, and school functioning in adolescence: A longitudinal follow-up. J Pediatr Psychol 2006; 31(1): 116-26.

[37]   Brown J, Bednar L, Sigvaldason N. Causes of placement breakdown for foster children affected by alcohol. Child Adolesc Social Work J 2007; 24(4): 313-32.

[38]   Moe V, Slinning K, Prenatal drug exposure and the conceptualization of long-term effects. Scand J Psychol 2002; 43: 41-7.

[39]   Glaser D. Child abuse and neglect and the brain - A review. J Child Psychol Psychiatry 2000; 41(1): 97-116.

[40]   Moe V. Foster-placed and adopted children exposed in utero to opiates and other substances: Prediction and outcome at four and a half years. J Dev Behav Pediatr 2002; 23(5): 330-9.

[41]   Henry J, Sloane M, Black-Pond C. Neurobiology and neurodevelopmental impact of childhood traumatic stress and prenatal alcohol exposure. Lang Speech Hear Serv Sch 2007; 38: 99-108.

[42]   Coggins T, Timler G, Olswang L. A state of double jeopardy: Impact of prenatal alcohol exposure and adverse environments on the social communicative abilities of school-age children with fetal alcohol spectrum disorder. Lang Speech Hear Serv Sch 2007; 38: 117-27.

[43]   Dixon D, Kurtz P, Chin M. A systematic review of challenging behaviors in children exposed prenatally to substances of abuse. Res Dev Disabil 2008; 29: 483-502.

[44]   Stade B, Stevens B, Ungar W, Beyene J, Koren G. Health-related quality of life of Canadian children and youth prenatally exposed to alcohol. Health Qual Life Outcomes 2006; 4(81). Retrieved June 3, 2009, from http://www.hqlo.com/content/4/1/81.

[45]   Mattson S, Roebuck T. Acquisition and retention of verbal and nonverbal information in children with heavy prenatal alcohol exposure. Alcohol Clin Exp Res 2002; 26(6): 875-82.

[46]   Roebuck-Spencer T, Mattson S. Implicit strategy affects learning in children with heavy prenatal alcohol exposure. Alcohol Clin Exp Res 2004; 28: 1424-31.

[47]   Cornoldi C, Vecchi T. Visuo-spatial working memory and individual differences. New York: Psychology Press; 2003.

[48]   Kaemingk K & Tanner-Halverson P. Spatial memory following prenatal alcohol exposure: More than a material specific memory deficit. Child Neuropsychol 2000; 6(2): 115-28.

[49]   Kalberg W, Provost B, Tollison S, et al. Comparison of motor delays in young children with prenatal alcohol exposure and with no prenatal alcohol exposure. Alcohol Clin Exp 2006; 30(12): 2037-45.

[50]   Bronson M. Self-regulation in early childhood: Nature and nurture. Baltimore: Guildford Press; 2000.

[51]   Vohs K, Baumeister R. 2004, Understanding self-regulation: An introduction. Quoted in Thorne J, Coggins T, Carmichael-Olsen H, Astley S. Exploring the utility of narrative analysis in diagnostic decision-making: Picture-bound reference, elaboration, and Fetal Alcohol Spectrum Disorders. J Speech Lang Hear Res 2007; 50: 459-74.

[52]   Banfield J, Wyland C, Macrae C, Munte T, Heatherton T. The cognitive neuroscience of self-regulation. In. R. Baumeister & K. Vohs (Eds.). Handbook of Self-regulation: Research, Theory, and Applications. New York: Guildford Press; 2004.

[53] Timler G, Olswang L, Coggins T. "Do I know what I need to do? " A social communication intervention for children with complex clinical profiles. Lang Speech Hear Serv Sch 2005; 36: 73-85.

[54] Thorne J, Coggins T, Carmichael-Olsen H, Astley S. Exploring the utility of narrative analysis in diagnostic decision-making: Picture-bound reference, elaboration, and Fetal Alcohol Spectrum Disorders. J Speech Lang Hear Res 2007; 50: 459-74.

[55] Schonfeld A, Paley B, Frankel F, O'Connor M. Executive functioning predicts social skills following prenatal alcohol exposure. Child Neuropsychol 2006; 12(6): 439-52.

[56] Kopera-Frye K, Dehaene S, Streissguth A. Impairments in number processing induced by prenatal alcohol exposure. Neuropsychologia 1996; 34(2): 1187-96.

[57] Burden J, Jacobson SW, Sokol RJ, Jacobson JL. Effects of prenatal alcohol exposure on attention and working memory at 7.5 years of age. Alcohol Clin Exp Res 2005; 29(3): 443-52.

[58] Lynch ME, Coles CD, Corley T, Falek A. Examining delinquency in adolescents differentially prenatally exposed to alcohol: The role of proximal and distal risk factors. J Stud Alcohol 2003; 64: 678-86.

[59] Coles CD, Kable JA, Taddeo E. Math performance and behavior problems in children affected by prenatal alcohol exposure: Intervention and follow-up. J Dev Behav Pediatr 2009; 30(1): 7-15.

[60] Streissguth AP, Barr HM, Kogan J, Bookstein FL. Understanding the occurrence of secondary disabilities in clients with fetal alcohol syndrome (FASD) and fetal alcohol effects (FAAE): Final report to the Centers for Disease Control on Grant NO R04/CCR008515 (Tech. Report No 96-16). Seattle: University of Washington, Fetal Alcohol and Drug Unit 1996.

[61] Streissguth AP, Bookstein FL, Sampson PD, Barr HM. The enduring effects of prenatal alcohol exposure on child development: Birth through seven years, a partial least squares solution. Ann Arbor, MI: The University of Michigan Press 1993.

[62] Adnams CM, Sorour P, Kalberg WO, *et al.* Language and literacy outcomes from a pilot intervention study for children with fetal alcohol spectrum disorders in South Africa. Alcohol 2007: 41: 403-14.

[63] Premji S, Benzies K, Serrett K, Hayden KA. Research-based interventions for children and youth with a fetal alcohol spectrum disorder: Revealing the gap. Child Care Health Dev 2007; 33: 389-97.

[64] Ryan A, Ferguson D. On, yet under the radar: Students with fetal alcohol syndrome disorder. Except Child 2006; 72(3): 363-3-79.

[65] McGee C, Bjorkquist O, Riley E, Mattson S. Impaired language performance in young children with heavy prenatal alcohol exposure. Neurotoxicol Teratol 2009; 31: 71-5.

[66] Kodituwakku P, Adnams C, Hay A, *et al.* Letter and category fluency in children with fetal alcohol syndrome from a community in South Africa. J Stud Alcohol 2006 67: 502-9.

[67] Coggins T, Friet T, Morgan T. Analyzing narrative production in older school-age children and adolescents with fetal alcohol syndrome: An experimental tool for clinical applications. Clin Linguist Phon 1998; 12(3): 221-36.

[68] O'Connor MJ, Frankel F, Paley B, *et al.* A controlled social skills training for children with fetal alcohol spectrum disorders. J Consult Clin Psychol 2006; 4: 639-48.

[69] Kable JA, Coles CD, Taddeo E. Socio-Cognitive Habilitation using the Math Interactive learning Experience (MILE) Program for Alcohol-Affected Children. Alcohol Clin Exp Res 2007; 31(8):1425-34.

[70] Swanson HL, Herman O. Math disabilities: A selective meta-analysis of the literature. Rev Educ Res 2006; 76(2): 249-79.

[71] Geary DC, Hoard MK, Byrd-Craven J, Nugent L, Numtee C. Cognitive mechanisms underlying achievement deficits in children with mathematical learning disability. Child Dev 2007; 78: 1343-59.

[72] Roebuck T, Mattson S, Riley E, Interhemispheric transfer in children with heavy prenatal alcohol exposure. Alcohol Clin Exp Res 2002; 26(12): 1863-71.

[73] Hegarty M, Kozhevnikov M. Types of visual-spatial representations and mathematical problem solving. J Educ Psychol 1999; 91(4): 684-9.

[74] Feuerstein R, Rand Y, Hoffman M, Miller R. Instrumental enrichment, an intervention program for cognitive modifiability. Baltimore: University Park Press; 1980.

[75] Taddeo E. Identification and analysis of deficient cognitive functions in children with fetal alcohol syndrome. Unpublished doctoral dissertation, Argosy University, Atlanta, Georgia 2006.

[76] Taddeo E, Kable JA, Coles CD. Identification and analysis of deficient cognitive functions in children affected by prenatal alcohol exposure. Manuscript submitted for publication 2009.

[77] Paour JL, Cebe S, Haywood HC. Learning to learn in preschool education. J Cognit Educ Psychol (online) 2000;1(1):3-24. Retrieved October 8, 2004 (www.iacep-coged.org).

[78] Feuerstein R, Feuerstein RS, Schur Y. Process as content in education of exceptional children. In Kozulin A, editor. The ontogeny of cognitive modifiability: Applied aspects of mediated learning experience and instrumental enrichment. Jerusalem, Israel: ICELP & HWCRI; 1997; pp.1-17

[79]   Kozulin A, Presseisen BZ, Mediated learning experience and psychological tools: Vygotsky's and Feuerstein's perspectives in a study of student learning. Educ Psychol 1995; 30(2): 67-75.

[80]   Peadon E, Rhys-Jones B, Bower C, Elliott, EJ. Systematic review of interventions for children with Fetal Alcohol Spectrum Disorders. BMC Pediatr 2009; 9 35-44.

[81]   Bohjanen S, Humphrey M, Ryan S. Left behind: Lack of research-based interventions for children and youth with fetal alcohol spectrum disorders. Rural Spec Educ 2009; 28 (2): 32-8.

[82]   Bertrand J. Interventions for children with fetal alcohol spectrum disorders (FASDs): Overview of findings for five innovative research projects. Res Dev Disabil 2009; 30: 986-1006.

[83]   Luster T, McAdoo H. Family and child influences on educational attainment: A secondary analysis of the high/scope Perry Preschool data. Dev Psychol 1996; 32: 26-39.

[84]   [O'Connor MJ, Paley B. Lessening the risk of social skill deficits in children exposed to alcohol prenatally: An evidenced based intervention in a community setting. Presented at 42nd Annual Gatlinburg Conference, New Orleans, LA 2009.

[85]   Streissguth AP. Fetal alcohol syndrome: A guide for families and communities. Baltimore, MD: Paul H. Brookes Publishing Co; 1997.

[86]   Frankel F. Parent-assisted children's friendship training. In Hibbs ED, S, Jensen P, editors. Psychosocial treatments for child and adolescent disorders: Empirically based approaches Washington, D.C.: American Psychological Association; 2005; pp. 693 715.

[87]   Coles CD, Strickland DC, Padgett LS, Bellmoff L. Games that "work": Using computer games to teach alcohol-affected children about fire and street safety. Res Dev Disabil 2007; 28: 518-30.

[88]   Strickland DC, McAllister D, Coles CD, Osborne S. An evolution of virtual reality training methodologies for children with autism and fetal alcohol spectrum disorders. Topics Lang Dev 2007; 27(3): 226-41.

[89]   Sobo EJ, Kurtin PS. Optimizing care for young children with special health care needs: Knowledge and strategies for navigating the system. Baltimore, MD: Brooks publishing; 2007.

[90]   Kalberg W, Buckley D. FASD: What types of intervention and rehabilitation are useful? Neurosci Biobehav Rev 2007; 32: 278-85.

[91]   Kalberg W, Buckley D, Educational planning for children with fetal alcohol syndrome. Ann Ist Super Sanita 2006; 42(1): 58-66.

[92]   Prather S. Demystifying inclusion: Implications for sustainable inclusive practice, Int J Incl Educ 2007; 11(5-6): 627-43.

[93]   Salend S, Duhaney G, The impact of inclusion on students with and without disabilities and their educators. Rem Spec Educ 1999; 20(2): 114-26.

[94]   Fuchs D, Mock D, Morgan P, Young C. Responsiveness-to-intervention: Definitions, Evidence, and implications for the learning disabilities construct. Learn Disabil Res Pract 2003:18(3):157-71.

[95]   Stecker P, Fuchs D, Fuchs L. Progress monitoring as essential practice within Response to Intervention. Rural Spec Educ Quart 2008; 27(4): 10-17.

[96]   Ardoin SP, Witt JC, Connell JE, Koenig JL. Application of a three-tiered response to intervention model for instructional planning, decision making, and the identification of children in need of services. J Psychoeduc Assess 2005; 3: 362–80.

[97]   Jenkins JR, O'Connor R. Cooperative Learning for Students with Learning Disabilities: Evidence from Experiments, Observations, and Interviews. In Swanson L, Graham S, Harris K, Eds. Handbook of Learning Disabilities. New York: Guilford; 2003, pp. 417-30.

[98]   Lancioni G, Reilly M. Self-management of instruction cues for occupation: Review of students with severe and profound developmental disabilities. Res Dev Disabil 2001; 22: 41-65.

[99]   Mennuti R, Christner R, Freeman A. An introduction to a school-based cognitive-behavioral framework. In Mennuti R, Freeman A, Christner R, editors. Cognitive-behavioral interventions in educational settings: A handbook for practice. New York: Routledge; 2006, pp. 3-19.

[100]   Hart T, Evans J. Self-regulation and goal theories in brain injury rehabilitation. J Head Trauma Rehabil 2006; 21(2): 142-55.

[101]   Zeki C. The importance of non-verbal communication in classroom management. Procedia: Social and Behavioral Sciences 2009; 1: 1443-9.

[102]   Zentall S. Theory and evidenced based strategies for children with attentional problems. Psychol Sch 2005;42(8): 821-36.

[103]   Roth WM. Gesture-speech phenomena, learning, and development. Educ Psychol 2003; 38(4): 249-63.

[104]   Rourke B, Ed. Syndrome of nonverbal learning disabilities: Neurodevelopmental Manifestations. New York: Guildford Press; 1995.

[105]   Tanguay P. Nonverbal learning disabilities at school: Educating students with nld, asperger syndrome, and related conditions. London, UK: Jessica Kingsley Publishers; 2002.

[106] Molenaar-Klumper M. Nonverbal learning disabilities: Characteristics, diagnosis, and treatment within an educational setting. London, UK: Jessica Kingsley Publishers; 2002.

[107] Wiggins G, McTigh J. Understanding by Design, 2nd Edition. Alexandria, VA: ASCD; 2005.

[108] Rasmussen C. Executive functioning and working memory in fetal alcohol spectrum disorder. Alcohol Clin Exp Res 2005; 29: 1359-67.

[109] Millians M. [Observations and results of a clinical tutoring program for children with FASD]. Unpublished raw data, 2008.

[110] [Stein J, Krishnan K. Nonverbal learning disabilities and executive function: The challenges of effective assessment and teaching. In L. Meltzer (Ed.). Executive function in education: From theory to practice. New York: Guildford Press; 2007.

[111] Hyrle D. A field guide to using visual tools. Alexandria, VA: ASCD; 2000.

[112] May P, Gossage P, Marais AS, *et al.* The epidemiology of fetal alcohol syndrome and partial FAS in a South African community. Drug Alcohol Depend 2007: 88: 259-71.

CHAPTER 6

Improving Outcomes in Adolescents and Adults with Fetal Alcohol Spectrum Disorders

Mary DeJoseph[*]

New Jersey/ Northeast FASD Education and Research Center, University of Medicine and Dentistry of NJ, Newark, NJ, USA

"Fetal Alcohol Syndrome is not just a childhood disorder; there is a predictable long-term progression of the disorder into adulthood...." **Ann Streissguth, JAMA 1991**

"I remember when I finished high school, everyone was talking about where they were going and what they were doing next. I spent all of high school trying to survive every day. I didn't think about planning ahead. At my graduation, I suddenly thought 'Oh my God, what do I do now?" **(Fran, an adult with FAS)**

Abstract: Fetal Alcohol Spectrum Disorders (FASD) are life long and do not disappear with maturity. As children who have been exposed prenatally reach pubescence, they will experience the typical physical and emotional issues associated with adolescence. Navigating the rocky waters of adolescence is particularly challenging to individuals whose developmental abilities are significantly less than what is expected of them according to their chronological age. In many instances, physical, psychological, behavioral and social problems become more serious and continue on into adulthood for those with FASD. Lifespan issues considered in this chapter are: routine health care; safety; sleep; oral and dental care; nutrition and fitness; sexuality; sexual abuse; work; and co-occurring disorders. Practical considerations are also suggested.

ADOLESCENCE: THE AGE OF ANGST

Progressing through the stages of adolescence into adulthood is challenging, even in the typically developing teen. Development is expected to include the achievement of predictable physical, mental, social, and behavioral milestones. While adolescence is generally considered to extend from 12 to 18 years, this range is not well defined as the onset of pubescence and the associated developmental stages may begin earlier and continue on into the early twenties. In addition, societal perceptions of when adolescence ends and adulthood begins, varies greatly. For example, several legal processes must be initiated by age 18. These include partial or complete guardianship and informed consent for medical treatment. Other rights, however, are not bestowed until the age of 21 (See Chapter 7).

During typical adolescence, teen-agers are expected to develop and master a broad range of abilities prior to entering adulthood. These include:

- comprehending abstract content such as higher order mathematics and moral and ethical standards, including rights and privileges;

- establishing and maintain satisfying personal relationships;

- moving gradually toward a more mature identity, purpose and independence;

- developing self-direction and pursue career interests;

- identifying more with peers than with parents.

The sudden and rapid physical changes that both genders experience during adolescence make this period one of extreme social awkwardness, self-consciousness and sensitivity. Simultaneously, rebellion, opposition and conflict with parents are appropriate developmental behaviors [1]. The amount and intensity of conflict that arises between

---

*Address correspondence to Mary DeJoseph: New Jersey/ Northeast FASD Education and Research Center, University of Medicine and Dentistry of NJ, Newark, NJ, USA; E-mail: marydejo@comcast.net

teen-agers and their parents is dependent to an extent on the support and stability of the childrearing environment [2]. Risk taking and exploration are behaviors associated with normal adolescent development [3]. Because good decision making skills generally lag behind physical size, strength and agility, safety and injury prevention are constant concerns in all adolescents. Information on injury, violence, poison prevention and other "critical adolescent health issues", from the American Academy of Pediatrics can be accessed at: http://www.aap.org/sections/adolescenthealth/critical lissues.cfm. One source for a review of developmental milestones in adolescence can be found at: http://www.nlm.nih.gov/medlineplus/ency/article/002003.htm

Adolescence presents difficult challenges for individuals with an FASD. Normal, hormonal-driven sexual and physiological changes will occur within the appropriate growth period while the person with an FASD will continue to function at much younger, intellectual, social and behavioral stages than that expected of their chronological age. As a result, developmental milestones may be delayed indefinitely or missed altogether. Some isolated maturation milestones might be achieved, but it is difficult to predict which will be achieved, which will be delayed, and which milestones will never be reached. Not equipped with the necessary developmental skills leaves persons with FASD incapable of navigating the complex world. Compounding this situation is that educational and many social support systems end when the individual with FASD reaches age 18 or 21, and then leaves the school system.

The biological processes inherent in adolescence do not stop the long term effects of prenatal exposure to alcohol. Although teens with FASD will experience growth spurts, postnatal growth retardation is likely to result in short physical stature. While neurological development continues into early adulthood, the amount of actual brain growth in persons with FASD will be affected [4]. As discussed in Chapter 3, the secondary disabilities associated with FASD become more pronounced [5]. Behaviors that may have been ignored, tolerated or enabled at earlier ages may now escalate to become dangerous and criminal. Cumulative stress from traumatic childhood experiences and primary brain damage increase the vulnerability of persons with FASD to develop significant co-occurring and psychosocial issues. [6-8]. Unfortunately, the point at which services are most needed to diagnose, intervene with and manage this population is exactly when services become most limited. Adolescents and adults may not have as distinct dysmorphia and growth deficits; the lack of diagnostic precision makes screening for FAS in adolescents, developmentally disabled adults, and institutional settings very difficult [9]. Without diagnosis, appropriate care teams cannot be organized. Clearly, decades of scientific research, as well as family and professional experience, demonstrate that the path to adulthood for a person with an FASD may be more difficult, convoluted, and perilous than in the typical person. There are many issues to be attended to for professional and personal care givers of the adolescent and adult with an FASD. One which has particular importance to long-term health, success, and quality of life is routine health care and preventive clinical services.

ROUTINE HEALTH CARE

Although there may be many immediate behavioral, mental, and emotional issues and/crises to deal on a daily basis, routine medical and dental care for the adolescent or adult with an FASD should not be ignored. This includes recommended history, physical exam, labs, and immunizations. Health care providers (primary care or specialists) who are also willing to deal with multiple, complex issues must be found and often educated. Concerns specific to the FASD must also be monitored and addressed. Some pediatricians may be willing to extend care with long-term patients, even into adulthood. This must be addressed with the individual pediatrician. Long-term care for adults and then geriatric care will have to be found and transitioned into.

 The American Academy of Pediatrics (AAP) Council on Child and Adolescent Health has a statement on the age limits of pediatrics: "The purview of pediatrics includes the physical and psychosocial growth, development, and health of the individual. This commitment begins prior to birth when conception is apparent and continues throughout infancy, childhood, adolescence, and early adulthood, when the growth and developmental processes are generally completed. The responsibility of pediatrics may therefore begin with the fetus and continue through 21 years of age. There are special circumstances (eg, a chronic illness and/or disability) in which, if mutually agreeable to the pediatrician, the patient, and when appropriate the patient's family, the services of the pediatrician may continue to be the optimal source of health care past the age of 21 years." Online access to this statement can be found at: http://aappolicy.aappublications.org/cgi/content/abstract/pediatrics;81/5/736

Recommendations for major preventive clinical services throughout adolescence and adulthood have been published by the United States Preventive Services Task Force (USPSTF), American Medical Association (AMA), American Academy of Pediatrics (AAP), American Academy of Family Physicians (AAFP), Healthy People 2010. The recommendations are similar; any one may serve as a guideline for a parent to check or clinician to use to organize history, physical, labs, and immunizations. A checklist for prevention materials and health maintenance guidelines for consumers/patients at any age is found at http://www.ahrq.gov/clinic/ppipix.htm. The specific checklist for women, for example, is found at: http://www.ahrq.gov/ppip/healthywom.htm.The Department of Health and Human Services, Office of Disease Prevention and Health Promotion provides access to multiple other nutrition and fitness resources This link can be found at: http://odphp.osophs.dhhs.gov/

Although dated, a still useful comparison of adolescent recommendations [10] has been adapted and is available in the adolescent health curriculum from the USC Keck School of Medicine. This link can be found at: http://www.usc.edu/student-affairs/Health_Center/adolhealth/content/a8.html

An expanded listing of national and international recommendations can be found at the links at the end of the chapter resources.

Adults with developmental disabilities in general may have significant health challenges and experience poorer health because of social circumstances, genetics, environment, individual behaviors, finances, nutrition, and health care access [11]. They may have multiple prenatal and postnatal exposures to environmental toxicants, which interact with individual genetic susceptibilities [12,13]. Comparative studies concerning people with intellectual disabilities have found a higher prevalence rate for epilepsy, diseases of the skin, sensory loss, and increased risk of fractures [14]. Women with a disability have a higher rate of some conditions, such as depression after trauma, when compared to men with the same disability or women with the trauma and no disability [15]. Depression impairs motivation in treatment and wound healing [16]. The life expectancy of people with mild intellectual disability does not differ from the general population. People with mild and moderate intellectual disabilities have longer life expectancy than 35 years ago; this presents a challenge to primary care and geriatric health care providers. People with profound disabilities continue to have shorter life expectancy [17].

Adolescents and adults with an FASD have additional health concerns. Diagnosis or continued monitoring of alcohol - related birth defects (ARBDs) is an ongoing health consideration. Growth deficiency that was initiated in utero with a combination of alcohol use and maternal undernutrition may persist into adulthood [17]. Marginal maternal deficiencies in nutrients like zinc may exacerbate alcohol related damage and lead to long-term problems in the offspring via epigenetic factors. Marginal zinc and iron deficiency may persist in the adolescent or adult with an FASD, despite an adequate diet postnatally [18]. Prenatal exposure to alcohol has detrimental effects on the developing immune system, immunecompetence [19], and the immunosuppressive effects of stress; adults and adolescents and adults with FASDs will need more frequent attention to infectious disease [20]. Some infectious diseases may increase in severity with an immune system that has been prenatally exposed to alcohol [21]. Alcohol also affects the developing hypothalamic-pituitary axis (HPA); alcohol can increase HPA tone in both mother and offspring. This leads to increased exposure to exogenous glucocorticoids and life-long impaired stress management [22]. Auto-immune diseases that are exacerbated by stress may be an increased concern. Research with adolescents and adults with FASDs on health risks specific to this disability needs to be done.

SAFETY

Safety is another primary health issue for adolescents and adults with FASDs. This population has a number of risk factors for accidents and injury: poor decision making; impulsivity; impaired motor co-ordination, working memory, attention, emotional and sensory regulation; and susceptibility to peer pressure. Even seemingly routine tasks like crossing the street safely may be impossible for those who are more severely affected.

One safety issue to highlight is driving. Many adolescents and adults with an FASD are able to complete requirements to get a driver's license and are consistently responsible and safe drivers. For others, driving safety may be adequate during routine driving and testing, but compromised under stress by impaired executive functioning and working memory, slowed problem solving, visual spatial deficits, and altered oculomotor control

[23-26]. Many ophthalmologic defects aside from visual acuity have been reported in people who have been prenatally exposed to alcohol [27]. The risk of serious eye malformations, however, may be limited to those with FAS, not those who have been heavily exposed without FAS [28]. Processing speed is decreased in children with both FAS and FAE [29]. A high prevalence of sensorineural, conductive, and central hearing deficits has been reported, which would interfere with driving safety [30]. Multiple imaging studies have demonstrated structural and metabolic abnormalities of a number of brain structures [31], including the corpus callosum [32], which are associated with prenatal exposure to alcohol. Abnormalities in the corpus callosum may affect coordination of motor planning and control, bimanual performance, and auditory interhemispheric transfer of information. Attention deficits are common in adolescents and adults [33].

Specific information about corpus callosal and other brain abnormalities is not accessible to the adolescent or adult with an FASD or the parents, Motor Vehicle Agency licensing officers, or primary care physicians completing driving physicals; this is just one example of potential safety risk from the "invisible disability" of FASD. These concerns also apply to adults and adolescents with an FASD who are operating heavy machinery. Decisions like driving and operating other machinery should be made with careful consideration of available data. It is important to remember that imaging studies of brain morphology and metabolism also indicate areas of the brain that may increase their activity to compensate and manage problem-solving successfully; this plasticity of the brain may benefit young adults with an FASD who are driving safely [34].

Other examples of possible safety and health concerns in adolescents and adults with an FASD are: remembering medication schedules; decisions about legal and illegal substances, including tobacco; risk-taking situations in which poor social problem solving [35], impulsivity, and peer pressure combine to compromise safety.

SLEEP

Another lifespan issue that affects the health of adolescents and adults with an FASD is sleep dysfunction. Sleep problems are described by most parents of children with an FASD; this is a problem that persists into adulthood and is often multi-factorial. Sleep problems in children and teens are associated with daytime impairment, altered psychomotor performance, behavioral disturbance, decreased social interest and physical activity, memory and learning deficits, and substance use. Behavioral and cognitive performance changes associated with shortened sleep duration early in life can persist for years [36]. Short sleep duration has also been associated with nightmares and suicidal behavior in adolescents; suicide attempts were inversely related to sleep duration [37]. Insomnia with daytime fatigue is a mental health problem that is chronic in many adolescents [38].

Normal sleep is a complex phenomenon that involves the interaction of intact brain structure/physiology with an internal and external environment that allow the normal progression and maintenance of sleep wake cycles. As with other lifespan issues, the adolescent or adult with an FASD may have a disruption of normal sleep at multiple points because of the primary brain damage.

Sleep is a state of unconsciousness in which the brain may be described as being more responsive to internal than external stimuli. Multiple brain areas are involved. Sleep is divided into rapid eye movement (REM) and non-REM (NREM) stages. Wakefulness, REM sleep and NREM sleep are three distinct states of existence. No single discreet "sleep center" has been identified in the brain; waking functions are actively turned off and sensory awareness is withdrawn during sleep initiation. Wakefulness is organized in the brain in multiple areas, including the reticular activating system, thalamus, and cortex; neurotransmitters like glutamate, acetylcholine, and norepinephrine are essential. The hypothalamus regulates autonomic body functions (heart rate, breathing, sweating, body temperature) during waking and sleep; chemical and pressure sensors throughout the body monitor blood pressure and oxygen levels during sleep and waking states. An intrinsic body rhythm called the circadian rhythm sets the timing for sleep initiation and is related to melatonin and the pineal gland. The hypothalamus will transmit inhibitory signals to arousal areas of the brain using the neurotransmitter GABA; serotonin and melatonin also facilitate sleep [39]. The limbic system is active during sleep, particularly stages where dreaming takes place. Normal sleep-wake organization appears to undergo significant reorganization during the transition to adolescence with shorter sleep, greater tolerance for sleep deprivation, and delayed sleep onset (later sleep and rise times) [40]. The circadian rhythm gradually moves sleep initiation earlier throughout adulthood. Aging results in a greater sensitivity to time zone or shift work.

Sleep disorders are described as intrinsic and extrinsic. Intrinsic sleep disorders are called dyssomnias; they include circadian rhythm disturbances. Common intrinsic problems are periodic leg movements of sleep (PLMS), restless leg syndrome (RLS), and the sleep apnea syndromes, including obstruction. Having ADHD symptoms or ADHD diagnosis is related to PLMS [41] Extrinsic factors that affect sleep are exercise, the sleep environment (noise, music, light, TV, computers, changes in altitude or location), medications, and other drug effects. These are called dyssomnias; they include circadian rhythm. Other sleep disturbances are parasomnias; this group includes nightmares, sleepwalking, nocturnal leg cramps, teeth grinding (bruxism) and bedwetting (nocturnal enuresis). The last group is sleep disorders which are associated with other medical/neurologic and psychiatric disorders.

Sleep research has demonstrated alterations in sleep duration and continuity and in sleep state organization in people prenatally exposed to substances. Differences in electroencephalographic sleep patterns between exposed and non-exposed infants have been demonstrated [42]. One study clearly demonstrated that prenatal alcohol exposure significantly increased the odds for having shorter sleep duration and lower sleep efficiency, independent of body size and postnatal maternal alcohol use [43]. Clearly, sleep dysfunction may initiate, aggravate, or mask disabilities that are assumed to be associated with an FASD.

An adolescent or adult with an FASD may have a combination of factors rather than a single cause of a sleep disorder. The sleep disorder can go on to cause or aggravate long-term health concerns. Some physical and brain changes that have been described in the person with an FASD may interrupt normal sleep onset, stages and duration. Breathing interruptions/snoring may be caused or exacerbated by: craniofacial dysmorphia, including mid-face hypoplasia, low nasal bridge, short nose; poor oral motor and pharyngeal tone; frequent sinus and upper respiratory congestion. These factors may lead to apneic episodes and frequent awakening. Chronic problems with obstructive apnea may cause acute and chronic hypertension and cardiac rhythm disturbances. The circadian rhythm in people with an FASD may be disrupted, as is serotonergic function [44].

All of the common sleep problems found in the general population of adults and adolescents can also be found in those who have been prenatally exposed to alcohol. Secondary sleep problems in the adolescent or adult with an FASD may be associated with co-occurring disorders and problems such as: ADHD, anxiety, depression and other psychiatric diagnoses, psychotropic and other medications, caffeine and other substance use, seizure disorders, and environmental disruptions.

Treatable factors should be ascertained through sleep diary, basic sleep hygiene, consideration of all secondary factors and review of medication schedule. Caffeine and alcohol use should be zero. Daily exercise can be a very high yield intervention for a number of problems. Formal sleep study in a sleep lab will diagnose treatable medical sleep conditions; adults with an FASD may be able to tolerate equipment such as continuous positive airway pressure (CPAP) for obstructive conditions if introduced to it gradually. Long term use of hypnotic medications can exacerbate the sleep dysfunction.

One school-based intervention used education, sleep diaries, and motivation with adolescents to address sleep problems. The goal was to identify and revise environmental causes of poor sleep and regularize bedtimes; significant behavioral change was reported [45]. Sleep problems are a critical problem to address in the adolescent or adult with an FASD because of the significant medical and psychiatric morbidity associated with them, including the potential for increased suicide risk; sleep evaluation should be considered a health maintenance and preventive measure.

ORAL AND DENTAL CARE

The next lifespan issue is oral and dental care. Dentists are in a position to view craniofacial structure, general growth, facial features and behavior in-depth over time. They may see both parents and offspring. They have access to informal screening regarding lifestyle, including alcohol use. Given all of the above, a dentist is in a position to identify an adolescent or adult with an FASD and refer for evaluation.

A number of factors may influence the development and maintenance of healthy dentition in the adult or adolescent with an FASD. Prenatal exposure to alcohol has been shown to affect the development of normal dentition through a number of mechanisms. Alcohol has a direct toxic effect on the ectodermal and mesodermal cells of the developing embryo; cranial neural crest cells which give rise to dentofacial structures are vulnerable [46]. Differential growth of the tooth germ and delay in dental root formation has been observed [47]. Serotonin and other neurotransmitters stimulate dental development and aid in cusp formation under the direction of multiple growth and transcription factors [48]; all of these neurochemicals may be altered with alcohol exposure during development. The result is a high incidence of dentofacial and temporomandibular joint disorders: soft enamel; small teeth; absent teeth, hypoplastic enamel; displaced or rotated teeth; mouth breathing caused by facial dysmorphia, which leads to dry mouth; malocclusions, crossbite, and overbite. Tooth eruption in children and emergence of adult dentition are delayed. Cleft lip with or without palate may be present. Poor dentition can lead to chronic low grade infections and poor nutrition. Cavities are more frequent because of enamel anomalies; high sugar diet and poor oral hygiene add to the problem. Cardiac Alcohol Related Birth Defects (ARBD) may be present, and antibiotic prophylaxis will be needed before cleaning to protect from endocarditis. More frequent hygiene visits will be needed if malocclusions aren't corrected. Hygiene at home will require patience and persistence.

Brushing, flossing, and routine dental exams and care can be very challenging as a lifespan issue for a person who has been prenatally exposed to alcohol. Sensory issues around lighting, equipment sounds, and unfamiliar sensations and smells can be a huge barrier. Unstable placements mean that adolescents may not have a regular dentist. If alcohol use is still an issue in the home, dental care may not be a top priority.

Establishment of a dental home similar to the model of a medical home can be a huge benefit. A pediatric dentist may consider extending ongoing care. Dentists can be educated during preliminary visits about FASDs in general and the specific needs of a particular adolescent or adult. As with gynecologic visits, equipment and procedures should be explained. The option to have a support person present should always be available. The adolescent or adult may need to watch a visit, cleaning or x-ray performed safely on a care giver. Appointments can be scheduled at the beginning or end of the day when the wait isn't as long. Pictures of what will take place at a visit can help. Rehearsal at home with keeping the mouth open and a variety of textures is one way to prepare. Sensory integration therapy with a therapist trained in sensory issues may be of benefit. Modifying lights and using sunglasses and headphones can make a difference. If no amount of preparation will help, sedation may be necessary.

NUTRITION AND FITNESS ISSUES

This author found no published studies on specific nutritional deficits or needs in adolescents and adults with an FASD. Animal studies on choline in the prenatal and postnatal period have been encouraging [49,50]; human studies are pending (see Chapter 2). As with other lifespan issues, the health care provider must apply what is known about nutrition, diet, and exercise to the adolescent or adult with an FASD. Exercise intervention research with persons who have disabilities is not specific to the person with an FASD. A mixture of aerobic and strength exercises have been studied in people with intellectual disabilities for key health outcomes such as pain/fatigue reduction and improved cardio-respiratory health. Weight training may be of benefit with sensory issues as well [51]. Physical activity guidelines may be found at: http://www.health.gov/paguidelines/

Basic recommendations and dietary guidelines across the lifespan are provided at the US Dept of Agriculture site introducing the new (2005) food pyramid and providing a wealth of information for consumers (http://www.mypyramid.gov/). The new pyramid emphasizes activity, moderation, a personal plan, proportional amounts of food groups, variety, and gradual improvement. The website offers a quick dietary overview and personal plan based on basic information entered. For more in-depth assessment and specific recommendations based on input of all foods and activity over 24 hours, the website offers MyPyramid Tracker (www.mypyramidtracker.gov). Both websites are useful tools. However, there are a few drawbacks for the adult or adolescent with an FASD. The recommendations cover multiple areas at once, don't allow for sensory issues, assume Internet access, and require basic reading and math skills. It may be prudent to look at recommendations in one food group at a time as a modification. The guidance of a nutrition professional to get started can be extremely helpful.

Because adults and adolescents with FAS or an FASD have such diversity in nutritional needs, a nutritionist or dietitian is a valuable part of the health care team. Dietitians and nutritionists both plan food and nutrition programs and help prevent and treat illnesses by promoting healthy eating habits and suggesting diet modifications. Dietitians run food service systems for institutions such as hospitals and schools.

A diet and activity diary should be prepared before an evaluation with a nutrition specialist. It should include: what is eaten over at least a three day period (quality, quantity, number of meals per day); basic physical activity; food preferences; sexual maturation/ menstrual history; known eating disorders; chronic medical conditions and meds; use of vitamins, supplements, alcohol, drugs, steroids; weight history, including failure to thrive. The nutrition specialist will need to know if the adolescent is taking "performance enhancing" supplements; these are combinations of amino acids (glycine, arginine, and methionine) that are supposed to facilitate production of ATP and increase muscle energy. They may not have any lasting effect on performance, and side effects. Steroids may also be available to adolescents and adults through a variety of sources; these are precursors to testosterone and can have effects on blood pressure, endocrine regulation, skin, and mood/emotional regulation.

The nutrition specialist also may need some basic education about FASDs. Together, the adolescent, nutritionist and care giver can then design a program of calories, percentages of fats, carbohydrates, and proteins. An adolescent who had failure to thrive as a toddler may catch up to normal weight and need significant revision of eating habits. It is important to remember that bone mass deposition is significant in adolescence, so calcium is a major nutrient. Iron deficiency is common in adolescents, and is important for growth and replacement in the menstruating female. Other deficiencies that may be found are vitamins A, B6, E, D, C and folate. If sufficient amounts cannot be maintained through foods, supplements may be recommended [52]. It is best to obtain nutrients from whole foods whenever possible while research on targeted supplementation needs is being completed [53]. For all adults, it is important to remember that cardiovascular disease processes begin early and are influenced over time by the interaction of genetic risk, and modifiable behaviors and environments. The major risks are diet, physical activity, and tobacco; these are all modifiable [54].

Another common dietary insufficiency in adults and adolescence is adequate fruit and vegetable intake; these foods provide vitamins, fiber, and calories. Fruits and vegetables are important in reducing risk of obesity, diabetes, cardiovascular disease, and certain types of cancer [55]. It is important to remember, however, that the Environmental Protection Agency considers diet an important source of organophosphate pesticide exposure. Detectable concentrations may even be found in frozen fruit. Significant postnatal organophosphate exposure has been associated with behavior problems, poorer short-term memory and motor skills and longer reaction times in children. Increased urinary excretion of organophosphate metabolites has been correlated with significant increase in incidence of hyperactive/impulsive subtype ADHD [56]. Pesticides are a potential source of neurodevelopmental damage that may co-occur with the prenatal damage from alcohol exposure in the adolescent or adult with an FASD. For example, lead and arsenic content from early pesticides may persist in the soil even if leaded paint has been removed from housing. Proper preparation of produce with washing or peeling is prudent, excessive produce should be avoided, and homes and properties should continue to be monitored.

School breakfast and lunch programs are mandated to meet standards for certain nutrients, although that only applies to the reimbursable school meals. After leaving school, meal choices are largely individual, except in residential settings. Preparing all meals at home is an added burden for care givers, but is necessary to insure a balanced diet [57]. This will be even more critical as more research highlights specific supplements helpful in individuals with an FASD.

Adequate nutrition in an adolescent or adult with an Intellectual or Developmental Disability requires ability to procure, safely prepare, chew, swallow, digest, and absorb a balanced diet. There may be problems for the affected person at any or multiple steps. Finances, executive function, working memory, and motor skills deficits can interfere with access to a variety of foods.

If a balanced diet is available, there are still many other considerations. Oral sensory and oral motor weakness may prevent certain foods from being eaten. Coordination of sucking or chewing and swallowing may need to be evaluated by a speech therapist. Poor dentition is a factor. Visceral sensation may be altered, and the affected adult or adolescent may not sense distended stomach or bowel. Alterations in intestinal organization, function and absorptive capacity have been demonstrated in rats. In one study, alterations in human intestinal mucosa were indicated by decreases in serum apoA-IV after prenatal exposure to alcohol; these changes may be linked to impaired digestion and absorption of nutrients [58]. These intestinal changes are a result of exposure of fetal intestinal mucosa to alcohol content in swallowed amniotic fluid (18 wks to delivery). Amniotic fluid levels of alcohol may be higher in women with under-nutrition and lower levels of enzymes to metabolize alcohol [59].

Hyperactivity with ADHD or manic behavior can interfere with focus and sitting still long enough to eat enough calories. Psychotropic medications can increase or decrease appetite and lead to weight change that must be addressed. Psychotropic medications can also alter metabolism, and have detrimental effects on weight and nutrition. Appetite and feeding behavior are regulated in the brain in multiple areas, including the hypothalamus and caudal brainstem; normal regulation of appetite and feeding behavior may have been affected by prenatal exposure to alcohol. The cortex and limbic system also have input regarding prior experience with food, reward, and emotion that affect eating and nutrition [60]. Social experience may interact with primary brain damage to further complicate the goals of adequate nutrition.

SEXUALITY

Another lifespan issue that must be considered is sexuality. Concentrating on the many complex medical, functional and behavioral issues associated with an FASD may preclude any attention to the anatomic, physiologic, emotional, and social aspects of the developing sexuality of the adolescent and adult with an FASD. Some of the urgent issues are puberty, hygiene, and physical maturation; gender identity; body image; relationships, intimacy, boundaries, future social aspirations; contraception; sexual preference; psychosexual development; sexual abuse and victimization; and prevention of sexually transmitted diseases. Murphy and Elias provide a comprehensive review of sexuality issues in children and adolescents [61]. The complete article can be found at: http://pediatrics.aappublications.org/cgi/reprint/118/1/398.

Sexuality is a profound component of our humanity in which human beings need each other; the capacity for giving and receiving love and affection remains throughout life, whether or not a relationship is ever expressed through genital sexual contact. Regardless of disability, all adolescents are sexual human beings and need comprehensive sexuality education. Parents and clinicians must keep in mind that one of the tasks of adolescence is to separate from parents and develop a sense of self-identity within the reality of cognitive ability. It may seem too abstract to explain, but an effort must be made to help the adolescent or adult with an FASD to understand that sexuality is not only a source of pleasure, it is the basis for human relationship and bonding.

Puberty in US children usually has an onset between 8.5 and 13 years of age. Early puberty can be a tremendous challenge for a child who may already be socially immature; it affects body image, self-esteem and increases the complexity of hygiene and self-care. Early puberty may increase the risk of sexual victimization and is associated with an increase of addictions in typically developing adolescents [62].

All females deserve appropriate gynecologic care, regardless of disability [63]; this may require several visits. If the adolescent is not sexually active, a pelvic exam may not be needed; recto-abdominal examination may suffice. Medical procedures and instruments should be presented. Positioning during pelvic exam should be modified if stirrups can't be managed. There should always be an option to have a care giver present during exams, but all adolescents must have the opportunity to speak privately with the health care provider. All adolescents must be approached with respect for personal privacy, whether or not the adolescent seems concerned. The young woman with an FASD may need an enema or laxative prior to a rectal exam to avoid embarrassment. The care giver may be concerned about abnormal uterine bleeding; this may be from normal anovulatory cycles for up two years after menarche. The clinician must consider other causes for irregular bleeding such as thyroid disease and some anticonvulsant and neuroleptic medications, so a complete medication list should be brought to each visit.

Adolescents and adults with an FASD should be well informed and consulted about decisions regarding abstinence, contraception and pregnancy. A pregnancy test should be given prior to any new medication being prescribed because of possible teratogenic effects on the developing fetus. In addition, some anticonvulsant medications for seizures and some psychotropics may affect liver enzymes and also decrease the effectiveness of oral and implanted contraceptives. Barrier devices for males and females can be used for safety and contraception; these include condoms, diaphragms, and cervical caps. However, their use requires motivation, cognitive understanding, and physical dexterity; the adolescent may become comfortable and reliable with these devices after considerable discussion, opened packages, anatomical models for demonstration, reminders, and practice. Even a typically developing adolescent may understand the rules and have the skills to use barrier devices, and not succeed in the actual situation.

Decisions about permanent sterilization procedures for both men and women should take into account all applicable local, state and federal laws. It is illegal to perform permanent sterilization procedures without consent or participation, regardless of the degree of impairment. Other factors to consider are the adolescent or adult's decision-making capacity, wishes, and feelings; ability to care for children; consequences of reproduction for the person and any children that might be born. Sperm and ova may be preserved for later use. Providing the adolescent or adult with practical experience with infants and toddlers, and the demands of child-rearing may be of assistance with informed decision making by all parties. There are countless ways to support pregnancy, delivery, and parenting by the adolescent or adult with an FASD. The young person may have questions about whether or not the FASD can be passed on to any offspring; care givers must clarify that only prenatal exposure to alcohol can cause an FASD.

Early and ongoing social experiences play a key role in psychosexual development. Adolescent tasks include having and maintaining intimate relationships, managing complex emotions and social situations, and developing independent thinking. The adolescent with an FASD may not achieve these milestones all at the same time, at the usual age range, or at all. Many adolescents with disabilities are delayed or prevented from achieving these goals by social isolation or a variety of functional limitations. Social skills may be broken down into manageable tasks, just as in every other area of instruction. This includes the basics first, such as: mastering appropriate greetings: eye contact; body language; personal space; self-advocacy skills; telephone and computer skills. A foundation in some or all of these basic skills will allow for the development of more complex skills. Mentors and peers may be very effective in this regard. Time spent and even small successes will bolster self-esteem. Providing the most routine of teen activities, like going to the mall or movies, will offer opportunities to practice. Age and situation appropriate clothing will be an invaluable help in easing the adolescent into situations. A number of social and friendship interventions for children have been successful [64]; research adapting these for adolescents will be beneficial.

Another critical component of social and sexual maturity is attaining independence in basic self-care and hygiene tasks. This includes the whole realm of showering, dental care, shaving, hairstyling, appropriate outfits, and managing menstrual flow. Adolescents and adults with an FASD may need frequent cues, supervision, formalized instruction, adaptive technology and frequent reinforcement well into adulthood or permanently to achieve and maintain successes. Parents and care givers must be encouraged to maximize independence, even if they are used to "helping" or completing tasks for the young adult.

SEXUAL ABUSE

Another important topic for discussion and education is the issue of sexual abuse. According to Murphy and Elias [61] (see link above), the National Center on Child Abuse and Neglect has reported that children with disabilities are sexually abused at a rate 2.2 higher than that for children without disabilities. The US Dept of Justice reports that 68-83% of women with developmental disabilities will be sexually assaulted in their lifetimes and less than half of them will seek assistance from legal or treatment services. Adolescents and adults with an FASD may be more vulnerable to abuse because of dependence on others for intimate and routine personal care, increased exposure to a larger number of care givers and settings, inappropriate social skills, poor judgment, inability to seek help or report abuse, and lack of strategies to defend themselves against abuse. Clues and symptoms of abuse occurring may be very non-specific, and difficult to recognize and report without specific skills training. Some behavioral clues include alterations in bowel/bladder patterns, sleep, mood, behaviors, and community participation. Sexual abuse has consequences for the victim in many different dimensions of health and behavior. Some problems associated with sexual abuse are: sexually transmitted disease and pregnancy; substance use and eating disorders; depression and other mood disorders; enuresis; runaway behavior and school failure; sexual dysfunction and sleep disturbances [63].

VOCATIONAL ISSUES

Another essential issue to consider during the adolescence and adulthood of people with an FASD is work and productivity; these areas rank high with social support and self-determination as key predictors in determining life satisfaction in people with any intellectual disability. Other quality of life determinants are life skills (independent living, social, and leisure skills) and vocational skills [65]. Young adults with a disability need advocacy and support with a variety of new agencies and support services throughout the transition and adult years. Some adults and families will choose sheltered workshops because of concerns about safety, transportation, long-term placement, work hours, maintaining disability benefits, social environment, and work skills issues [66]. The majority of adults with an intellectual disability prefer integrated employment over sheltered workshop, regardless of disability severity [67].

The transition years prior to high school are critical to vocational success. There are a number of things that should happen during transition planning that a parent or care giver might need to facilitate, such as introduction to the relevant service providers and transfer of information to those agencies. A life skills curriculum should include: how to use the internet to search for employment and employment enhancement services; awareness of issues associated with safe work environments; interviewing strategies; appropriate use of medication; managing finances; dealing with workplace routines and expectations; being cautious about at-risk situations; and knowing when to ask for help [68].

Some of the general barriers to successful work for people with disabilities are external: stigma, employer and co-worker attitudes and preconceptions; transportation; completing applications and job testing; social skills and support at interviews. Other barriers are internal, and need to be addressed early on in the vocational arena: self-esteem and self-worth; fear of success; self- sabotage; realistic view of strengths and career goals. All of these internal factors affect career choice, self-presentation at the interview and the job, and ultimate vocational success. Addressing these issues through counseling and skill building prior to standard vocational tasks is efficacious [69,70]. The intersection of racial, cultural and disability identity are concepts that may seem too abstract to explore, but may also affect vocational outcome. These aspects of self-identity may impact presentation and success at interviews in African- American and Native American adolescents and adults with disabilities [71,72].

Adults and adolescents with an FASD have the additional barriers of school disruption and dropping out; cognitive and language deficits disproportionate to their IQ and academic performance; poor working memory; impulsivity; social skills that lag behind chronological age; safety issues mentioned earlier; multiple sensory processing challenges [73]; and co-occurring mental illness. Their most important obstacle is the lack of identification, diagnosis, and appropriate interventions for their primary brain damage associated with prenatal exposure to alcohol. Vocational Rehabilitation will be an important service to maximize.

Vocational Rehabilitation (VR) should be viewed as a multidisciplinary team process. It may be up to the parent or care giver to co-ordinate information. The team may include: a physician for medical and health issues; occupational therapist/ physical therapist; psychologist for counseling to address some of the above issues; teachers; case managers; job placement agencies [74]. VR programs may be public (state-federal agencies), private-for-profit (insurance-based), private-not-for-profit (Goodwill Industries). VR personnel in all sectors are asked to provide assessment, counseling, job development and placement, and case management for people with disabilities. There is both direct and indirect empirical evidence from a variety of levels to support the efficacy of pre-vocational counseling, skills training, and social and coping skills [75]. When individuals first apply for VR services, VR counselors will classify their primary disabilities as being one of 19 impairment codes (for example, sensory, physical or mental impairments). Each impairment code is assigned one of 37 "cause codes" (cancer, accident, developmental disability, unknown) [76]. Assessment and counseling should proceed simultaneously. Assessment may be optimized by combining standardized tests of strengths and preferences with naturalistic assessments; this might include interviews, portfolios and productivity samples, on-the-job assessment, person-centered planning to clarify aspirations and supports, narrative and graphic organizers such as journal [77].

Consumer choice and self-determination have been taken into account in the Workforce Investment Act (WIA) of 1998, with the description of an Individualized Plan for Employment (IPE). Information about the WIA and disability-related laws and regulations can be found at: http://www.doleta.gov/disability/rlar.cfm

The "Plain English" version of the WIA can be accessed at: http://www.doleta.gov/usworkforce/wia/Runningtext.cfm

An example of a state vocational services manual is from New York State; their regulations state that an IPE must be developed that is "consistent with the strengths, resources, priorities, concerns, abilities, capabilities, interests, and informed choice of the individual"(http://www.ocfs.state.ny.us/main/cbvh/vocrehab_manual/06_IPE.htm). Goals must be set regarding placement in independent employment, supported employment, or sheltered workshop. Taking the time and effort to consider all of these steps increases the likelihood of positive outcomes [78].

The WIA also includes provisions for access for people with disabilities to employment and training programs provided through the nation's One-Stop Career Centers [79]. One guide to these centers and the laws governing them can be found at: http://www.doleta.gov/usworkforce/wia/act.cfm

An Internet search for a local One-Stop Center (for example, NJ is: http://lwd.dol.state.nj.us/labor/wnjpin/findjob/onestop/services.html) may provide links to the State Department of Labor and Workforce Development, the Division for VR Services, and specific state initiatives for development of customized employment for people with disabilities.

Many adolescents and adults with an FASD may arrive at VR services by way of a psychiatric diagnosis or substance use disorder. Historically, people with psychiatric disability are underemployed; this is especially prominent in those with psychotic disorders. Some factors that showed promise in the success of VR with this population were completing a readiness inventory, VR counselors with training and experience with psychiatric disabilities, and professionals outside the VR system who advocate for successful participation [80] For those with psychiatric and substance use disorders, long-term rehabilitation must include vocational services. Employment appears to be an effective intervention to facilitate positive recovery outcomes. However, it has been found that less time may be spent in planning and matching for long-term employment in this population with multiple disabilities [81], which could hinder success.

In adolescents and adults with an FASD and co-occurring psychiatric and substance use disorders, productivity and work may initially work as a tool to enhance recovery rather than recovery being a tool to improve employment outcome. Work has the multiple benefits of income, responsibility, socialization, opportunities to use any skills and improved self-esteem.

One area of research in VR is cognitive remediation. Adults and adolescents with an FASD struggle with work because of numerous cognitive difficulties. Cognitive impairments are also obstacles to receiving the full benefit from VR. Cognitive remediation may include computerized tasks, problem-solving tasks, strategy coaching, and any methods for improving attention. Combining any of these strategies with VR may improve outcome [82]. Other areas of research in the VR of people with an intellectual disability focus on technology use to support employment activities and virtual reality programs to enhance a variety of skills [83, 84].

CO-OCCURRING ISSUES IN ADOLESCENTS AND ADULTS WITH AN FASD

Health, vocational, and lifespan developmental issues are essential to monitor in the overall care of the adolescent and adult with an FASD. Unfortunately, families and clinicians often are forced to delay attention to these areas because of more urgent co-occurring disorders and issues. The term "Co-occurring Disorders" is most commonly used when a person has distinct primary mental illness with primary addiction. "Co-occurring issues" may include: a disability such as an FASD; symptoms of mental illness; significant physical illness; trauma; language and cultural issues; environmental and social challenges like homelessness or lack of food or heat; family disruption, and criminal behavior. In the multi-axial diagnostic system used in psychiatry (DSM-IV-TR), these would be noted under Axis 1 (Other conditions that may be the focus of clinical attention) or Axis IV (Psychosocial and Environmental Problems). Co-occurring medical issues may be physical ARBDs, traumatic brain injury, sensory processing disorders, and neurological diagnoses associated with prenatal alcohol exposure like seizures.

Symptoms of mental illness are often found in people who have been prenatally exposed to alcohol. This is a particular concern when the prenatal exposure is in a binge pattern [85]. Clinicians and families struggle with the problem of diagnostic challenges and appropriate interventions [8, 86]. Some individuals will have symptoms of mental illness as a primary or secondary disability of the FASD itself. Others will have a distinguishable primary mental illness that co-occurs with the FASD. Mental illness and an FASD can co-occur with or without sufficient criteria to make two independent diagnoses. It is often difficult or impossible to differentiate these clinical scenarios; however, we must realize that treatment efficacy and successful client outcomes depend on our recognizing the presence of co-occurring issues.

Ideally, the medical diagnosis of an FASD would be made first; symptoms that are not explained by the primary FASD would then be further evaluated. Prenatal exposure to alcohol must be considered as a risk factor specifically in the initial evaluation. A standard adult psychiatric evaluation or a structured diagnostic interview like the Practical

Adolescent Diagnostic Interview [87] will not suggest the presence of a co-occurring FASD. FASDs are not usually recognized as a co-occurring disorder for a variety of reasons: they are not considered mental health disorders; mental health treatment for affected people is not reimbursed; and psychiatrists may not be trained to diagnose an FASD or modify treatments.

It is likely that a high percentage of people with an FASD have at least one co-occurring mental health disorder [5,88]. Multiple studies have identified ADHD as the most common co-occurring mental disorder with an FASD [89]. Other disorders co-occurring with an FASD or as a primary feature of the FASD are reviewed in Chapter 3.

People who are prenatally exposed to alcohol have a number of risk factors for mental illness. For example, some psychiatric diagnoses have a strong genetic link (schizophrenia, major depression, bipolar spectrum disorders, and ADHD). Profile of birth mothers demonstrated significant percentages of these and other DSM diagnoses [90]. Psychiatric diagnoses with a strong genetic link also have a high rate of substance use. It is estimated that about 50% of people with mental illness use substances. Information about co-occurring mental illness and substance abuse and dependence may be found in the Treatment Improvement Protocol (TIP) # 42 [91]. TIPS are best practice guidelines for the treatment of substance abuse. They are published by the Substance Abuse Mental Health Services Administration Center for Substance Abuse Treatment (SAMHSA/CSAT). A discussion about these reports and online access links to the TIPS referenced in this chapter may be found in the chapter reference section.

Other risk factors for people with prenatal alcohol exposure to develop mental illness have to do with the detrimental effect of alcohol on the developing brain. Prenatal exposure to alcohol is associated with smaller brain volume and with possible damage to the frontosubcortical nuclei implicated in the regulation of mood [92]. Cells in the brain that produce neurotransmitters to regulate mood and thinking may be absent, disconnected or non-functional. This will alter the amount or activity of neurotransmitters like GABA and serotonin, which are critical in mental health and mood regulation.

Alcohol also has negative effects on the developing hypothalamic-pituitary axis (HPA). Dysregulation of the HPA has been implicated in the consistent finding of mood and anxiety disorders in children and adults with prenatal alcohol exposure [93]. The HPA is a pathway that produces cortisol, which normally helps us to manage stress throughout our lives. Prenatal alcohol impairs the person's ability to manage stress in a healthy way. Individuals with an FASD experience multiple stressors often combined with poor coping skills. The combination of increasing stressors and decreasing coping abilities as well as underlying genetic vulnerabilities may cause mental illness to develop into full disorders. Additional stress is caused by the language processing disorders the person with an FASD will experience throughout the evaluation and management process. Straightforward treatment of a primary mental illness may fail in the person with an FASD; methods to address the whole picture must be developed. This would include understanding the baseline stress level, reducing stresses, improving coping mechanisms, and modifying the standard treatment as needed.

Before any differential diagnosis or intervention process can be considered, it is important to assess the safety of the person with an FASD; this is a population at significant risk of suicide at all ages studied [94]. Suicide in the general population is the third leading cause of death 15-24 year olds; fourth leading cause of death in 25-44 year olds; eighth leading cause of death in 45-64 year olds. General information about suicide can be found at: **http://www.cdc.gov/violenceprevention/pdf/Suicide_DataSheet-a.pdf**

The finding of suicide risk in those with an FASD is not surprising, given the combination of co-occurring mental illness, risk of substance abuse, poor coping skills, impulsivity, and impaired understanding of consequences in some people who have been prenatally exposed to alcohol. It is especially important to remember that a person with an FASD may not appear to plan or execute a suicide attempt effectively; this is not indicative of the seriousness of the intent. The true lethality of the attempt in the adolescent or adult with an FASD may not be an accurate indicator of the intent to die; ineffective planning is common in the person with an FASD. Suicide assessment and intervention protocols need to be modified for those with an FASD because of cognitive differences and communication impairments. Standard suicide contracts should be avoided because of the high degree of impulsivity. Some steps to take to reduce suicide risk are: address basic needs and increase stability; teach distraction techniques; remove access to lethal means; increase social supports; treat depression; build reasons for living; monitor closely; strengthen positive relationships [94]. Competencies for addressing suicide risk, thoughts, and behaviors are detailed in SAMHSA TIP 50, "Addressing suicidal thoughts and behaviors in substance abuse treatment" [95].

Starting on a long term program of therapy without first addressing safety issues is futile and potentially dangerous; the clinician must first evaluate physical safety for the adolescent or adult with an FASD and others. This includes issues of violence, harmful intent, victimization, adequate housing/food and other issues of self-harm such as self-mutilation. People with FASDs are at risk of becoming homeless because of difficulty managing money, inability to follow multiple directions to complete multiple tasks governed by multiple rules. They are often naïve and gullible, which puts them at risk for manipulation and abuse and they lack ongoing supports.

Once safety has been evaluated and the FASD and other co-occurring issues have been diagnosed, there are placement and intervention considerations to keep in mind. In typical adolescents and adults, psychiatric severity can be significantly reduced when co-occurring issues are treated together and mental health services and drug treatment are provided as an integrated program [96].

Substance abuse is another significant secondary disability in the adolescent or adult with an FASD. The person who has been prenatally exposed to alcohol has multiple risk factors for addiction [97]. A woman drinking during pregnancy may be alcoholic, and pass on the genetic vulnerability to alcoholism; poor stress management and cumulative trauma may further predispose the individual to expression of these genes. Poor decision making and peer pressure may initiate unhealthy drinking patterns early in adolescence; these are prominent features of the adolescent who has been prenatally exposed. Adolescents who engage in heavy drinking at an early age may become dependent on alcohol later in life and experience adverse health outcomes. According to the National Institute on Alcohol Abuse and Alcoholism (NIAAA), consuming alcohol during adolescence may have lasting effects on brain development [98]; this further impairs decision making.

The adolescent with an FASD is also at risk for the same factors which are associated with alcohol use in typical teens. A permissive environment for alcohol use, deviant behavior, and poor school performance have all been found to predict drinking initiation in teen years; these are factors common to many adolescents with an FASD. Cigarette smoking is highly correlated with adolescent drinking [99,100]. Early puberty is associated with risk for drinking at an early age [62]. The pregnant adult or adolescent is influenced by the drinking behavior of their male partners and the couples' knowledge about healthy pregnancy behaviors [101,102].

Research demonstrates that there may be a biologic origin to early drinking in adolescence by teens that were prenatally exposed to especially higher doses of alcohol [103-105]. The chemical senses are among the first to develop; prenatal exposure to alcohol may lead to an altered response to alcohol odor and contribute to later abuse risk [106]. Finally, a low level of response (LR) to alcohol is one of several genetically influenced phenotypes related to alcoholism risk. Most of the studies demonstrating this trait had been carried out in male subjects but a low LR to alcohol is seen in women with a family history of alcoholism [107]. This is another risk factor for adults and adolescents whose maternal drinking during pregnancy may have been due to alcoholism; obtaining a history of LR to alcohol may help identify women with an FASD who are at higher risk of affecting the next generation with prenatal exposure to alcohol.

Women with substance use disorders in general are less likely to enter substance abuse treatment; those with a co-occurring psychiatric disorder may require specific program modifications to experience treatment effectiveness [108]. Women with an FASD who are being evaluated and treated for addiction may not be recognized and diagnosed as a person with a co-occurring disorder. They will often need more intensive and longer term services, including addiction treatment that welcomes mother and child (ren). The pregnant, alcohol dependent adolescent or adult with an FASD must be assessed for severity of withdrawal first; once medically supervised detoxification has been completed, a level of treatment must be determined. This requires a collaboration of the obstetrician, addictionologist, and patient [109]. The management plan may utilize medications that require the additional support of a psychiatrist. Short-term abstinence leading to the ultimate goal of long-term recovery will require a multidisciplinary team [110].

People impaired by substance use have a difficult time entering and participating in treatment. This situation is aggravated when the primary brain damage from prenatal exposure to alcohol combines with frontal lobe dysfunction from repeated exposure to substances. Support, education, motivational interviewing and "socially sanctioned coercion" have all been applied to assist people in making a decision for treatment [111]. More than 770 drug courts in the US mandate treatment of drug and alcohol dependence; they have gathered significant data that demonstrate that insight does not have to be present at the outset of drug treatment to be successful [111]. Motivational interviewing principles have also been applied successfully to a wide range of behavioral changes; the FRAMES model may augment success and positive interactions [112]. The specific needs of women in substance abuse treatment are detailed in TIP 51, "Substance Abuse Treatment: Addressing the Specific Needs of Women" [113]. The effectiveness of motivational Interviewing and other Brief Interventions have not yet been well studied among individuals with an FASD.

Addiction treatment programs can be a critical resource in prevention of alcohol exposed pregnancies as well as treatment of drug and alcohol dependence. Screening and admitting staff should ask about prenatal alcohol use in all assessments; this includes the client as well as client offspring. Twelve step meetings may be an important part of treatment and recovery from addictions and Twelve Step Facilitation (TSF) may provide a foundation for a newly abstinent person with an FASD. Project MATCH compared success rates of TSF, Motivational Enhancement Therapy (MET), and Cognitive Behavioral Therapy (CBT), but didn't look at adolescents or adults with an FASD specifically. All three treatment modalities were successful in different populations [109]. The CDC publication "Reducing Alcohol Exposed Pregnancies: A Report of the National Task Force on Fetal Alcohol Syndrome and Fetal Alcohol Effects" offers an in-depth review and discussion of this topic. It is available online at: **http://www.cdc.gov/ncbddd/fasd/documents/121972RedAlcohPreg+Cov.pdf**

The person with an FASD will need support to participate in a twelve step program successfully. Many areas of the country have "Double Trouble" meetings; these are 12 step self-help groups designed to meet the special needs of people with addiction and mental health issues [114]. Double Trouble meetings may be more flexible about impulsive behaviors than routine meetings. Double Trouble in Recovery is listed in the National Registry of Evidence-Based Programs and Practices (NREPP). This may be accessed at: **http://www.doubletroubleinrecovery.org/** Resources and links for other 12 step meetings are found in the resource list at the end of this chapter.

Another significant resource for people with an FASD and co-occurring issues is the recovery movement in the mental health field. Recovery centers which were previously called "drop-in" centers offer a variety of supports, groups, and meetings in some areas. "Developing a Recovery and Wellness Lifestyle: a Self-Help Guide" is an example of resources available from SAMHSA/ CMHS. It is available online at: **http://download.ncadi.samhsa.gov/ken/pdf/SMA-3718/SMA-3718_lifestyle_11p.pdf**

Workbooks for recovery from substance abuse and mental illness are not designed specifically for adolescents and adults with an FASD but they may be helpful if enough motivation and support are available [115].

When considering placement options for addiction treatment programs, the core disabilities from the FASD must be kept in mind. General program characteristics for substance abuse treatment for adolescents are detailed in SAMHSA TIP 32: Treatment of Adolescents with Substance Abuse Disorder [116]. Guidelines for treatment of those with co-occurring disorders are covered in previously discussed TIP 42 [91] and in the American Society of Addiction Medicine (ASAM) Service Intensity Criteria for Individuals with Co-Occurring Disorders [117]. Communal recovery housing settings are options for long term support in maintaining abstinence, especially for ex-offenders, people with co-occurring psychiatric disorders, and others who are homeless [118].

PRACTICAL CONSIDERATIONS FOR THE CARE OF ADOLESCENTS OR ADULTS WITH CO-OCCURRING ISSUES

This section offers a variety of practical strategies and suggestions for an adolescent or adult with an FASD who is struggling with one or multiple co-occurring issues. These strategies have been found useful and are often cited by a variety of clinicians in the field for managing of the affected adolescent and adult. However, no evidence based research has been published to validate their efficacy. Additional links may be found in chapter resources

Primary disabilities may cause difficulties for individuals with an FASD in any structured program. Adolescents and adults with an FASD may be sporadic in keeping appointments, struggle with completing tasks independently, consistently get into difficulty with others, and may be viewed as manipulative, unmotivated, or non-compliant. They often have problems in programs that rely on verbal receptive language skills, information processing outside of sessions, making realistic decisions and following up independently, and asking for help when needed. Treatment staff must be prepared for a client who may wander off, daydream, or talk inappropriately in group situations. Individual support, attention, and repetition may be required.

One diagnostic error that is made in individuals with an FASD is that one of the co-occurring disorders is not identified. Another error is an actual misdiagnosis. These errors drive interventions that may not be successful and lead to frustration, discouragement, and poor outcomes. When interventions fail, it is important to remember that a single behavior will have different causes and effective interventions depending on the actual diagnosis. Following is an example to illustrate [119]:

An adolescent who is antisocial and acting out more than the typical adolescent may have an FASD, adolescent depression or adolescent bipolar disorder. The cause of the behavior in the adolescent with an FASD may be misreading social cues, modeling behavior, or difficulty communicating thoughts and feelings; the intervention might be role playing or a mentor to model more social behavior. The adolescent with unipolar or bipolar mood disorder may have the acting out and antisocial behavior because of depression or mania. Intervention for the same behavior would be psychotherapy and appropriate medication.

Chapter 3 contains a table that will assist in sorting out causes and interventions for sample behaviors. Tables like this are useful to remind care givers and treatment professionals to look at underlying causes for behavior and develop interventions to address the root problem. However, the adolescent or adult with an FASD may have multiple issues, so interventions are rarely straightforward.

Outcomes for the client with an FASD can often be improved by using a strengths based approach. The provider needs to factor in strengths in the family, the community (including cultural strengths) and what are the strong points in the provider and program themselves. Treatment providers may need to make a philosophical shift in responsibility. "We must move from viewing the individual as failing if s/he does not do well in a program to viewing the program as not providing what the individual needs in order to succeed" [119].

Lack of follow-through by the adolescent or adult with an FASD may not indicate lack of motivation and reward based systems such as point systems may need to be modified to provide more immediate reinforcement. Many practical strategies from school programs, vocational programs, and organizations for FASD on a national, state, and private level have been published. A sample of these is found in the resources section.

There are numerous issues that must be dealt with on a daily basis by those who deal personally and professionally with clients who have been prenatally exposed to alcohol and have significant co-occurring issues. Individual care givers, professionals, and treatment programs can only go so far toward insuring optimal outcomes.

FUTURE DIRECTIONS

It is clear from this overview chapter that research is needed in all aspects of lifespan issues affecting the adult or adolescent with an FASD. Some states have networks for diagnosis and case management [120,121]; this system could provide a foundation on which to build prevention, education, and treatment networks. Lack of resources prevents needed research and service delivery. Research and service delivery needs include: screening, diagnosis and interventions for adolescents and adults; role of family; effectiveness of programs in health, education, and vocations; prevention of multigenerational incidence; and delivery of effective lifelong services.

One document that details these issues is the "Consensus Statement on Fetal Alcohol Spectrum Disorder (FASD) - Across the Lifespan" [122]. This statement was developed by the Institute of Health Economics in Alberta, Canada (www.ihe.ca). The direct link to the pdf of the Consensus Development Conference Statement can be found at: http://www.ihe.ca/publications/library/2009/consensus-development-conference-statement-on-fetal-alcohol-spectrum-disorder-fasd---across-the-lifespan/

Another publication with future directions needed is the "Call to Action: Advancing Essential Services and Research on Fetal Alcohol Spectrum Disorders- A Report of the National Task Force on Fetal Alcohol Syndrome and Fetal Alcohol Effects" http://www.cdc.gov/ncbddd/fasd/documents/08_121973CallActionBk+Cov.pdf

CHAPTER RESOURCES

Routine Health Care

For specific adolescent issues, the American Academy of Pediatrics has a list of position papers: http://www.adolescenthealth.org/Position_Papers/612/2210.htm

The Society for Adolescent Health and Medicine (SAHM) website provides information on adolescent issues and providers: http://www.adolescenthealth.org//AM/Template.cfm?Section=Home

The AMA section on Adolescent Health may be accessed at: http://www.ama-assn.org/ama/pub/physician-resources/public-health/promoting-healthy-lifestyles/adolescent-health/guidelines-adolescent-preventive-services.shtml

The AMA "Guidelines for Adolescent Preventive Services" may be found at: http://www.ama-assn.org//ama1/pub/upload/mm/39/gapsmono.pdf

AAP Bright Futures Guidelines for ages 0-21: http://brightfutures.aap.org/

AMA Guidelines for promoting Adolescent Healthy Lifestyles: http://www.ama-assn.org/ama/pub/physician-resources/public-health/promoting-healthy-lifestyles/adolescent-health.shtml

American Academy of Pediatrics website may be searched: http://www.aap.org/

United States Preventive Services Task Force website: http://www.ahrq.gov/clinic/uspstfix.htm

American Academy of Family Practice Clinical Recommendations: http://www.aafp.org/online/en/home/clinical/clinicalrecs.html?navid=clinical+recommendations

The Canadian Task Force on Preventive Health Care is currently updating recommendations: http://www.aafp.org/online/en/home/clinical/clinicalrecs.html?navid=clinical+recommendations

World news on child and adolescent health: http://www.who.int/child_adolescent_health/en/

TREATMENT IMPROVEMENT PROTOCOLS

SAMHSA Treatment Improvement Protocols can be found online at: http://www.ncbi.nlm.nih.gov/bookshelf/br.fcgi?book=hssamhsatip

A discussion about TIPS: http://www.ncbi.nlm.nih.gov/bookshelf/br.fcgi?book=hssamhsatip&part=miscinfo

TIP 51 Substance Abuse Treatment: Addressing the Specific Needs of Women: http://www.ncbi.nlm.nih.gov/bookshelf/br.fcgi?book=hssamhsatip&part=tip51

TIP 42 Substance Abuse Treatment for Persons with Co-Occurring Disorders: http://www.ncbi.nlm.nih.gov/bookshelf/br.fcgi?book=hssamhsatip&part=A74073

TIP 32 Treatment of Adolescents with Substance Abuse Disorders: http://www.ncbi.nlm.nih.gov/bookshelf/br.fcgi?book=hssamhsatip&part=A56031

TIP 29 Substance Use Disorder Treatment for people with Physical and Cognitive Diisabilities: http://www.ncbi.nlm.nih.gov/bookshelf/br.fcgi?book=hssamhsatip&part=A52487

PRACTICAL CONSIDERATIONS AND STRATEGIES

Information about 12 Step programs and meeting lists can be found at http://www.12step.org/

AA can be found at http://www.aa.org/. This site also links to a meeting locator and online meetings.

A larger listing of other self-help/ mutual aid groups for additional problems can be found at: http://www.selfhelpgroups.org/

City of Edmonton and area members of Region 6 Fetal Alcohol Spectrum Disorder Child and Youth Sub-Committee. FASD Strategies not Solutions. Access on line: http://www.region6fasd.ca/pdf

Alberta Learning Publication. Special Programs Branch. Teaching students with fetal alcohol spectrum disorder: Building strengths, creating hope 2004 downloaded 8/1/2010 from http://education.alberta.ca/media/377037/fasd.pdf

Lutke, J, Antrobus, T. Fighting For a Future. FASD and 'the system: adolescents, adults, and their families and the state of affairs. Proceedings from a two-day Forum: June19020, 2004. Can be accessed on line at: http://www.fasdconnections.ca/HTMLobj-1807/fighting_for_a_future.pdf

The National Organization on Fetal Alcohol Syndrome information, research, links to other FASD- related organizations. It can be accessed on line at: http://www.nofas.org/resource/links.aspx

SAMHSA FASD Center for Excellence website (http://www.fasdcenter.samhsa.gov/ has multiple resources, with a specific factsheet about living independently: http://www.fasdcenter.samhsa.gov/documents/WYNKIndLiving_6_colorJA_new.pdf

CDC National Center on Birth Defects and Developmental Disabilities also has resources, publications and support. It can be accessed at: http://www.cdc.gov/ncbddd/fasd/index.html

REFERENCES

[1]   Flisher A, Kramer R, Hoven C, *et al*. Risk behavior in a community sample of children and adolescents. J Amer Acad Child Adolesc Psychiatry 2000; 39(7): 881-887.
[2]   Rutter M. Psychopathological development across adolescence. J Youth Adolescence 2007; 36: 101-110.
[3]   Eaton D, Kann L, Kinchen S, *et al*. Youth risk behavior surveillance- United States 2005. MMWR Surveill Summ Jun 2006; 55(5):1-108.
[4]   Riley E, McGee C, Sowell E. Teratogenic effects of alcohol: A decade of brain imaging. Am J Med Gen Part C Semin Med Genet 2004;127C: 35-41.
[5]   Streissguth A, Bookstein H, Barr HM. Risk factors for adverse life outcomes in fetal alcohol syndrome and fetal alcohol effects. J Dev Behav Pediatr 2004; 25: 228-238.
[6]   Anda R, Felitti V, Brenner JD, *et al*. The enduring effects of abuse and related adverse experiences in Childhood. Eur Arch Psychiatry Clin Neurosci 2006; 256: 174-186.
[7]   O'Connor M, Paley B. Psychiatric conditions associated with prenatal alcohol exposure. Dev Disabil Res Rev 2009; 15: 225-234.
[8]   Chudley AE, Kilgour AR, Cranston, M, Edwards, M. Challenges of diagnosis in fetal alcohol syndrome and fetal alcohol spectrum disorder in the adult. Am J Genet Part C Semin Med Genet 2007; 145C: 261-272.
[9]   Burd L, Klug M, Martsolf J, Kerbeshian J. Fetal Alcohol Syndrome: Neuropsychiatric phenomics. Neurotoxicol Teratol 2003; 25: 697-705.
[10]   Elster AB. Comparison of recommendations for adolescent clinical preventive services developed by national organizations. Arch Pediatr Adolesc Med 1998; 152: 193.
[11]   Krahn GL, Hammond I, Turner A. A cascade of disparities: health care and health care access for people with intellectual disabilities. Ment Retard Dev Disab Res Rev 2006; 12(1): 70-82.
[12]   Tyler CV Jr, White-Scott S, Ekvall S, Abulafia L. Environmental health and developmental disabilities: A lifespan approach. Fam Community Health 2008; 31(4): 287-304.

[13]   Mendola P, Selevan S, Gutter S, Rice D. Environmental factors associated with a spectrum of neurodevelopmental deficits. Ment Ret Dev Disabil 2002; 8: 188-197.

[14]   Jensen DE, Krol B, Groothoff JW, Post, D. People with intellectual disability and their health problems: a review of comparative studies. J Intellect Disab Res Feb 2004; 48(Pt 2): 93-102.

[15]   McDermott S, Moran R, Platt T, Dasari S. Health conditions among women with a disability. J Women's Health 2007; 16(5): 713-720.

[16]   Doering L, Moser D, Lemankiewicz W. Depression, healing, and recovery from coronary artery bypass surgery. Am J Crit Care 2005; 14: 316-324.

[17]   Patja K, Iivanainen M, Vesala H, Oksanen H, Ruoppila Life expectancy of people with intellectual disability: a 35-year follow-up study. J Intellect Disabil Res Oct 2000; 44(Pt 5): 591-9.

[18]   Shankar K, Hidestrand, M, Liu X, *et al.* Physiologic and genomic analyses of nutrition-ethanol interactions during gestation: Implications for fetal ethanol toxicity. Exp Biol Med 2006; 231: 1379-1397.

[19]   Thomas J, Zhou F, Kane C. Proceedings of the 2008 annual meeting of the Fetal Alcohol Spectrum Disorders Study Group. Alcohol 2009; 43: 333-339.

[20]   Gauthier T, Drews-Botsch C, Falek A, Coles C, Rrown L. Maternal alcohol abuse and neonatal infection. Alcohol Clin Exp Res 2005; 29(6): 1035-1043.

[21]   McGill J, Meyerholz D, Edsen-Moore M, *et al.* Fctal cxposure to ethanol has long-term effects on the severity of influenza virus infections. J Immunol 2009; 182: 7803-7808.

[22]   Zhang X. Sliwosk J, Weinberg J. Prenatal alcohol erxposure and fetal programming: Effects on neuroendocrine and immune function. Exp Biol Med 2005; 230: 376-388.

[23]   Spadoni A, Bazinet A, Fryer S, Tapert S, Mattson S, Riley E. BOLD response during spatial working memory in youth with heavy prenatal alcohol exposure. Ahcohol Clin Exp Res 2009; 33(12): 2067-2076.

[24]   Green CR, Mihic AM, Armstrong IT, *et al.* Oculomotor control in children with fetal alcohol spectrum disorders assessed using a mobile eye-tracking laboratory. Eur J Neurosci.2009; 29: 1302-1309.

[25]   Connor P, Sampson P, Streissguth A, Bookstein, F, Barr, H. Effects of prenatal alcohol exposure on fine motor coordination and balance: A study of two adult samples. Neuropsychologia 2006; 44: 744-751.

[26]   Domellof E, Ronnqvist, L Titran M, Esseily, R, Fagard, J. Atypical functional lateralization in children with fetal alcohol syndrome. Dev Psychobiol 2009; 51: 696-705.

[27]   Stromland K, Hellstrom A. Fetal alcohol syndrome-An ophthalmological and socioeducational prospective study. Pediatrics 1996; 97(6): 845-850.

[28]   Flanagan E, Aros S, Bueno M, *et al.* Eye malformations in children with heavy alcohol exposure in utero. J Pediatr 2008; 153: 391-395.

[29]   Dalen K, Bruaroy, Wentzel-Larson T, Langreld L. Cognitive functioning in children prenatally exposed to alcohol and psychotropic drugs. Neuropediatrics 2009; 40(4):162-7.

[30]   Church M, Eldis F, Blakeley B, Bawle E. Hearing, speech, vestibular, and dentofacial disorders in fetal alcohol syndrome. Ahcohol Clin Exp Res 2006; 21(2): 227-237.

[31]   Guerri C, Bazinet A, Riley E. Foetal alcohol spectrum disorders and alterations in brain and behavior. Alcohol Alcohol 2009; 44(2): 108-114.

[32]   Xiangyang M, Coles C, Lynch M, *et al.* Evaluation of corpus callosum anisotropy in young adults with fetal alcohol syndrome according to diffusion tensor imaging. Ahcohol Clin Exp Res 2005; 29(7): 1214-1222.

[33]   Mattson S, Calarco K, Lang A. Focused and shifting attention in children with heavy prenatal alcohol exposure. Neuropsychology 2006; 20(3): 361-369.

[34]   Sowell F., Mattson S, Kan E, Thompson P, Riley E, Toga A. Abnormal cortical thickness and brain-behavior correlation patterns in individuals with heavy prenatal exposure. Cerebral Cortex 2008; 18(1): 136-144.

[35]   McGee C, Fryer, S, Bjorquist O, Mattson,S, Riley, E. Deficits in Social problem solving in adolescents with prenatal exposure to alcohol. Am J Drug Ahcohol Abuse 2008; 34: 423-431.

[36]   Touchette E, Petit D, Seguin J, Boivin M, Tremblay R, Montplaisir J. Associations. Between sleep duration patterns and behavioral/cognitive functioning at school entry. Sleep 2007; 30(9): 1213-1219.

[37]   Liu X. Sleep and adolescent suicidal behavior. Sleep 27 (7) 2004: 1351-1358.

[38]   Roberts R, Roberts CR, Chan W. Sleep disturbance in adolescents. Sleep 2008; 32(2): 177-184.

[39]   Harris C. Neurophysiology of sleep and wakefulness. Respir Care Clin N Am 2005; 11(4): 567-586.

[40]   Sadeh A, Dahl R, Shaha G, Rosenblatt-Stein, S. Sleep and the transition to adolescence: A longitudinal Study. Sleep 2009; 32(12): 1602-1609.

[41]   Gau S, Chiang, H. Sleep problems and disorders among adolescents with persistent and subthreshold attention-deficit/hyperactivity disorders. Sleep 2009; 32(5): 671-679.

[42]   Stone K, LaGasse L, Lester B, *et al.* Sleep problems in children with prenatal substance exposure: the maternal lifestyle study. Arch Pediatr Adolesc Med 2010; 164(5): 452-456.

[43]   Pesonun A, Raikkonen A, Matthews K, *et al.* Prenatal origins of poor sleep in children. Sleep 2009; 32(8): 1086-1992.

[44]   Zhou F, West J, Blake C. General discussion at the fetal alcohol syndrome symposium. Exp Biol Med 2005; 230: 407-412.

[45]   Moseley L, Gradisar, M. Evaluation of a school- based intervention for adolescent sleep problems. Sleep 2009; 32(3): 334-341.

[46]   Sant'Anna L, Tosello, D. Fetal alcohol syndrome and developing craniofacial and dental structures- a review.Orthod Craniofacial Res 2006; 9:172-185.

[47]   Imai,R, Miake T, Yanagisawa T, Yakushiji M. Growth and formation of the tooth germ in a rat model of fetal alcohol syndrome. J Hard Tissue Biol 2007; 16(2): 61-70.

[48]   Moiseiwitsch J. The role of serotonin and neurotransmitters during craniofacial development. Crit Rev Oral Biol Med 2000; 11(2): 230-239.

[49]   Thomas J, Biane J, O'Bryan K, O'Neill T, Dominguez, H. Choline supplementation following third trimester equivalent alcohol exposure attenuates behavioral alterations in rats. Behav Neurosci 2004;121(1): 121-130.

[50]   Zeisel S. The fetal origins of memory: The role of dietary choline in optimal brain development. J Pediatr 2006; 149(5) Supplement: S131-S136.

[51]   Rimmer J, Chen M, McCubbin J, Drum C, Peterson, J Exercise intervention research on persons with disabilities: What we know and where we need to go. Am J Phys Med Rehabil 2010; 89: 249-263.

[52]   Larson, N, Neumark-Sztainer, D. Adolescent Nutrition. Pediatr Rev 2009; 30: 494-496.

[53]   Lichtenstein A, Russell R. Essential nutrients: Food or supplements? Where should the emphasis be? JAMA 2005; 294(3): 351-358.

[54]   Hayman L. Starting young: Promoting a healthy lifestyle with children. J Cardiovasc Nurs 2010; 25(3): 228-232.

[55]   O'Connor T, Watson K, Hughes S, *et al.* Health professionals' and dietetics practitioners' perceived effectiveness of fruit and vegetable parenting practices across six countries. J Am Dietetic Assoc 2010; 110(7): 1065-1071.

[56]   Bouchard M, Bellinger D, Wright R, Weisskopf, M. Attention deficit/Hyperactivity disorder and urinary metabolites of organophosphate pesticides. Pediatrics 2010; 125 (6): e1270-e1277.

[57]   Kramer-Atwood, J, Dwyer J, Hoelscher D, Nicklas T, Johnson R, Schultz, G. Fostering healthy food consumption in schools: Focusing on the challenges of competitive foods. J Am Dietetic Assoc 2002; 102(9): 1228-1233.

[58]   Traves C, Coll O, Cararach V, Gual A, DeTajada B, Lopez-Tejero M. Clinical approach to intestinal maturation in neonates prenatally exposed to alcohol. Alcohol Alcohol 2007; 42(5): 407-412.

[59]   Shankar K, Ronis M, Badger T. Effects of pregnancy and nutritional status on alcohol metabolism. Alcohol Res Health 2007; 30(1): 55-59.

[60]   Berthoud H, Morrison C. The brain, appetite, and obesity. Ann Rev Psychol 2008; 59: 55-92.

[61]   Murphy N, Elias E for the Council on Children with Disabilities. Sexuality of children and adolescents with developmental disabilities. Pediatrics 2006 118(1): 398-403.

[62]   Faden V, Newes-Adeyl G, Chen C. The relationship of Tanner Stage, age and drinking in adolescent boys and girls. Alcohol Clin Exp Res 2006; 30(6) Supplement: 55A.

[63]   Greydanus DE, Omar HA. Sexuality issues and gynecologic care of adolescents with developmental disabilities. Pediatric Clin North Am 2008: 55(6): 1315-35.

[64]   Bertrand J. Interventions for children with fetal alcohol spectrum disorders (FASD): Overview of findings for five innovative research projects. Rev Dev Dis 2009; 30: 986-1006.

[65]   Miller S, Chan F. Predictors of life satisfaction in individuals with intellectual disabilities. J Intellec Dis Res 2008; 52(part 12): 1039-1047.

[66]   Migliore A, Grossi T, Mank, D, Rogan,P. Why do adults with intellectual disabilities work in sheltered workshops? J Voc Rehabil 2008; 28: 29-40.

[67]   Migliore A, Grossi, T, Mank D, Rogan, P. Integrated employment or sheltered workshops: Preference of adults with intellectual disabilities, their families, and staff. J Voc Rehabil 2007; 26: 5-19.

[68]   Winn S, Hay I. Transition from school for youths with a disability: Issues and challenges. Disabil Soci 2009; 24(1); 103-115.

[69]   Leon L, Matthews L. Self-esteem theories: Possible explanations for poor interview performance for people experiencing unemployment. J Rehabil 2010; 76(1): 41-50.

[70]   Fabian E, Ethridge G, Beveridge S. Differences in perceptions of career barriers and supports for people with disabilities by demographic background and case status factor. J Rehabil 2009; 75(1): 41-49.

[71]   Mpofu E, Harley D. Racial and disability identity: Implications for the career counseling of African Americans with disabilities. Rehabil Counsel Bull 2006; 1: 14-23.

[72] Rowley D, Rehfeldt R. Delivering human services to Native Americans with disabilities: Cultural variables and service recommendations. N Am J Psychol 2002; 4(2): 309-316.

[73] Duquette C, Stodel E, Fullarton S, Hagglund K. Secondary school experiences of individuals with foetal alcohol spectrum disorder: Perspectives of parents and their children. Int J Inclusive Educ 2007; 11(5-6): 571-591.

[74] Gobelet C, Luthi F, Al-Khodairy A, Chamberlain, M. Vocational rehabilitation: A multidisciplinary intervention. Disabil Rehabil 2007; 29(17): 1405-1410.

[75] Pruett S, Rosenthal D, Swett, E, Lee, G, Chan, F. Empirical evidence supporting the effectiveness of vocational rehabilitation. J Rehabil 2008; 74(1): 56-63.

[76] Cimera R. The national costs of supported employment to vocational rehabilitation: 2002-2006. J Voc Rehabil 2009; 30: 1-9.

[77] Hagner D. The role of naturalistic assessment in vocational rehabilitation. J Rehabil 2010; 76(1): 28-34.

[78] Beveridge S, Fabian, E. Vocational rehabilitation outcomes: Relationship between Individualized Plan for Employment goals and employee outcomes. Rehabil Counsel Bull 2007; 50(4): 238-246.

[79] Luecking R, Cuozzo L, Leedy M, Seleznow E. Universal one-stop access: Pipedream or possibility? J Voc Rehabil 2008; 28: 181-189.

[80] Rogers ES, Anyhony W, Lyass A, Penk W. A randomized clinical trial of vocational rehabilitation for people with psychiatric disabilities. Rehabil Counsel Bull 2006; 49(3): 143-156.

[81] Donnell C, Zheng Y, Mizelle N. Consumers of vocational ehabilitation services diagnosed with psychiatric and substance use disorders. J Rehabil 2009; 75(3): 41-49.

[82] McGurk S, Wykes T. Cognitive remediation and vocational rehabilitation. Psychiatric Rehabil J 2008; 31(4): 350-359.

[83] Wehmeyer M, Palmer S, Smith S, Parent, W, Davies, D, Stock, S. Technology use by people with intellectual and developmental disabilities to support employment activities: a single-subject design meta analysis. J Voc Rehabil 2006; 24: 81-86.

[84] Standen P, Brown D. Virtual reality in the rehabilitation of people with intellectual disabilities: A review. Cyber Psychol Behav 2005; 8(3): 272-282.

[85] Barr H, Bookstein F, O'Malley K, Connor P, Huggins J, Streissguth A. Binge drinking during pregnancy as a predictor of psychiatric disorders on the structured clinical interview for DSM-IV in young adulthood. Am J Psychiatry 2006; 163(6): 1061-1065.

[86] O'Connor M, Paley B. Psychiatric conditions associated withprenatal alcohol exposure. Dev Disabil Res Rev 2009; 15: 225-234.

[87] Hoffman N, Bride B, MacMaster S, Abrantes A, Estroff T. Identifying co-occurring disorders in adolescent populations. J Addict Dis 2004; 23(4): 41-53.

[88] Clark E, Lutke J, Minnes P, Quellette-Kuntz H. Secondary disabilities among adults with fetal alcohol spectrum disorder in British Columbia. J FAS Int 2004: 2 e13 Oct 2004: 1-12

[89] Burd L, Carlson C, Kerbeshian J. Fetal alcohol spectrum disorders and mental illness. Int J Disabil Hum Dev 2007; 5(4): 383-396.

[90] Astley S, Bailey D, Talbot C Clarren S. Fetal alcohol syndrome (FAS) primary prevention through FAS diagnosis: I. Identification of High risk birth mothers through the diagnosis of their children. Alcohol Alcohol 20003; 5(5): 499-508.

[91] Center for Substance Abuse Treatment. Substance Abuse Treatment for Persons With Co-Occurring Disorders. Treatment Improvement Protocol (TIP) Series 42. DHHS Publication No. (SMA) 05-3922. Rockville, MD: Substance Abuse and Mental Health Services Administration, 2005.

[92] O'Connor M, Paley B. The relationship of prenatal alcohol exposure and the postnatal environment to child depressive symptoms. Disabil Rehabil Psychol 2006 31: 50-64.

[93] Hellemanns K, Verma P, Yoon E, *et al.* Prenatal alcohol exposure increases vulnerability to stress and anxiety-like disorders in adulthood. Ann NY Acad Sci 2008; 1144: 154-175.

[94] Huggins J, Grant T, O'Malley K, Streissguth A. Suicide attempts among adults with fetal alcohol spectrum disorders: Clinical considerations. Mental Health Aspects of Dev Disab 2008; 11(2): 33-41.

[95] Center for Substance Abuse Treatment. Addressing Suicidal Thoughts and Behaviors in Substance Abuse Treatment. Treatment Improvement Protocol (TIP) Series 50. HHS Publication No. (SMA) 09-4381. Rockville, MD: Substance Abuse and Mental Health Services Administration, 2009.

[96] Hser Y, Grella C, Evans E, Huang Y. Utilization and outcomes of mental health services among patients in drug treatment. J Addict Dis 2006; 25(1): 73-85.

[97] Enoch M. Genetic and environmental influences on the development of alcoholism: Resilience vs. risk. Ann NY Acad Sci 2006; 1094: 193-201.

[98] Alcohol research: A lifespan perspective. US Dept of Health, NIH: NIAAA publications 2008; 74.

[99] Archie C, Anderson M, Gruber E. Positive smoking history as a preliminary screening device for substance use in pregnant adolescents. J Pediatr Adolesc Gynecol 1997;10: 13-17.

[100] Grucza R, Bierut L. Cigarette smoking and the risk for alcohol use disorders among adolescent drinkers. Alcohol Clin Exp Res 2006; 30(12): 2046-2054.

[101] Perreira K, Cortes K. Race/Ethnicity and nativity differences in alcohol and tobacco use during pregnancy. Am J Public Health 2006; 96(9): 1629-1636.

[102] Chang G, McNamara T. Orav E, Wilkins-Haug L. Alcohol use by pregnant women: partners, knowledge, and other predictors. J Study Alcohol 2006; 67(2): 245-251.

[103] Alati R, Clavarino A, Najman J, *et al.* The developmental origin of adolescent alcohol use: Findings from the mater study of pregnancy and its outcomes. Drug Alcohol Dependence 2008; 98: 136-141.

[104] Spear N, Molina J. Fetal or infantile exposure to ethanol promotes ethanol ingestion in adolescence and adulthood: A theoretical review. Alcohol Clin Exp Res 2005; 29(6): 909-929.

[105] Alati R, Al Mamun A, Williams G, O' Callaghan M, Najman J, Bor W. In utero alcohol exposure and prediction of alcohol disorders in early adulthood: A birth cohort study. Arch Gen Psychiatry 2006; 63: 1009-1016.

[106] Youngentob S, Kent P, Sheehe P, Molina J, Spear N, Youngentob L. Experienced-induced fetal plasticity: The effect of gestational ethanol exposure on the behavioral and neurophysiologic olfactory response to ethanol odor in early postnatal and adult rats. Behav Neurosci 2007; 121(6): 1293-1305.

[107] Eng M, Schuckit M, Smith T. The level of response to alcohol in daughters of alcoholics and controls. Drug Alcohol Depend 2005; 79: 83-93

[108] Greenfield S, Brooks A, Gordon S, *et al.* Substance abuse treatment entry, retention and outcome in women: A review of the literature. Drug Alcohol Depand 2007; 86: 1-21.

[109] Christensen C. Management of chemical dependency in pregnancy. Clin Obstetr Gynecol 2008; 51(2): 445-455.

[110] Helmbrecht G, Thiagarajah S. Management of Addiction disorders in pregnancy. J Addict Med 2008; 2: 1-16.

[111] Nace E, Birkmayer F, Sullivan M, *et al.* Socially sanctioned coercion mechanisms for addiction treatment. Am J Addict 2007; 16: 15-23.

[112] AGOG Committee on Health Care for Underserved Women. Motivational interviewing: A tool for behavior change. ACOG Committee Opinion Number 423; 2009.

[113] Center for Substance Abuse Treatment. Substance Abuse Treatment: Addressing the Specific Needs of Women. Treatment Improvement Protocol (TIP) Series 51. HHS Publication No. (SMA) 09-4426. Rockville, MD: Substance Abuse and Mental Health Services Administration, 2009.

[114] Vogel H, Knight E, Laudet A, Magura S. Double trouble in recovery: Self-help for people with dual diagnoses. Psychiatry Rehabil J 1998; 21(4): 356-364.

[115] Daley D. Dual diagnosis workbook: Recovery strategies for substance use and mental health disorders, revised edition. Herald House/ Independence Press; Independence, Missouri. 1994, 2003.

[116] Center for Substance Abuse Treatment. Treatment of Adolescents with Substance Abuse Disorders. Treatment Improvement Protocol (TIP) Series 32. DHHS Publication No. (SMA) 05-3922. Rockville, MD: Substance Abuse and Mental Health Services Administration, 1998.

[117] Minkoff K, Zweben J, Rosenthal R, Ries R. Development of Service Intensity Criteria and Program Categories for Individuals with Co-Occurring Disorders. Published in: Addiction Treatment Matching: Research Foundations of the American Society of Addiction Medicine (ASAM) Criteria. Gastfriend, D ed. Co-published simultaneously as J Addictive Dis, Vol 22, Supplement Number 1 2003.

[118] Jason L, Olson B, Ferrari J, LoSasso A. Communal housing settings enhance substance abuse recovery. Am J Public Health 2006; 96(10): 1727-1729.

[119] Dubovsky D. Powerpoint presentation: "Working with Individuals with an FASD and Mental Health Concerns". Presented in Sault Ste Marie Michigan 2010.

[120] Astley S. Profile of the first 1400 patients receiving diagnostic evaluations for fetal alcohol spectrum disorder at the Washington State Fetal Alcohol Syndrome Diagnostic and Prevention Network. Can J Clin Pharmacol 2010; 17(1): e132-164.

[121] Brimacombe M, Adubato S, Cohen D, Wilson A, Lamendola M. Comprehensive approaches to the diagnosis, screening and prevention of fetal alcohol syndrome in New Jersey. J. FAS Int 2005; 3: e4.

[122] Consensus Statement on Fetal Alcohol Spectrum Disorder(FASD) – Across the Lifespan. Institute of Health Economics Consensus Statements 2009; 4: 1-14.

CHAPTER 7

Fetal Alcohol Spectrum Disorders and the Law

Kathyrn A. Kelly[*]

Project Director, FASD Legal Issues Resource Center, Fetal Alcohol and Drug Unit Department of Psychiatry and Behavioral Sciences, School of Medicine, University of Washington, USA

> *"We can envision few things more certainly beyond one's control than the drinking habits of a parent prior to one's birth"*
>
> **Florida Supreme Court *Dillbeck v. State* (1994)**
> **643 So. 2d 1027, 1029**

Abstract: Legal standards and legal institutions have a great impact on the lives of individuals with Fetal Alcohol Spectrum Disorders (FASD). Most individuals with FASD need and are eligible for a range of special services and programs. Frequently, however, it is difficult to obtain that assistance because the application processes are complex and because program officials are not familiar with FASD. The programs and services of particular importance include an appropriate education, Social Security benefits, and state programs for individuals with developmental disabilities. Approximately 60 % of individuals with FASD get in trouble with the law. Officials in the criminal justice system rarely recognize or understand FASD, and the system often treats defendants with this disability in a manner that is ineffective. Parents of and advocates for individuals with FASD need to better understand how to deal with the criminal justice system, and officials in that system need to be trained about FASD and about more appropriate corrective and other legal responses.

INTRODUCTION

Law, legal standards and legal institutions are of central importance to individuals with Fetal Alcohol Spectrum Disorders (FASD). First, for much of their lives most of these individuals will be dependent, often increasingly so, on a range of government services and programs. Because FASD cannot be treated medically--the underlying organic brain damage cannot be repaired—the quality of life of these individuals depends to a substantial degree on how society, particularly government agencies and programs, treat them. Obtaining access to needed services and programs requires understanding and meeting the legal rules that govern eligibility, as well as becoming familiar with the legal procedures and obstacles that stand in the way. As one parent of a child with FASD poignantly noted, no one who needed these services could possibly master the application process. Also, at some point in their lives, most of those with FASD are going to get in trouble with the law. When they do, legal standards and procedures establish the framework for deciding whether they will get assistance from the courts, will be punished (and if so, how severely), or will simply end up back on the streets [1-3].

These issues, and the importance of the law, are likely to increase as an individual with FASD grows from infancy to adulthood. When children with FASD are young, parents may be able, and might even be in the best position, to help deal with the behavioral problems associated with FASD. But as the children grow older, the ability of parents to deal with these problems will often decline. The problems of adolescents and adult children often cannot be solved by their parents. Parents may find older children harder to deal with, and, as their offspring age, the capacity of parents to intercede on their behalf will be reduced. Also, at some point parents have to worry about how these sons and daughters will function when the parents can no longer be active in their lives.

Individuals with FASD usually fare poorly when they have come into contact with the law. Legal rules, standards and procedures were not written to deal with FASD as such. The officials involved in the administration of those rules, standards and procedures—agency officials, lawyers, judges, and others—often are unfamiliar with FASD and have no idea when an individual might have that disability. The overarching task for parents, advocates, and

---

[*]Address correspondence to Kathryn A. Kelly: Fetal Alcohol and Drug Unit, 180 Nickerson Street, Suite 309, Seattle, Washington, 98109, USA; E-mail: faslaw@u.washington.edu

Susan A. Adubato and Deborah E. Cohen (Eds)

attorneys representing individuals with FASD is to bridge this gap. They must learn and articulate how the behavioral patterns of individuals with FASD can be seen to fit appropriately into the relevant legal structure and standards. At times this means that parents who understand the problems of their son or daughter, but not why the government or attorneys are being unhelpful, must somehow communicate with officials and attorneys who understand the law but are frustrated with the behavior of that son or daughter and his or her inexplicably overprotective parents.

At times, the same event may look entirely different to parents or advocates on the one hand, and to judges, lawyers and agency officials on the other. For example, an individual with FASD who is on probation may frequently fail to keep appointments with a probation official. The probation officer will probably see that problem as indicating the need for punitive action in order to teach the probationer the responsibility to keep appointments and the adverse consequences of failing to do so. A parent, on the other hand, would be likely to see that behavior as the inability of the individual with FASD to remember appointments and to manage and keep track of time. What seems an attitude problem to the probation official would be a symptom of the disability to the parent.

The problems that arise from the interplay of FASD and the law are numerous and complex. There is, however, one step useful in almost all these arenas: obtaining a medical diagnosis of FASD. To those involved in the administration of the law, there often will seem to be nothing terribly wrong with an individual with FASD, no problem to which the law should, or even could, respond. A medical diagnosis—even if its exact meaning may not be clear—can be uniquely effective in persuading agencies and courts, lawyers and bureaucrats that there is more to the situation before them than meets the eye.

A variety of useful materials in relation to obtaining a diagnosis can be found at the Web site of the Fetal Alcohol Unit of the University of Washington: **http://depts.washington.edu/fadu/legalissues/** and at the Web site of FASD Ontario Justice Committee: **http://fasdjustice.on.ca/**

ELIGIBILITY FOR SOCIAL PROGRAMS

Most individuals with FASD need—although they may not receive—special services and assistance to cope with their disability. The relevant programs, such as the state agencies for the developmentally disabled or Social Security benefits do not ordinarily provide automatic eligibility to those with FASD; indeed, in many instances the existence of FASD as such may not be relevant. To obtain the needed services and assistance it must be demonstrated that the symptoms and manifestations of that disability fall within the particular standards utilized for the program in question. Understanding the eligibility rules and mastering the procedures of each agency for establishing eligibility are of critical importance. Agencies can be quite idiosyncratic in their requirements regarding the information and documents to be provided or the tests to be administered; what matters is not what might be convincing to a parent or advocate, but the established agency method of proceeding. The burden of doing so is usually the responsibility of the individual, the family or an advocate seeking admission to the program in question; precisely because of the disabling effect of FASD, the burden of meeting these standards and navigating those procedures falls on family members or other advocates. As the father of one individual affected by FASD reflected "No one who needs these services could possibly apply for them".

Frequently the documents needed to begin an application process—application forms, instructions, standards, lists of needed supporting material—can be found on the Web site of the agency in question.

Individuals with Disabilities Education Act

The Individuals with Disabilities Education Act (IDEA) requires that public schools provide for any student with a disability an Individualized Education Program (IEP) tailored to the specific needs of the student. Most schools and school districts are familiar with this requirement and have a range of approaches for dealing with this legal obligation.

Many teachers and schools, however, are unfamiliar with the particular needs of students with FASD and with the specific teaching techniques that are likely to be effective for those students. There is a substantial amount of material about those needs and techniques, and it may be helpful for parents or advocates to identify or provide those materials to the school officials responsible for preparing the IEP. The federal government supports an office that provides useful information about FASD, the SAMHSA (Substance Abuse Mental Health Services Administration) FASD Center for Excellence. Materials at that office's Web site dealing with education problems can be accessed at: http://www.fasdcenter.samhsa.gov/grabGo/factSheets.cfm

Education officials at the Yukon Department of Education in Whitehorse, Canada have developed a detailed teaching curriculum for students with FASD, which can be accessed at the Web site of FASD Connections: http://www.fasdconnections.ca/ieh2.htm

Social Security

The Social Security Administration administers several assistance programs for which individuals with FASD may be eligible.

Supplemental Security Income (SSI) are financial benefits for adults whose disabilities are so severe that they cannot work full time and who do not have substantial other income or financial assets. To be eligible an applicant must be unable to work full time at any job, not merely unable to work full time at his or her past or preferred job. There is an exception for individuals who work full time in special job programs for individuals with disabilities. To establish eligibility an applicant must be able to show both that he or she has a disability and that the disability is the reason he or she cannot work full time. The Social Security Administration (SSA) recognizes that FASD is a disability, and that it is a disability that can prevent an individual from working full time. It is not enough, however, merely to show that an applicant has FASD; there must also be a demonstration of the effect of the disability on the applicant's ability to work. Under certain circumstances an individual can continue to receive SSI benefits even though he or she is working; the rules governing whether an individual can do so are set out on the SSA Web site: http://www.socialsecurity.gov/pubs/10095.pdf

SSA also provides assistance for children with disabilities if their disabilities cause "marked and severe limitations" and the parent or parents of the child have very limited income and assets.

Additional information about these programs can be obtained by calling the Social Security Administration's toll free line, 1-800-772-1213. Much information is also available on line at http://www.ssa.gov

The process of applying for either of these programs involves submitting a detailed application. If an initial application is denied, the applicant can seek review of that decision, and is entitled to a hearing [2]. The process of working through this system is described at the Social Security Administration Web site, and in the article available at: http://depts.washington.edu/fadu/legalissues/

An attorney is not required to handle the initial stages of this application process, although one may be helpful. Pursuing a legal appeal of a denial of benefits usually does require a lawyer. There is a national organization of attorneys and others who represent individuals applying for Social Security benefits, the National Organization of Social Security Claimants Representatives (NOSSCR). That organization's Web site can be accessed at: http://www.nosscr.org/

It is possible to arrange for Social Security benefits to be paid to a designated third-party payee. That may be an important safeguard for the individual with FASD who has difficulty handling money.

State Developmental Disabilities Programs

All states have some program to assist individuals with developmental disabilities (DD). The nature of those DD programs vary widely. Some are limited to assisting clients in obtaining access to the programs of other agencies, federal, state, local or even private. Other DD programs provide services, housing, a permanent counselor or advocate, or financial assistance to individuals. An official of a DD agency, for example, might be a designated payee for a client receiving Social Security. In general, any and all of these types of programs can be of considerable value to individuals with FASD [3].

The eligibility standards for state DD programs also vary greatly from state to state. Most of these programs were originally limited to individuals with a full scale IQ score of 70 or less, and were expressly denoted as programs for persons with intellectual disabilities. This restriction is a serious problem for individuals with FASD, many of whom have a tested IQ score above 70, but actually function at a level typical of individuals with a significantly lower IQ.

In recent years, a number of state programs have modified eligibility criteria to include individuals who have an IQ of more than 70 but who demonstrably suffer from certain identifiable impairments. These alternative eligibility standards have a variety of labels, such as "a condition similar to mental retardation (now referred to as intellectual disabilities)." States with such alternative standards look to different criteria to supplement the showing of disability based on IQ alone, factors such as impaired adaptive behavior or educational achievement (which might be based on years of schooling completed or based on skills and knowledge as measured by standardized testing).

In order to establish eligibility for DD services for an individual with FASD, it is essential to understand the eligibility requirements in the particular state. Some standards may be identified from the Web site of the state DD agency, but that may not always be possible. Establishing DD eligibility generally requires that the individual take one or more tests; sometimes a knowledgeable parent or advocate must provide information. Each DD agency has its own requirements regarding which tests must be taken. Some agencies administer the tests themselves; others require the DD applicant to obtain (and, likely, pay for) tests by outside experts. Some insurers will cover the cost of these tests. Generally a call to or meeting with officials at a local DD office will be necessary to learn what the eligibility standards are, the type of testing that is required, and who must administer the tests.

All DD agencies use some type of application form, usually available on the agency's Web site. Generally, someone assisting the applicant is required to fill out the form. The requisite forms may provide a convenient initial guide to the governing standards and procedures.

When an individual who may need DD services is involved in the criminal justice system, an effort should be made to obtain assistance from the judge or a probation official in establishing eligibility. An agency which might move slowly, or not at all, in response to a regular application may respond with alacrity if an application is endorsed by a letter or a phone call from a judge or probation official.

Many DD agencies are currently experiencing severe financial problems because of the recession. In some instances those agencies may have established a waiting list, possibly a long one, and may not be accepting any new clients in the foreseeable future.

Protection and Advocacy Programs

Congress has established a national Protection and Advocacy (P & A) System to aid individuals with disabilities and their families. There is a federally mandated P & A office in every state which offers advice and assistance on a wide range of issues including special education, community living, financial entitlements, health care, shelters and other employment and residential facilities. P & A offices can provide information about the criminal justice system, although they do not represent defendants in criminal cases. Assistance in obtaining vocational rehabilitation is provided under a related system of national offices, the Client Assistance Program (CAP). CAP and P & A agencies are often located in the same facility. Lawyers in P & A and CAP agencies can provide legal representation and other advocacy services to all people with disabilities.

Information about the location and telephone number for the P & A and CAP office in each state can be obtained at the Web site for the National Disability Rights Network, an organization of those agencies. That Web site also explains in greater detail the work of those agencies and other programs for individuals with disabilities. The link to the information about each state is at: **http://.www.napas.org/aboutus/pwd.htm**

CRIMINAL JUSTICE ISSUES

Getting in Trouble with the Law

A study for the Centers for Disease Control and Prevention (CDC) found that approximately 60% of individuals with FASD become involved in trouble with the law. For about two-thirds of those individuals, that incident occurred first (or only) when that individual was under the age of 18. Many of the offenses were relatively minor with shoplifting being the most common offense. Among the individuals with FASD in this study who got in trouble with the law, 28% had been in jail (either following arrest or as the result of a short sentence), 19 % had been held in a juvenile facility, and 4% had been in prison, a sentence typically limited to individuals serving more than a year in custody. However, because almost 80% of the subjects in this study were under 21, the study likely understates the seriousness of the problem. Since the study included comparatively few individuals over 21, it unavoidably understated the numbers of individuals with FASD who first got into trouble over that age. The small number of studied individuals who had been sentenced to jail terms stems, to some extent, from the fact that juvenile offenders are not sentenced to prison except in extraordinary circumstances [3-5].

A Canadian study of Juvenile Court defendants ordered to undergo a forensic psychiatric assessment found that 23.3% were diagnosed with an FASD while another study in a Canadian Prison confirmed an FASD diagnosis in 10% of the studied inmates. An additional 18% had evidence of significant central nervous system (CNS) deficits or brain dysfunction but no available history of prenatal exposure to confirm or rule out a diagnosis [5-7].

The high frequency with which individuals with FASD get in trouble with the law is theorized to be the result of several different factors rooted in this disability. Individuals with FASD tend to be impulsive, and will act without thought of the consequences. Shoplifting, typically of items of minor value taken for immediate personal use, exemplifies this problem. Individuals with FASD do not completely grasp the accepted norms of behavior, standards which would lead individuals without disabilities to avoid on normative grounds behavior that may be criminal in character. They may also fail to realize the serious consequences of engaging in certain forms of criminal behavior because of a lack of familiarity with the nature of criminal sanctions and because of limited ability to understand cause and effect. They may not really understand that a particular action, for example, could result in a lengthy prison term. Because individuals with FASD are eager to please others and highly suggestible, they can readily be manipulated into taking part in a criminal enterprise, often being given the most dangerous part of the undertaking with little or perhaps no understanding of what they are being asked to do and why. The consequences of this behavior may be particularly serious because of the gravity of the offenses (e.g. drug trafficking). It also is possible that the more sophisticated criminals apprehended may quickly make a deal for a light sentence leaving the major blame, and sentence, for their colleague with a disability. This sort of plea agreement is not merely unjust to the defendant with FASD; it also results in the most dangerous offender quickly getting out on the streets to commit more crimes [5].

Although the offenses committed by individuals with FASD vary widely, they often are associated with the underlying cognitive and behavioral problems. A telltale sign of FASD would be an inexplicably inept crime, as occurred with a patient of the Fetal Alcohol and Drug Unit who stole a piece of jewelry from a neighbor and then wore it to the victim's house a few days later.

As the Canadian Bar Association has pointed out, "The criminal justice system is based on normative assumptions that a person acts in a voluntary manner, makes informed choices with respect to the decision to commit crimes, and learns from their own behavior and the behavior of others….These normative assumptions and the sentencing principles such as specific and general deterrence are not valid for those with FASD…." [5].

Getting in trouble with the law is a danger, but it also can be an opportunity. This may be the only time an individual with FASD—particularly an adult--is in contact with a government agency that might have a genuine interest in helping that individual obtain needed services and assistance. Officials in the criminal justice system may be uniquely able to arrange for services and assistance from federal, state and local agencies. Parents and advocates need to encourage court officials to help in this way, stressing that they may have access and leverage that the parents do not. Lawyers representing a defendant with FASD can act as effective advocates, arguing that getting that assistance will advance the court's interest in preventing recidivism. The significant respect most individuals with FASD have for authority figures can also be turned to a good purpose. A defendant with FASD might be particularly responsive to admonitions and supervision by a judge, who may be able to guide the defendant's actions—and encourage him or her—in a way that the parents or others could not.

On the other hand, getting in trouble with the law can be extremely destructive. If a defendant with FASD is incarcerated for a long period of time, the infrastructure that sustained him or her prior to the conviction may be destroyed and cause more psychological damage. Individuals with FASD are particularly likely to be victimized while incarcerated, with psychological consequences that may significantly impair their future behavior. At times the inability of these individuals to avoid socially inappropriate forms of behavior may lead to assaults which, in turn, may prompt prison officials to place the individuals in solitary confinement for their own protection, causing even more psychological harm. Individuals with FASD who are sent to jail or prison may, when released, return to the community more impaired and dysfunctional than they were when initially incarcerated [8].

There is enormous variation in the degree to which lawyers, prosecutors, judges, probation officers and other court officials know about FASD, or understand how it might have affected the past conduct of an individual or could impact his or her future behavior. Obtaining the right treatment of a defendant with FASD—and avoiding recidivism—may depend, to a significant degree, on the ability of an advocate (e.g., a lawyer dealing with a judge, or a parent talking to a lawyer or police officer) to offer a convincing explanation of FASD and its connection to involvement in trouble with the law [8, 9].

The United States Department of Health and Human Services (USDHHS) has published a number of credible specific accounts of these issues and the best ways of dealing with defendants with FASD. Those publications can be of considerable value in persuading officials in the criminal justice system to recognize FASD as a very real, distinct and important disability. Those valuable accounts include "Fetal Alcohol Spectrum Disorders and Juvenile Justice: How Professionals Can Make A Difference," "Fetal Alcohol Spectrum Disorders: When Your Child Faces the Juvenile Justice System", and "Fetal Alcohol Spectrum Disorders and The Criminal Justice System." They are available at: <u>http://www.fasdcenter.samhsa.gov/grabGo/factSheets.cfm</u>

Dealing with Attorneys

One of the recurring problems that arises when an individual with FASD gets in trouble with the law is the often difficult relationship between that individual's parents and the individual's attorney. Unless an effective, cooperative relationship can be established, there is little likelihood that the criminal justice system will deal appropriately with the defendant.

Attorneys are the key method of presenting information and arguments to the court system, of identifying or developing the kind of information the court system cares about, and putting it in a form that will be effective. Most attorneys, however, do not know anything about FASD: what it is, how to detect it, or why it might be relevant to a criminal case. In practice, only family members or close family friends usually are aware that a defendant has or may have FASD, are able to see a connection between FASD and the alleged criminal conduct, and can articulate the likely consequences of possible sentences (or plea agreements) for the defendant. The attorney representing the defendant with FASD needs information and advice from the defendant's parents or other family members, and those family members are often exceedingly anxious to provide that assistance [2].

Most attorneys, however, are wary of taking advice about legal tactics from family members. Time and again defense attorneys have had to fend off ill considered advice or misinformation from a defendant's family. The parents of even guilty defendants routinely tell the attorney that their child is innocent or, at the least, misunderstood. This may be the case for a defendant with FASD, but defense attorneys instinctively shun such advice and assistance. It is common for the parents of a defendant with FASD, acting in what they perceive to be the best interests of their child, to so offend or annoy the attorney that the lawyer either resigns or refuses to talk further with the parents. The challenge then is for family members or other advocates to find a way to overcome this barrier to helping the defendant's attorney understand FASD and its relevance.

Several steps by parents can enhance the likelihood of a constructive relationship with the attorney representing their child or adult offspring. First, collect relevant documents in order to provide the attorney with confirmation of the life-long disability. The lawyer will be more persuaded by documents revealing some atypical history than by pleading phone calls from a parent. The lawyer, moreover, needs documents to persuade a prosecutor to accept a more favorable plea agreement, or to obtain a better sentence; the lawyer cannot rely on stories or explanations that he or she has heard from the defendant's parents. The key documents to provide to the attorney would be (a) an FASD diagnostic report, (b) special education or other illuminating school records, (c) social welfare agency records indicating that the defendant has some type of cognitive problem, and (d) birth records indicating that the mother was intoxicated at the time of the birth or that the baby was impaired in some way. Copies of these materials should be provided to the lawyer in a notebook or folder, with the originals retained.

Second, it is important to recognize that the lawyer, by training, does not want non-lawyer family members and friends deciding legal tactics. Provide all relevant documents or other information to the attorney, but don't offer direction to the lawyer as to how to use it. Remind the attorney that the parents are willing to work cooperatively with probation officials or the court to support a supervision plan designed for a defendant with FASD.

Juvenile Offenders

Unlike the adult criminal justice system, the juvenile justice system is generally focused on steps to prevent future offenses and to assist a juvenile offender, rather than trying to inflict punishment. Juvenile court officials will generally be more willing to respond to suggestions from parents and family members about the steps that should be taken in dealing with a juvenile offender. If a child with FASD becomes involved with the criminal justice system, the parents should be aggressive in identifying the programs and services the child needs—including programs and services that will continue into adulthood. They should press the juvenile court officials for help in establishing eligibility for those programs and services [10].

The methods that will be effective in preventing recidivism by children with FASD will often be significantly different than the approaches that would work best for children who do not have this disability. Judges, attorneys and probation officials should be alerted to the nature of the disability, and urged to consider alternative corrective methods. Many of the considerations relevant to adult defendants will also be applicable to juvenile defendants. However, because the juvenile justice system is, in comparison with the adult criminal justice system, more oriented towards treatment than punishment, it will at times make sense for juvenile justice officials to try using such alternative approaches for a child suspected of having FASD, without insisting on or waiting for a formal diagnosis. The concept is "treat, as if" the individual had been diagnosed. If the alternative strategies prove to be ineffective, a new approach can be employed. Juvenile probation officials in particular need to be trained to recognize, and respond appropriately to, FASD.

One important factor that should be considered in dealing with juvenile defendants is that juveniles with FASD have great difficulty making appropriate friends, since they often lack key social skills. Cut off from developing friendships with most of their peers, adolescents or young adults with FASD may by default associate with other juveniles with behavioral problems. Or, more sophisticated, non-disabled peers may "befriend" them in an effort to exploit them. Individuals with this disability are insufficiently socially skilled to discern when they are being "used" and can be drawn into new law-violation in a futile attempt to follow the directions of their "friends". An approach, proposed but not published by Streissguth, to assist these young people in developing relationships with pro-social peers and, also, to avoid recidivism involves identifying a peer advocate or mentor (either volunteer or paid) who can provide companionship for a juvenile with FASD. Churches, volunteer groups, school counselors who can identify potential student volunteers, college student employment offices are all possible sources for these mentors. They can also provide tutoring and educational support.

Contingency management techniques may be effective tools to induce juveniles with FASD who have been in trouble with the law to act in a more constructive manner. Contingency management provides small material inducements for good behavior, such as providing clean drug tests or regular school attendance. Gift cards for coffeehouses, bookstores, department stores, grocery stores and other, similar incentives have all been utilized in drug treatment programs and in court. These techniques have proven to be highly effective and could be used to reinforce compliance with probation requirements [11].

Culpability under the Law

Whether FASD may support a defense of diminished capacity depends on the state law standard for that defense, and on the nature of the underlying offense. Individuals with FASD are impulsive, and have difficulty thinking ahead to plan and organize their activities. The existence of this disability could be highly relevant to whether a defendant had premeditated an act, or was actually innocent of an act which would have required significant planning and preparation. In most cases these issues are not litigated at trial. Rather, the attorney for the defendant relies on this type of information and legal reasoning to negotiate a more favorable plea agreement.

Sexual Offenses

One of the most difficult problems arises when adults with FASD have sexual contact with non-disabled individuals under the age of 18. The appropriate legal response to such situations should take into account the fact that individuals with FASD often function—in terms of their understanding, maturity and abilities—at a level far below their chronological age. In one study a group of individuals with FASD who had an average age of 17 years were functioning at an average age of only 7 years. It would not be surprising if a 28 year old individual with FASD was functioning at the level of a child of less than 18 [2,3].

In evaluating claims of unlawful sexual contact, the competence and understanding of the individuals involved is ordinarily, and properly, a major consideration. Individuals are regularly prosecuted for having sexual contact with someone who, despite a chronological age of more than 18, was too impaired to give meaningful consent to sexual activity. State law generally treats adults with such serious impairments in the same way it protects minors. The cognitive impairments caused by FASD, like intellectual disabilities, may preclude the requisite consent. Where the other party to the sexual contact knew that a disabled adult lacked the ability to provide such consent, criminal charges have been filed, despite the fact that the victim with FASD was over 18 [12].

Most prosecutors would not file charges of sexual contact with a minor against an individual who was the same age of the victim. Some state statutes do not apply in such cases. Even if they did, there would be no grounds for determining on the basis of age which of the 15 year old participants was the victim and which should be charged with a crime. Where an individual with FASD is sufficiently impaired that he or she would be treated like a child if there were sexual contact with an adult, it seems inappropriate to treat that individual as an offender for having sexual contact with a minor whose maturity level was as great, or greater, than the individual with a disability.

False Confessions

Individuals with FASD, because of their disability, are likely to confess to crimes which they did not commit, or crimes which did not even occur. There are several reported court decisions in which this occurred, and more cases which are unreported. This problem occurs in part because individuals with FASD are very suggestible as well as extremely anxious to please interrogators or other authority figures. They may confuse events which actually occurred with stories recounted to them by the police or others. Even when an individual with FASD does understand that the confession he or she is being asked to sign is not correct, he or she may do so with the naïve misunderstanding, perhaps fostered by the police, that there will be no consequences to the confession. Those two problems are interconnected; a non-disabled person who wanted to please a police officer, but was mindful of the consequences, might be exceptionally polite to a police officer, but would not confess to a crime that he or she did not commit. Similarly, a person who did not have FASD would not believe a police officer's assurance that he or she could just go home without any further consequences after confessing to a serious crime [13].

This situation is illustrated with painful clarity by the prosecution of Gabriel B., who was diagnosed as a teenager with FASD. Mr. B, then 18 years, pled guilty to, and was convicted of, a serious arson at his high school in Washington state. A state psychiatric hospital subsequently examined him and concluded, in part because he seemed unwilling to acknowledge his culpability, that he was a threat to the community. Two years after B.'s conviction, another individual came forward and confessed to the crime, exhibiting knowledge of events that only the arsonist could have had. Mr. B. was exonerated; prosecutors admitted that they had made a mistake, dropped the charges, and asked the court to overturn his conviction. The transcript of the police interrogation made crystal clear that, when asked about the offense, Mr. B. was entirely unable to describe the manner or location in which the fire had been started; only when the police repeatedly corrected his mistaken descriptions did B. finally give the correct answers. The police officers seemed to have been oblivious to the fact that—in a taped interview—they were feeding the answers to the suspect. The officers seemed more motivated by a desire to be helpful to a perpetrator they perceived as having a poor memory than to obtain a confession from him at all costs. Mr. B. later explained that he knew at the time that he had not started the fire, but told the police what they wanted to hear so he could go home as he had been promised.

Competence to Stand Trial

The competency of a defendant with FASD to stand trial, and to assist with his or her own defense, is not simply a matter of IQ. Individuals with FASD generally function at a level below that typical of others with the same IQ. Assessment of this issue should focus, not merely on general competency, but on three problems likely to affect a defendant with FASD:

First, does the defendant have a clear enough grasp of the distinction between reality and fiction that he or she can assist counsel in evaluating and responding to testimony or argument about what occurred?

Second, does the defendant have a sufficient grasp of cause and effect that he or she understands the effect of actions that he or she wants the attorney to take?

Third, does the defendant understand what is taking place in the courtroom? For a defendant with FASD to understand what is transpiring during the hearing and the implications, the court may need to take regular recesses to allow for "interpretive" assistance to be provided to the defendant. An effective "interpreter" might be a Special Education teacher or other experts who have been trained in communicating with the cognitively disabled [8, 14].

Sentencing

The relevance of a diagnosis of FASD to sentencing, and to plea bargaining, depends at the outset on the nature and elements of state sentencing statutes. As a practical matter, FASD might be very relevant to sentencing:

a) Individuals with FASD may be less culpable under state standards. They may not fully understand the relevant norms of conduct; ignorance of the law may not be a defense, but an incomplete ability to understand the standards of conduct bears on culpability. Some offenses by individuals with FASD may be the result of impulsive behavior, over which the offender had less control than non-disabled defendants.

b) The existence of FASD may be important in determining what role a defendant played in an offense. Individuals with FASD are often manipulated by sophisticated criminals into taking part in offenses they may not understand, fully or at all. They may also, when questioned by investigators, accept responsibility for performing a more active role in the offense than actually occurred. They may believe this will ingratiate them with their codefendants or hide their disability from the questioner.

c) The existence of FASD may be critical in designing a sentence or sentencing alternative that will reduce the risk of recidivism, and will avoid causing far greater harm to a defendant with FASD than would be inflicted on a non-disabled defendant. Sentencing a defendant with FASD to prison will not teach the defendant a lesson likely to deter future offenses if the defendant does not fully understand why he or she has been incarcerated.

The Canadian Bar Association has observed that traditional "sentencing options available to courts are often ineffective in changing the behavior of those with FASD…" and that incarceration may serve "…no rehabilitative or deterrent purpose…. [T]hose with FASD [are] judged on a standard that they are incapable of meeting because of their disability" [5].

Sentencing an individual with FASD to jail or prison can be destructive and counterproductive. These individuals usually have considerable difficulty functioning competently in society; they typically depend on a variety of support structures—such as sheltered housing, a solicitous landlord, occasional work for an understanding employer, a network of friends and relatives—to manage from day to day, to sleep in a safe place and to get enough to eat. A term of incarceration can destroy those support structures; once established arrangements may be impossible to recreate, helpful individuals may move on, move away, or refuse to deal with a former inmate. Lacking that previous assistance, the offender with FASD may be more likely to end up living on the streets, or falling under the sway of manipulative offenders [8,15,16].

The latter danger is particularly great because imprisonment places a highly credulous individual with the disability into close and repeated contact with hardened offenders whom the individual with FASD may come to regard as his friends, and who will use that supposed friendship to lure the individual into criminal schemes. In this respect, placing an individual with FASD—whose maturity level may be 12 or 14— in a jail or prison is like imprisoning a child of that age, something that the law absolutely forbids and that no sensible judge would ever consider doing. One possible way to argue against such incarceration would be to arrange for a full battery of testing to assess the level of maturity of a defendant and point to state laws setting the minimum age of persons who can be held with the adult population in a penal facility [8].

Individuals with FASD are extremely impressionable. They are prone to modeling themselves on those with whom they have contact and to replicating behavior—including criminal behavior—that they see, hear about, or experience. Because of their impairments, individuals with FASD would be very vulnerable to physical and sexual abuse in prison, resulting in harms that could translate into further behavioral deterioration upon release. Placing an individual with FASD in an institution in which many of the contacts will be with hardened criminals runs a substantial risk that the individual will pose a greater danger to society after incarceration than before. That danger is all the greater if the individual develops relationships with sophisticated criminals with whom he might be in contact after his release. As stated previously, individuals with FASD can often be manipulated by others to engage in illegal conduct [8].

Probation and Parole

Individuals with FASD often fare poorly on probation or parole if the supervising official does not understand and fails to take into account the disability.

Parolees and probationers with FASD generally have great difficulty keeping their appointments with the supervising officer, or with others such as drug testing agencies. That problem stems not from an unwillingness to meet these obligations, but from a significant incapacity to remember these obligations or to manage time in a way that permits the individual to appear as directed. Punishing these individuals for their inability to keep these appointments is generally pointless; fear of punishment will not eliminate the disability that prevents an individual from complying. The more appropriate and effective method for dealing with this problem is for the supervising officer or others to provide reminders to the individual of what he or she is supposed to do and when [15,16].

Similarly, individuals with FASD often have difficulty complying with other conditions of probation or parole because they simply do not understand, or remember, what they have been directed—and forbidden—to do. Here, too, repeated reminders, including written lists that an individual (and family members or other advocates) can keep and review regularly, can be helpful.

Individuals with FASD generally benefit from a greater and more prolonged period of supervision, on probation or on parole, than might ordinarily be provided to or warranted for other defendants. These individuals have significant ongoing need for structure, guidance, and monitoring. Community based supervision with the greatest possible structure and oversight often proves to be the most effective approach and the one that best prevents reoffending. If electronic monitoring is available, this can be a highly useful component of a supervision plan. Continuing, long term drug testing can be a valuable reminder for individuals with memory impairment, and in fact can be actively sought and depended upon by those with FASD. Appointment reminders, explicit directions, concrete language, repetition of expected behaviors and flexibility in responding to violations can all yield greater supervision success [17].

RELEVANT SOCIAL AND FAMILY ISSUES

Addiction

Studies show that more than 30% of those with FASD have problems with addiction. This common problem is often the cause for their involvement in trouble with the law. The disposition of their case may involve referral to a drug treatment program as well as opting into a Drug Court program [3,18]. However, the approaches to drug treatment that are most effective for individuals with FASD differ significantly from the methods that might be used for other clients. Traditional talk therapy tends to be ineffective for individuals with FASD, who are generally not as introspective as others. Group meetings can be overwhelming because it is often difficult for the individual with FASD to fathom all the information and emotion that is being shared in the group. Traditional 12-step programs such as Alcoholics Anonymous (AA) require a degree of insight and writing skill that individuals with FASD often do not possess. To be successful in AA, someone with FASD will often need a level of support from an advocate far beyond that which an AA sponsor generally offers. Treatment staff will work more effectively with the individual with FASD if they have participated in training to help them understand the limitations and strengths of those with this disability.

Useful strategies include close, one to one supervision by a drug counselor who can simplify treatment goals, involve the family in the treatment plan, find a peer advocate for the individual and intercede on the individual's behalf with the treatment program's participants and staff. A peer advocate might be a family member, a friend, or a member of a church community. Since those with FASD generally respond well to the authority of a court, a judge can play a significant role in providing ongoing positive support of treatment goals. Drug testing, when ordered, is helpful since it is a concrete reminder of the court's requirement of abstinence. Many individuals with FASD request such testing because it provides a very practical and immediate incentive to avoid drug use. More frequent drug testing for a longer period of time will usually be the best tactic. Relapse Prevention techniques for those with FASD need to be modified to be effective in helping the individual maintain sobriety. Repetition, continuing reinforcement, concrete concepts and language are all helpful. In a residential drug treatment program the rules for patients will likely have to be taught and re-taught [17].

The SAMHSA FASD Center for Excellence has developed a FASD curriculum for addiction professionals and a training manual for those working in the addiction treatment field. They are available at: http://www.fasdcenter.samhsa.gov/educationTraining/courses/CapCurriculum/competency5/professional5.cfm and http://ncadistore.samhsa.gov/catalog/productDetails.aspx?ProductID=17776

Vulnerable Victims

The disabilities of individuals with FASD, both as children and as adults, render them easy prey for criminal conduct. They are likely to accept criminal abuse, or to refrain from complaining to authorities, because they do not fully understand the inappropriateness of the treatment, or because they want to avoid displeasing the offender. A child with FASD might easily fail to grasp the importance of parental admonitions against sexual contacts with adults, and might fail to recognize the dangerousness of a situation. Some 72% of adolescents and adults with FASD have been physically or sexually abused [3,13].

Prosecuting an offender for victimizing an individual with FASD may be complicated by the difficulties of preparing and relying on testimony from the victim. As witnesses, as in other aspects of their lives, individuals with FASD are both credulous and very eager to please. A victim-witness with FASD may believe that the correct response to a question must be whatever answer the questioner may appear to want, whether or not the response is factually true. Thus police and prosecutors must exercise greater care in interviewing these victims, taking pains not to lead them in any particular direction but, rather, inducing them to tell their own stories [12].

Loss of Parental Rights

Most if not all states have statutes under which authorities can bring some form of lawsuit to terminate the parental rights of parents who are unable to care for their children. The standards under which parental rights can be terminated by a court vary to some degree. If the courts terminate the parental rights of the individual or individuals with parental rights, the child may then be sent to foster care or freed for adoption.

In proceedings to terminate parental rights, FASD may be relevant in either or both of two different ways. First, if the parent or parents involved have FASD, the court may regard that as evidence of—or an explanation of—their inability to care for the child. Second, if the child in question has FASD, the court may regard that as demonstrating that the child has special needs which require a heightened level of parenting skills. State court decisions regarding these problems are one of the largest categories of judicial opinions dealing with FASD.

There is, however, no distinct legal issue applicable in this context to parents or children with FASD. Rather, FASD is simply a factual circumstance which may affect the abilities of the parent or parents or the level of needs of the child. FASD thus represents the source of certain types of practical problems. Those problems often have significant and effective practical solutions.

There are a number of programs and a substantial body of experience which courts and attorneys should look to in dealing with children with FASD. These children can be more challenging to raise; they have special needs, and the best ways of coping with those needs are often far from obvious. Parents of children with FASD should not forfeit their parental rights simply because they cannot personally devise on their own all the creative approaches and strategies that clinicians and other parents have developed.

Similarly, although some parents with FASD may experience difficulty raising a non-disabled child, there is a similar body of experience regarding how to assist and guide those parents in caring for their children. The Parent-Child Assistance Program (P-CAP), which began in Washington State and has been replicated in a number of other states and many sites in Canada, provides assistance to these parents with disabilities. There are helpful articles to be found on the SAMHSA FASD Center for Excellence Web site: **http://www.fasdcenter.samhsa.gov/** and on the Fetal Alcohol and Drug Unit Web site: **http://depts.washington.edu/fadu/** (At this Web site, click on P-CAP).

Guardianship

In some states it is possible for a parent or a state agency (such as the Division of Developmental Disabilities) to be named the guardian of an adult child with FASD. Whether that is the right thing for a parent to do, or even attempt to do, is a difficult question. Depending on state law, a guardian might be able to make medical decisions, manage funds, or have the right to be involved in the decision-making in a criminal proceeding. On the other hand, being placed under the supervision of a guardian could offend or demoralize some individuals. Parents and family-members are often concerned as to a guardian's liability for the actions of the individual with FASD; whether and when that might be the case would vary with state law. In assessing the right choice, the degree to which the individual with FASD is disabled would undoubtedly be a major consideration. The laws as to guardianship differ from state to state.

Recently Illinois state law was modified to add FASD to the list of the conditions that would warrant creating a guardianship. That statute expanded the definition of "disabled person," for whom guardianship can be ordered, to include a person who "is diagnosed with fetal alcohol syndrome or fetal alcohol effects" [19].

New Directions for Research

Given the complex interplay among law, FASD, and public policy, there are several areas in which future research can have a major impact on the lives of individuals with FASD.

First, it would be very important if prevalence studies could identify particular subpopulations within which the incidence of FASD is particularly high. Because diagnosing FASD is quite expensive, it may not be cost effective for a school, court, or other agency to screen for and seek to diagnose FASD so long as those with this disability may be only a small proportion of the clients served. Finding and dealing more effectively with such a small fraction of the population served will have only a very modest impact on the agency's ability to carry out its mission. Thus for many agencies screening for and detecting FASD may well be a fairly low priority. However, if the group served by a particular agency could be shown to have an FASD incidence of 10-20% or more, then the practical impact of identifying those with this disability will be far greater. (Recent studies of the adolescents in juvenile courts in Colorado and Minnesota found a prevalence rate of 14%-16% while a prevalence rate of 23% was found in a population of juvenile offenders court-referred for a psychiatric evaluation in British Columbia). A demonstrably high rate of incidence of FASD would tend to drive public policy. There is little reliable information about the comparative level of FASD among various population groups or agency clientele. It seems sensible to look in particular at the incidence level among groups in need of relevant social services—e.g., juvenile defendants, students in special education, or the homeless—or within a population among whom the level of alcohol abuse is high.

Second, research is needed to validate anecdotal information that individuals with FASD function at a higher level after the age of 30 than they do at 18 or 25. Although those anecdotes are certainly not conclusive, the way in which agencies deal with individuals with FASD would be far different if there was evidence that after the age of 30 the ability of those individuals to function in society improved significantly. We need to know what types of skills and behaviors (if any) improve after that age, whether this improvement is more common among some subgroup of individuals with FASD, and what techniques or environmental factors appear to facilitate that improvement.

Third, among the individuals with FASD who get in trouble with the law, a very small fraction commit sexual offenses. Although there is no evidence that the level of such offenses is higher among these individuals than within the general population, the occurrence of these offenses causes very serious harm, and also has serious consequences for the offender. Those harms and consequences could be prevented to some degree if there were an understanding of the phenomenon and its possible causes.

REFERENCES

[1]   Streissguth AP. Fetal alcohol syndrome: A guide for families and communities. Baltimore: Paul H. Brookes Publishing Company; 1997.

[2]   Streissguth AP, Barr HM, Kogan JK, Bookstein FL. Secondary disabilities in people with FAS and FAE. In: Streissguth AP, Kanter J, editors. The Challenge of Fetal Alcohol Syndrome: Overcoming Secondary Disabilities. Seattle: University of Washington; 1997.

[3]   Streissguth AP, Barr H, Kogan J, Bookstein FL. Understanding the Occurrence of Secondary Disabilities in Clients with Fetal Alcohol Syndrome (FAS) and Fetal Alcohol Effects (FAE). Final Report to the Centers for Disease Control and Prevention. Grant #R04/CCR008515. Seattle: University of Washington School of Medicine; 1996.

[4]   LaDue R, Dunne T. Legal issues and the Fetal Alcohol Syndrome. The FEN Pen Fall 1995; 6-7.

[5]   Canadian Bar Association, Resolution 10-02-A, Fetal Alcohol Spectrum Disorder in the Criminal Justice System, passed August 14-15, 2010.

[6]   Conry JL, Fast DK, Loock CA. Youth in the criminal justice; identifying FAS and other developmental disabilities. Vancouver BC: Final Report to the Ministry of the Attorney General 1997.

[7]   MacPherson P, Chudley AE. FASD screening and estimating incidence in an adult correctional population. Presented at the 2nd International Conference on Fetal Alcohol Spectrum Disorders, Victoria, BC, March 7-10, 2007.

[8]   R. v. Harper, 2009 YKTC 18. Territorial Court of Yukon, His Honour Judge Heino Lilles.

[9]   Cox LV, Clairmont D, Cox S. Knowledge and attitudes of criminal justice professionals in relation to fetal alcohol spectrum disorder. Can J Clin Pharmacol 2008; 15; e306-e313.

[10]   LaDue R, Dunne T. Issues in the legal realm: Fetal Alcohol Syndrome and the decision to decline or retain. The FEN Pen Spring 1996; 2-6.

[11]   Prendergast M, Podus D, Finney J, Greenwell, L, Roll, J. Contingency management for treatment of substance use disorders: A meta-analysis. Addiction. 2006; 101: 1546-1560.

[12]   U.S. v Root, 2009. U.S. District Court, District of Colorado, Hon. John L. Kane

[13]   Kelly KA. The victimization of individuals with Fetal Alcohol Syndrome/Fetal Alcohol Effects. TASH Connections Aug/Sept 2003; 29-30.

[14]   LaDue R, Dunne T. Capacity concerns and Fetal Alcohol Syndrome. The FEN Pen Winter 1996; 2-3.

[15]   LaDue R, Dunne T. Fetal Alcohol Syndrome: Implications for sentencing in the criminal justice system. The FEN Pen Fall 1996; 2-3.

[16]   LaDue R, Dunne T. Fetal Alcohol Syndrome: Implications for sentencing in the criminal justice system. The FEN Pen Spring 1997; 2-3.

[17]   U.S. Department of Health and Human Services, Substance Abuse and Health Services Administration, Center for Substance Abuse Prevention. Fetal Alcohol Spectrum Disorders: curriculum for addiction professionals, Level 2, Facilitator's manual. 2007.

[18]   Marlatt GA, Parks GA, Kelly KA. Monograph Series 9 National Drug Court Institute. Quality improvement for drug court: Evidence-Based Practices. National Drug Court Institute 2008; 23-32.

[19]   Illinois Compiled Statutes, ch. 775, section 5/11a-2.

CHAPTER 8

Families Living with FASD: Up Close and Personal

Kathleen T. Mitchell[1,*] and Mary DeJoseph[2]

[1]*National Organization on Fetal Alcohol Syndrome 1200 Eton Court, NW, Third Floor, Washington, DC 20007; USA and* [2]*UMDNJ-NJMS, New Jersey FASD Education and Research Center, Newark, NJ*

> *"Never doubt that a small group of thoughtful, committed citizens can change the world; indeed it's the only thing that ever has"*
>
> **Margaret Mead**

Abstract: This chapter contains a series of unedited stories from family members and people affected by prenatal alcohol exposure. There is an entire spectrum of family needs, just as there is a spectrum of effects. All families share the grief of lost dreams for their children and the shocking transition to a whole new journey in parenting. All families are stretched beyond expectation emotionally, mentally, spiritually, and financially. Health, marital, and safety challenges are common. The chapter includes contributions from both adoptive and birth families, mothers and a father, affected people and siblings, with and without alcoholism in the family.

INTRODUCTION

Raising a child with Fetal Alcohol Spectrum Disorders (FASD) can be both challenging and rewarding. Today, there are FASD family support groups scattered across the United States and on-line. Many states have trained FASD Coordinators and diagnostic centers. The National Organization on Fetal Alcohol Syndrome (NOFAS) and other agencies provide information, support, and advocacy to families, healthcare professionals, educators and policy makers. There is an abundance of materials and information available for both parents and public health agencies (See suggested readings at the end of this chapter). Family centered care should remain at the heart of diagnosis, management and follow-up for affected individuals and their families.

Receiving a diagnosis of an FASD is never easy for families. Adoptive families may have a different response than birth families do. Adoptive or foster parents may experience anger as their first emotion. Their anger is often towards the birth mother initially. Later they may direct their anger towards the adoption or foster care agency for the lack of disclosure. Birth families, however, experience initial shame and remorse. Recognizing that your child lives with a disability because you drank during pregnancy is a sad realization that often is compounded by late diagnosis for the child. The diagnosis of an FASD will likely trigger a period of grief for all families, both adoptive and birth. Forgiveness is an important step in healing and moving forward.

Both alcoholism and FASD remain highly stigmatized disorders. Being a birth mother is like being branded with a *Scarlet Letter (I'm a Bad Mother)* that both she and her family must carry for the rest of their lives. Long after recovery from alcoholism, mothers and their families face continuing shame and stigma from neighbors, children's teachers and friends, extended family members, physicians, etc. Stigma is a major issue and causes problems on many levels. Faced with the prospect of stigma, women who drink during pregnancy may deny they have a problem and be reluctant to pursue a diagnosis. Some physicians are reluctant to diagnose an FASD because of the labeling and stigma that ensues for mothers and children. Stigma and shame can lead to relapse, escalation in drinking, and medical complications.

One does not have to be an alcoholic to give birth to a child with effects from drinking while pregnant, but it is clearly understood that women with addictive disorders, such as alcoholism, are the highest risk group for having children with an FASD. Alcoholism should be viewed as a progressive disease and should be diagnosed and treated

---

*Address correspondence to Kathleen T. Mitchell:** National Organization on Fetal Alcohol Syndrome 1200 Eton Court, NW, Third Floor, Washington, DC 20007, USA; E-mail: Mitchell@nofas.org

Susan A. Adubato and Deborah E. Cohen (Eds)

within a disease management and recovery model, but must consider general societal attitudes and beliefs towards drinking. This would reduce stigma and thereby increase the likelihood of preventing FASD. Many addicts have themselves been exposed to alcohol prenatally; identification of these adults in our systems of care could result in a reduction in recidivism and obtaining appropriate support and services. Whether or not alcohol is identified as the mother's primary substance of abuse, assessment and screening should include asking questions about amounts and frequency of alcohol use, and should explore the possibility of prenatal alcohol exposure in the adult client and her pregnancies. Knowing that an adult client has been exposed to alcohol prenatally, or who may have prenatally exposed their children to alcohol would be important information to make appropriate referrals and to the on-going treatment planning process. Comprehensive, long-term case management for both the mother, effected child (ren), and other family members should be considered [1,2]. A platform that includes research and implementation is needed to inform the broader health care and educational system about addiction and FASD [3-5].

To address the issues of stigma, trauma and to support birth families, the NOFAS Circle of Hope (COH) was formed in 2004 and in 2005 the Substance Abuse and Mental Health Services Administration (SAMHSA) FASD Center for Excellence funded NOFAS to support the Circle of Hope-Birth Mothers Network (COH-BMN). The COH-BMN is an international FASD birth mom peer mentoring network. There are regional COH-BMN coordinators located throughout the United States. The coordinators are available to connect with and support birth mothers who have used alcohol during pregnancy and/or have a child (ren) with FASD. Its mission is "to increase understanding and support and strengthen recovery for women who drank during their pregnancy(s), and their families." The goals are to improve and strengthen the lives of birth families, provide peer support for birth families, and decrease the stigma, blame, and shame that birth families may experience. The COH-BMN accomplishes its mission and goals by educating agencies that serve high-risk women, educating policymakers and agency directors. The COH-BMN speakers' bureau provides trained speakers who are available to provide personal testimony and training on FASD. All of these activities support the values guiding the network which are confidentiality, honesty and integrity of all members, reducing the stigma of FASD, and assuring a safe environment for women. The COH-BMN seeks to create momentum and cohesiveness for national action to prevent FASD. To contact the Circle of Hope Birth Mothers Network (COH-BMN) go to http://www.nofas.org/coh/default.aspx

HERE ARE OUR STOIRES

A Survivor from the Beginning: An Adult's Story of Living With Fetal Alcohol Syndrome

I'm 50 years old and I live in Fort Lee, New Jersey. I've rented a room in the home of an 87 year old woman who is an angel. She's like a grandma to me. I've lived there for about 7 years and we have really gotten to love each other; I'm there for her and she's there for me. Her age is really starting to catch up with her- she's had some serious falls. Now I do all the food shopping, driving, giving her medicine and calling to remind her when to take it.

I work at a CVS as a cashier and it is really hard and overwhelming for me. I work 35 hours a week so I can keep my benefits. I've moved from a bigger store to a smaller one and I hope it helps, because I'm not sure how much longer I can hang in there. Some days I don't want to do it anymore, but I don't have a choice. Maybe I could qualify for disability, but I don't know how to do that.

I am one of 4 children- mom had the first three a year apart, then 7 years later she had me. She was 31 years old when she had me. I've gotten bits and pieces of the story- her alcoholism got much worse during the 7 years before she had me. She definitely drank while she was pregnant with me. My brother and sisters are fine. The FAS made me different. I was born tiny and premature. My doctors and family thought I wasn't going to make it. I guess I was a survivor from the very start! I watched my mom turn to skin and bones, drinking all the time and too drunk to get out of bed. Her alcoholism was our big family secret. She died when I was 11 and she was 42.

My mom was never really involved with me. My sister raised me. I remember another angel in my life: my brother's wife. She always included me in their family when I was growing up. She shared her home, her new baby, and her weekends with me. She taught me how to drive and took me on summer vacations. She died of cancer when she was only 29 years old.

School was very hard for me; I remember thinking how hard I had to focus all the time. I didn't have any friends; it was very lonely. I still tend to isolate. My worst subjects were math and history. Even today at work, if there is any counting to do, I have to use a calculator. I can't get a pharmacy certification, because there's a lot of math on the test and the pressure is too overwhelming.

I remember when I finished high school everyone was talking about where they were going and what they were doing next. I didn't have all those plans. I spent all of high school trying to survive every day. I didn't think about planning ahead. At my graduation, I suddenly thought "Oh my God, what do I do now?" My family wanted me to go to business school so of course I did what they expected of me. They had high expectations of me. I was terrified of disappointing them. I went to a business college in Manhattan for about half a year. Then I realized it couldn't work and I walked out. I still got up every day and left the house and pretended as if I were going to school. Then I just walked around or sat somewhere all day. They found out and I got my first job.

I've always had trouble with keeping jobs, but I had that first job for 6 yrs. A good friend of my dad's hired me as a file clerk at an insurance company. It was good until they started promoting me. When they made me a typist, I hit another wall because I couldn't spell and there was a lot of pressure. I quit before I was fired.

When my father retired, he was planning on remarrying and moving to the Catskills. He said I could stay on at our home and try to make it on my own. I had grown up most of my life in Washington Heights, Manhattan; I figured I could stay and rent out some rooms and take care of myself. Some really weird and scary people stayed with me. One was even in my room in the middle of the night. I figured that was enough of that.

My brother invited me to come and stay with him in New Jersey and find a job. I lived there for a couple years and found some jobs here and there in retail and a drug store. A lot of people helped me with jobs, but I didn't really know what I wanted, and I had no idea about the FAS. I just knew something was different, something was wrong with me. At this point, I started to drink. I really wanted to die, but I was afraid to die. At this point, I got help and started to see a therapist. Slowly and gently she helped me to realize that I am from an alcoholic family. I got clear that my mom drank while she was pregnant. I stopped drinking and have been going to the 12 Step program Al-Anon for 17 years. I go to 3 meetings a week and retreat twice a year. I love it there and have lots of friends.

After that, I lived with my sister and her husband. When they were getting ready to move, I couldn't move with them. I thought maybe getting a medical diagnosis of FAS would help me get some support. I made a lot of phone calls and talked to (Dr.) Ann Wilson at The Arc of New Jersey. I went for all the FAS testing at Dr. Susan's clinic (the Northern NJ FAS Diagnostic Center at UMDNJ-New Jersey Medical School); she is another angel who is always there for me. The testing was really hard, but she helped me through it and made me feel comfortable and told me I could stop if it was too much.

Along with FAS, I have Osteogenesis Imperfecta (OI). I always had soft bones and a lot of broken bones. In my early 30's, I had back pain and hearing loss and osteoporosis. A doctor finally noticed that I had blue sclera and told me I have OI. I am in a support group for OI- it is a small group, but every month we get together for a meeting or a picnic. I am the only one in the group who drives and is mobile, I have a mild case. This gives me a whole network of friends. I also struggle with an eating disorder and with anxiety and depression. The medicine helps but it has to be changed a lot.

For fun, I like to do yard work and gardening. It is very calming to be outside. I love animals- I walk dogs and take care of cats for neighbors when they call me. It is my dream to be a service or companion dog trainer, but that's not in the picture right now.

Here's what I would tell others with FAS: There is hope and help out there. I wouldn't have survived if I didn't fight for myself, even with all the shame and embarrassment. If your family is not supportive, go to friends who are. I look for people who accept and love me for who I am.

-Reviewed and submitted by Fran (dictated to Mary D)

From Victim to Warrior Mom: Creating a Circle of Hope

Who knew that drinking a "little wine" now and then when I was pregnant back in 1972 would cause my daughter to have lifelong brain damage? Certainly, not me. I mean, alcohol was just about the only legal drug I used back in those days. I went to rock and roll concerts, smoked pot, dropped *Purple Haze* acid and drank Boones Farm Apple wine. Alcohol was like the magic potion that made me suddenly thin, sexy and pretty.

Growing up in an alcoholic family, my view of alcohol was quite warped. Alcohol, especially beer and wine, were in the food group, as innocuous as peanut butter and jelly sandwiches. Alcohol was the common thread for all of our family social gatherings and was causing chaos and emotional pain within our family, but we had no idea our family problems were due to my dad's alcoholism. My parents were successful "pretty" people who had seven children that all attended parochial schools. We lived in a beautiful home that sat adjacent to the tenth hole of a private golf County Club. We grew up with secrecy and shame, but really had no clue that our dad was suffering with a treatable disease: alcoholism. We thought alcoholics were the homeless people we would see in the city when we visited our grandmother, certainly not our well-dressed daddy that drove a Cadillac convertible. I found early on that alcohol seemed to "cure" my insecurities and fears. Alcohol became my coping mechanism and by the time I was in middle school, I was drinking every weekend. My memories of the tenth grade consist of cutting class and daily alcohol and other drug use. I began to experience frequent black outs so it was no surprise that I ended up pregnant, and dropping out of school. I married the father of my baby; he was cute and had long hair. As soon as I discovered I was pregnant, I stopped "partying", and got clean - I was a good mommy. Unfortunately, no one yet understood that alcohol was a teratogen that could cause cell death and result in permanent birth defects. So, during pregnancy, I ate my veggie-burgers, made my macramé hemp plant holders, and went to my prenatal care appointments at the "free-clinic" for welfare moms - oh and drank wine.

I had a blond haired, blue eyed little boy! He was perfect, just beautiful! Life progressed further and so did my alcoholism. When my son was nine months old, I found myself pregnant again. In 1972 being barefoot and pregnant at seventeen was not that bad of a lifestyle. We were hippies, and material things were not on the priority list, drugs were. Karli was born in 1973, ironically the year that Smith and Jones coined the term Fetal Alcohol Syndrome (FAS) [6]. I had Karli in a high risk clinic for welfare moms. The doctor handed me my six pound baby girl, perfectly healthy!

Karli had surgery for a double hernia at six weeks of age. About that time she developed an ear infection. That ear infection (otitis media) lasted for three years; no anti-biotic seemed to work for her. I was told by her pediatrician that she had colic due to allergies. For years her doctors told me that her ear problems had caused her to be slightly delayed, but reassured me that *she would grow out of it*. I had no clue that alcohol was the culprit. So I continued to drink in subsequent pregnancies. After Karli I had another little girl. She was beautiful, fat and happy. I loved my children so very much, and was convinced I was the world's best Mommy. My only goal in life at that time was to be the best Mommy I could be.

I left my husband because of his drug use. His addiction prevented me from seeing my own addiction. I spent all of the years I was with him, focused on his use and trying to change him. It did not take me long to find another man whose life was crippled by alcoholism. He became husband number two. My life rapidly spiraled in a downward direction. Evictions, broken cars, homelessness, and desperation became a normal state. I would promise my children that Mommy would not drink or eat pills, and everyday I broke my promise. My addiction had taken me into a world that I knew was wrong, but I could not stop; the compulsion to use and the physical withdrawal would win every time. I overdosed several times, and was miraculously saved by family members and hospitals.

When I found myself pregnant the forth time, I somehow thought that the pregnancy would *fix* me. "This is a good thing, this will force me to keep things together and to be a better mom," I would tell myself. I had tried over and over to get clean. When I went for professional help, I was told that I would need to be on narcotics the rest of my life. They enrolled me in the maintenance methadone program where they treat addicts with a daily dose of a synthetic narcotic. I drank cheap wine, probably everyday, and I smoked. I went into labor about 2 months early. I gave birth to my son and I said goodbye to my son the day he was born. He was too small, his lungs were not developed.

I was the world's biggest victim; life had been harsh to me. *Poor me, poor me... Pour me a drink,* as they say in Alcoholics Anonymous (AA). I had lost everything, and actually looking back, I had never had much to begin with.

Alcohol had robbed me of most of life's rewards. But, I did have my three beautiful children. They were the only thing that mattered in life. About a year after my son died, I became pregnant again. I was scared to death to have a second baby while on methadone. The methadone treatment required that you stay on the drug if you became pregnant. I was afraid; I had already buried a son. I went to a university hospital in Washington, D.C. and walked into the office of an obstetrician. I begged him to talk with me and give me advice. My desperation came through loud and clear, and he talked with me. We made a deal: he would provide me with free care and I would allow him to discuss my case history with his students.

I went to all of my appointments, I loved this doctor. I continued to drink and to smoke cigarettes. He tried to convince me to stop smoking, and I did try often and even managed to cut down. He never asked me about my alcohol use. In February of 1982 I gave birth to a gorgeous baby girl! She was like a ray of sunshine on a dark gloomy day. Laughter had come back into the lives of my children and me. I had quit going to the methadone clinic (abruptly) and I was trying to detox myself at home using pills and booze. My sweet little 10 year old son had become the parent and he tried his best to take care of me and his sisters. After 2 months of painful withdrawal from the methadone, I was finally beginning to get strength back. But, just when hope had arrived, our entire world came crashing around us. One sunny April afternoon, I entered my baby's room, and found her lifeless body lying in her crib. I went into severe shock, and many of the memories of that day remain foggy. An autopsy finding later reported that my daughter died of Sudden Infant Death Syndrome (SIDS).

I had a very strong internal nudge the day I became pregnant with my daughter, that she was going to change our lives significantly. Her birth and sudden death miraculously altered life as we knew it for my children and me. My father had just completed a thirty-day stay in an addiction treatment center and was in early recovery the day my daughter passed away. He understood that I was suffering from alcoholism, not just a rebellious nature. Eventually he convinced me to admit myself into treatment for my addiction. Although it took one thirty day stay in treatment and another ten month stay in a therapeutic residential center, I finally surrendered! I was indeed an alcoholic. Sure, my diagnosis read "heroin addict" on my admitting papers, but there was no doubt about it. It all began with alcohol and the drug use just went hand in hand with the alcohol.

How could a person who puts needles in her arms not understand that she is an addict? They teach you in 12 step recovery that addiction is cunning, baffling and powerful. I look back over my years of addiction and wonder why none of the doctors, nurses, or social workers (not even child protective service workers!) ever addressed my addiction. Did they avoid the question because they were afraid of the answer? Did they believe that I was a hopeless case, or just not worth the trouble? Did they not ask about my alcohol use because they were so focused on the drugs? Were they that ill-informed about addiction, or did they believe there was no treatment available so why bother? I believe it may have been a little of each.

My daughter, Karli, continues to pay the tab for those years of addiction. She has a lifelong disability: Fetal Alcohol Syndrome (FAS). At 36 years of age, she still lives at home and plays with her collection of baby dolls and sticker books. Her brain is forever impaired because I drank wine occasionally while pregnant with her. Karli was not diagnosed with FAS until she was 16 years old. She probably would never have been diagnosed if I had not figured out that alcohol had caused her delays and brought it to the attention of her physicians. My alcohol use also was the reason for the deaths of my last two children.

Through divine intervention, I found my way from a life of addiction to a life in recovery. Today, my life is happy, joyous and free. Recovery has brought me many blessings, including five beautiful grandchildren. I am grateful to know that not one of those babies was prenatally exposed to alcohol - what a miracle! I managed to obtain a master's degree and actually contribute to society. I am the vice-president and national spokesperson for the National Organization on Fetal Alcohol Syndrome (NOFAS). It has been over 25 years since my last drink or drug and it saddens my heart to know that women are not being clearly informed about the facts on drinking during pregnancy.

In 2005 the United States Surgeon General re-issued the warnings regarding the use of alcohol during pregnancy. "There is no known safe level of alcohol during pregnancy," and if a woman is pregnant "she should stop to avoid further risks on the developing fetus."

(Visit http://www.cdc.gov/ncbddd/fasd/documents/SurgeonGenbookmark.pdf).

FASDs are preventable lifelong disabilities. While pregnant, **there is no safe amount of alcohol, no safe time to drink alcohol, and no safe type of alcohol**. And if you don't believe me, just ask Karli.

-Kathleen Mitchell - Vice President and International Spokesperson for the

National Organization on Fetal Alcohol Syndrome (NOFAS)

A Commitment of Love: One Dad's Perspective

I have been Kathy's partner for twenty-four years. We married in 1992. I met the children when they were still quite young. Karli is our middle child; she has fetal alcohol syndrome (FAS). Although raising a child with a developmental disability has not been easy, it has been very worthwhile. I believe that my life has been enriched and I am a much better person for having the experience. Karli rarely has a bad day; she always has something nice to say about everyone. Life is not perfect, and some days can be frustrating, but you really can't get too upset with her. All she wants is to be loved. We have learned to be patient with her process and try hard not to overwhelm her. She needs to be prepared for all transitions and changes to her schedule.

Our family has worked together to focus on her strengths and accept her weaknesses. We are careful to educate all service providers and everyone in her daily life about her disability. All of her activities are designed to enhance her self esteem. We have been blessed to have great support for Karli. She was very close with her grandparents, and for the first thirty years of her life, she spent a lot of time with them. Karli loved being there and her grandparents loved having her. Her grandparents are now deceased and her brother and sister help us out often. Typically she spends at least one night over at each of their homes. She is able to help them with their children and home chores, and they provide her with fun activities and involvement with their families. She has a few visits a year with her biological father as well. All of this support gives us a break and helps to keep us from getting burnt out. Caring for Karli takes a devoted team, and it all works perfectly for us.

When I married Kathy, I knew I was committing to two people. When I married Kathy and promised to always be there for her, I made those same promises to Karli. I knew she would always need us, and that we had the job of ensuring that her life was happy and safe. Anyone that knows Karli, absolutely, without a doubt, falls in love with her. She's so giving and she is a great teacher in how to live life and treat others. If we could all be like Karli, the world would be a better place.

-Michael Mitchell - stepfather of Karli and husband to Kathleen T. Mitchell

A Birth Mom's Story: A "Social Drinker" Learns the Hard Way

I grew up on a dairy farm in the Midwest, the 8th of 10 children, with a large, Catholic, extended family. I graduated 2nd in my high school class in 1973, and attended a private Catholic college. I partied some in high school, mostly beer-drinking, the beverage of choice at that time in the Midwest. I partied less in college, as I was a serious student, graduating cum laude.

My first job out of college was working at a group home with delinquent teenaged boys. I worked there for 3.5 years, met my husband in that town, and got married at age 25, in 1980. I started working on my Master's Degree in Counseling Psychology, finishing my program in 1982.

From 1982-1984, my husband and I worked at a residential facility for 42 abandoned, abused and neglected children, ages 3-12. The children had many behavioral challenges, including sexual acting out, as most had suffered sexual abuse. At that time, I became aware of Fetal Alcohol Syndrome, and although many of the children had been pre-natally exposed to alcohol, none had the formal diagnosis. I was stretched and challenged in this setting, but thoroughly enjoyed this "parenting" experience.

From 1985 – 2000, I specialized in providing treatment foster care, while my spouse worked as an educator and co-foster parent. We "fostered" 25 children over the course of 15 years. Why did these children enter into the "system"? We had two teen moms and their newborn babies. Many of the children had parents with chemical dependency and/or mental health issues. Others were adolescents with behavioral and mental health challenges. Some of the children had suffered neglect, abuse, and/or abandonment. I now wonder how many of those parents were pre-natally exposed to alcohol/drugs themselves. Three of the 25 children had the FAS diagnosis, but now that I have a greater understanding of FASD, I realize that the majority of the 25 children probably suffered from some level of undiagnosed FASD. I was a very effective foster mom who took my role seriously.

While I really enjoyed being a foster mother, I longed to have children of my own. I became an adoptive parent at the age of 31. We then attempted to deal with infertility unsuccessfully *via* the medical route. I became pregnant, but miscarried at ten weeks, so we pursued a second adoption. When our second child was 2.5 months old, I became pregnant unexpectedly.

Because I wasn't planning to get pregnant, I continued my pattern of social drinking- 4-6 servings of beer or wine per week.

After I realized I was pregnant, I spoke with my doctor, asking him directly about FAS, and if it was safe to use alcohol during pregnancy. He assured me that moderate use of alcohol was not problematic, that it took large amounts of alcohol to cause FAS. I reduced my consumption somewhat, but didn't eliminate my alcohol use. If only I had known then what I know now!! Unplanned pregnancies and social drinking result in prenatal exposure to alcohol at a rate much higher than most people care to consider. And many health care providers still don't give women a strong, clear message about avoiding alcohol use during both the preconception and prenatal periods.

My Son's Story: Unintentional Consequences

In 1989, my only "biological" child was born. He was on target developmentally from birth - 2. "Temperament" problems became apparent from ages 2.5 – 5. My son was very stubborn, strong-willed, and "inflexible". He was "home-schooled" until age 10, along with his three adopted siblings. During the elementary years, he was unwilling to participate in ice skating lessons, T-ball, Vacation Bible School, and swimming lessons, even though his brother and "home-schooling" friends were avidly involved in these activities. He frequently hid himself to avoid activities that we were encouraging him to participate in. In retrospect, he must have been struggling with high anxiety.

My son displayed oppositional behaviors that were non-compliant vs. defiant. "Refusals" were a challenge multiple times daily. Although my son was very "bright" (superior IQ), he had significant reading struggles and was very much an underachiever as a home-schooler, compared to my other children who learned how to read at a typical pace. This son of mine saw the world through different eyes, with a perspective that didn't match others' perceptions.

My son began attending public school in 4th grade. His teacher became very frustrated with him at times. At the end of the year she cried while having a final meeting with me and my son, as she felt she had been ineffective. Some felt his issues were the result of being home-schooled...... the old "blame the parent" routine. He was sent to the behavior room many times during 4-6th grades, and was "expelled" from the school during sixth grade for using a pencil as a "weapon." He threw a pencil across the "time-out" room, and it accidentally hit the teacher on her forehead as she turned around to look at him while leaving the room. The resulting school change was traumatic for him and he was expelled three weeks later from the next school.

During 7th grade, my son began "using". I was not aware of his use until the end of 8th grade. During this time, he was very engaged in the "graffiti" culture, and often didn't come home from school. He became very loyal to his "using" peer group and continued to disregard parental authority. By fall of 9th grade, he had "dropped out" of school. While partying on Halloween, he jumped through a fire to liven up the party. His pants caught on fire and he ended up with 2nd degree burns on the calf of his leg. Several weeks later, he was assaulted while very intoxicated. He ended up at the emergency room, then detox, then his first round of inpatient Chemical Dependency treatment. He began attending a "sober" high school after treatment. He relapsed several times, repeating treatment three more times during the course of high school.

During a period of sobriety, he got involved in a fight at a party, resulting in a peer having a broken jaw. Felony assault charges were filed against him three months later and a warrant was issued for his arrest. He "ran away," as a peer told him he was going to be charged with attempted murder. The "run" resulted in a 6 week long binge, followed by treatment, and a residential placement for ongoing truancy issues. The following summer (age 17), he was placed at a correctional facility for 120 days for the "assault" (brawl at a party, although he was the only one charged) that had occurred the previous summer. While at the correctional facility, he breezed through the General Education Development (GED) process, scoring very high on all of the subtests. We were all relieved that his period of mandatory education was over, as school had always been a challenge and poor fit for him.

He was placed at a group home after leaving the correctional facility. While there, he got a job at a local fast food restaurant which also happened to be the local drug trafficking vicinity. His boss bought him alcohol for his 18th birthday and he was kicked out of the group home for possession of prescription drugs that didn't belong to him. The county sent him back to treatment for violating probation by bringing drugs into the group home. This was a 4-month hard core adult treatment. He "absented" from treatment with only 14 days to go as he was determined to attend a friend's wedding. This resulted in a new warrant, and after 3 weeks, he was arrested. He fled arrest on foot, hid and a police dog eventually sniffed him out, resulting in a deep dog bite to his shoulder and upper arm. After 2 weeks in Juvenile Detention, he was released from juvenile jurisdiction and allowed to begin tech school in a community 60 miles from home. He attended class for 3 weeks, then quit going. As parents, we felt he should be given the same opportunity to pursue higher education as his two older siblings, but we weren't surprised when it fell apart.

I was so relieved when he made it to age 18. For years, my prayer for him had been "keep him alive 'til 25", as he was always engaged in very high-risk behaviors. Life continues to be a challenge for him, although he has recently gotten back on a sober path. He has been holding a part-time job for 8 months, hired by one of his close friends.

The Challenge of Getting the Diagnosis

When my son was going through intake for CD treatment, I informed the interviewer that he had been prenatally exposed to alcohol. This information was disregarded. Because my son is very bright and articulate, people (CD and mental health service providers) disregarded my concerns when I indicated that prenatal exposure may be the cause of many of his mental health and behavioral challenges. This happened at 3 or 4 different intake sessions for different services. It was as though the practitioners didn't know how to respond to a birth mother who was readily admitting to having used alcohol during pregnancy. This disregard was very frustrating for me. Instead of referring us for an FASD evaluation, we were referred for an ASD evaluation (Autism Spectrum Disorder)..... The results indicated he didn't fall on that spectrum.

Eventually, our "in-home" therapist heard my concerns, and acknowledged that many of his challenges were "red flags"- common characteristics of those with one of the Fetal Alcohol Spectrum Disorders (FASD). The therapist recommended to the judge that he be "ordered" to have an FASD evaluation. That evaluation confirmed my suspicion that the prenatal alcohol exposure had caused permanent damage to my son. He was diagnosed with Alcohol Related Neurodevelopmental Disorder (ARND). He is on the higher functioning end of the spectrum.

THE SUMMARY

My ignorant decisions, based on inaccurate information from my doctor, have resulted in unintended lifelong consequences for my family and especially my son. We saw multiple mental health providers over the years who never inquired about possible prenatal exposure. Everyone else "missed" the signs, but inside my heart and mind, I held myself accountable. My son knows it was not my intention to hurt him. He doesn't hold this against me. His behavioral challenges have "stretched me" in countless ways, making me a stronger person. He keeps me on my knees. But overall, the joy he has brought me outweighs the misery......at least for today............

-Submitted anonymously

An Adoptive Mom's Reflections on Raising Two Pre-teen Girls with Prenatal Exposure to Alcohol

(Note: These two girls have never been formally diagnosed for an FASD. However, these reflections mirror the difficulties faced by adoptive parents who are not given accurate information about the behaviors often associated with prenatal exposure to alcohol.)

We had been waiting a long time to adopt again after receiving our son, Tyler, from Korea so we decided to do foster care.

Alexis was abandoned by her mom at the Hospital when she was one day old. They thought she was about 4-6 weeks early and weighed less than 5 lbs. Her Mom used alcohol and had a cocaine addiction and gave birth to Alexis outside the hospital and was rushed to the hospital. We were told she didn't have the best Apgar score and was cold when she arrived at the hospital. She remained there until she was 18 days old when she came home to us. We were lucky that she did not need machines to check her breathing so we were very relieved. She was a very fussy baby. I remember the nurse told me that she was fuzzy and cried often at the hospital. To help with this, they told us to keep her wrapped up very snuggly and this really helped keep her calm. As she grew older and this didn't work, she became a very fussy baby and eventually we learned we had to let her cry herself to sleep which was difficult on everyone. She learned to rock herself to relax and would even hold her hand above her head and stare at her hand as she rocked. She still has a difficult time falling asleep and rocks. She continues to rock every time she stirs at night. When we brought this to the doctor's attention, she was tested and we learned that she has sleep apnea. She needs clonidine and melatonin every night to fall asleep while she rocks.

Tessa was born at the hospital after her mom arrived in labor. They thought she was about 4-6 weeks early and less than 5 lbs too. When she was delivered they learned that she had cocaine in her system and her birth mother probably drank as well, so they put Tessa into foster care. I was told she went to her first home after 3 days in the hospital. Except for drops they gave her for her eyes, she appeared ok to the first foster parents taking care of her. When she was five months old, she came home with us. The first time they put her in my arms, I felt something was wrong. She was a very limp baby and too flexible. I mentioned it to our doctor and, on her second checkup, they told me call to call early intervention for a check-up. She had weak muscle tone but responded very well to treatment and was walking by about 14 months. She never did crawl; she used to scoot by keeping her legs beneath her while she used her arms to bring herself forward. She was a very content baby and hardly ever cried long or hard. We had many challenges and setbacks as they grew.

We have been having Family Based counseling for about 6 months now. I believe however that it has helped me more than the girls. This brings me to the whole story of what works for the girls. We have had counseling for the girls for years now. They had counseling at the ages of about 4-6 and we took a break. We began again at about age 8 and went from wrap around counseling to family based. I have had a very good relationship with each of the therapists involved and it helps me most of the time but I honestly wonder how much it helps the girls.

Currently, Tessa is on Focalin XR 5mg; she took 10mg during school. We recently put her on 25 mg of Zoloft with what I think has helped her so much. In the past she would get so upset and argue and cry from anywhere from 5 minutes to up to 90 minutes at times. You can imagine how exhausting this is for the whole family! This has improved so much since adding the Zoloft! She takes allergy meds for seasonal allergies. She has also been on lactulose syrup since she was about 5 years old. She was difficult to toilet train and suffered from constipation until we added the lactulose to her medicines.

Lexy has really been on many meds too. She has always since birth actually been a very difficult child. She cried excessively since birth and is full of anxiety. She wants to be in charge of everyone in our house and makes it difficult for all of us. She was on a few ADHD meds but none of them ever helped. I have always been slow to give her medicine just because I worried so much about the difficulties they might present later in life as many of the medicines are not usually given to children or that is what I believed. Currently, she takes Clonidine HCL ½ of.1 MG, 20mg Celexa, 5mg of Abilify and 40 MG of protonix. She has been seeing a GI specialist. She had an endoscopy which showed no problems but continues to have many stomach aches. Currently, we are trying to have her use the Protonix and Miralax combined with Metamucil. She resists and fights, using the last two meds almost every day; she doesn't believe that they help. Many people have told her to give them a chance. I think a lot of it is just the fact that it has been months of the stomach aches and her anxiety which compounds the whole problem. We also have two other breathing tests.

So it has been tough and the girls have totally different personalities. Lexy tries to act like an adult and rule everyone and Tessa is very childlike. They even choose to dress completely opposite. So, of course, that is an everyday challenge. I can honestly say that they have been a bit better the last few weeks. I have insisted that they stay in and try to get along when they are both being kept in for their behaviors. We adopted a contract with outlines of what cannot be accepted and the result of that behavior about 2-3 months ago. Of course, they argue about that too but we are seeing tiny steps in the right directions. My biggest difficulty is the times I have to remember and use them (which are constantly) and the exhaustion it causes. I sometimes feel like a warden instead of a Mom.

I also wanted to tell you about the Adoption Conference I attended in June, 2009, with the children. It was wonderful; the children were with other children all day being well supervised. They were happy to go because some of my best friends from my adoption group came with their children. I had 2 ½ days with my best friends and many classes to attend. What I most wanted to talk about were two important subjects. I heard that the state (New jersey) was considering stopping wrap around services because they did not feel that they were helping the children as much as they hoped that they would. From my point of view, living it, I can agree. Even though there are many competent workers I feel that they are like cheerleaders keeping the parents going but the kids really don't get that much from the services they offer. I have had many conversations with friends where it is discussed that the children can behave while they are there, but 2 minutes after they leave, things can fall apart over anything and the whole string of their everyday behaviors takes over. Many times we have discussed that the workers would understand so much better the challenges that we faced if they lived with the children. We have tried so many routes to changing behaviors - charts, rewards, time outs, and I constantly thank them for good behaviors but that can fall apart seconds later because so many things set our children off. It can be a noise, something that touches them, a remark from someone or the lack of a remark from someone; it can be, and is, everything.

When I have attended many other meetings, families who have fostered children for years almost always say that wrap around doesn't help. Of course, everyone has their own thoughts and situations but I can understand them feeling the way that they do. I did mention to Lexy's psychiatrist last week that I attended the conference and I told her what I heard about the wrap around services and she told me that she had heard it too.

I was also impressed by another class I attended called Attachment Disorder: Children with Fetal Alcohol and Drug Exposure. Bottom line, they have come to believe that neurofeedback has helped them help their patients the most. I had explored trying this in the past but, of course, neither our family nor state insurance the girls have would pay for it. Presently, both of my girls go to psychiatrists that do not take insurance or they only take one and we have a co-pay. Insurance is a whole other factor that makes it difficult or impossible for many adoptive families. When I saw the psychiatrist last week, I asked her if she had heard of good results from the neurofeedback. She told me that many of her patients have had it and have had good results. She then said that once the therapies ended the results seem to be lost.

I've had many thoughts and experiences I felt I needed to share. Also, since this is sometimes a very difficult road to walk, I want to be as optimistic as I can to families about what to expect but it is also tough to tell them the difficulties they will face. There are so many families just like ours that are desperate for help.

-Helen Smith, (Philadelphia FASD Task Force)

An Unexpected Diagnosis – Fetal Alcohol Syndrome

For many reasons my husband and I chose to add our first child to our family through adoption. After attending seminars, doing lots of research, lots of prayer and weighing the options of domestic versus international adoption, we chose to adopt internationally. When we were given our son's limited medical history and sixty second video, we immediately had concerns. He was the fifth pregnancy to a supposed older birth mom who had never parented any of her children. His growth and developmental milestones were significantly delayed. We made our wishes known to the director of our adoption agency that we wanted a child as healthy as can be. (We were obviously naive to the tragic effects post institutionalization alone would have on any child,) We did not even want a child with correctable medical issues, (*i.e.* cleft palate). Did I not feel equipped or did I just want what every parents want, a healthy child? It's irrelevant now.

Our son was born anywhere from six to ten weeks premature. He had been back and forth between the hospital and the orphanage four different times in his first year of life. As most parents do prior to accepting the referral of our son, we sent both the limited medical history and short video clip to two different international adoption specialists to review and consult with us. One specialist was very pessimistic and had significant concerns about our son's poor growth history and lots of questions about his birth mother's history of alcohol/drug use since this information was unavailable to us. The second specialist was very optimistic and had no concerns about our son having physical indications of alcohol exposure. (Mind you he was 10 months old at the time). We were thrilled and very hopeful. We accepted the referral of our son and traveled to Astana, Kazakhstan in June 2002. Dominic became our son on July 4, 2002. Huge concerns about Dominic's limited fine and gross motor skills, lack of eye contact, extremely low tone, inability to suck or chew plagued our minds and hearts during the two weeks we visited daily with Dominic. Ringing in the back of our minds were the words of the director of the adoption agency back in Indiana "Do not go to court if you have any concerns!" The decision for us was made the moment we accepted the referral of our son. To us, it was as if we had given birth and were going to the nursery to see him for the first time. Not following through with the adoption despite huge concerns was not an option for us. He was our SON.

Within two months of arriving home to the US, Dominic was seen by a local international adoption specialist, a urologist, a gastroenterologist, a nutritionist, an attachment specialist, an ophthalmologist, a developmental pediatrician, and a psychologist. He was already receiving six hours of therapy (Occupational, Physical, Speech, Developmental) per week. Yes- a few of my strengths are that I am proactive, solution-focused and thorough. These were all to my newly adopted, significantly-delayed, son's advantage. Everything, I mean EVERYTHING was work with Dominic. He did not want to use his hands, he could not sit, push up on his arms when on his belly, could not suck or chew, was extremely gaggy, had significant attachment issues, and had severe sensory integration dysfunction. He was most content being left alone and laying on his back rocking side to side like he had been doing for the first twelve months of his life. I was heartbroken. I was flooded with grief both for my broken dreams and for the tragic neglect my son suffered prior to being adopted. Coping strategy number ONE: I began seeing a psychotherapist to help me safely process all my feelings and frustration.

Other than having global delays, Dominic did not receive any official diagnosis until he was two years old. The diagnosis was made during a visit to a second developmental pediatrician who also practiced as a geneticist and had access to the previous evaluations. Upon seeing my son, he very casually said "Your son has fetal alcohol syndrome." What? How could that be? No other specialists had said this.

Another year went by and Dominic had begun in the early intervention preschool program in our state, continuing to receive all the above therapies. At about the age three, Dominic began hitting, pinching, biting, and pulling hair. He had great verbal skills. He could tell you exactly what he had done wrong and what he should do instead, but the behaviors continued despite redirection and many interventions (*i.e.*, time out, behavior modification program). I was reading everything I could get my hands on. What was wrong with our son? Why did he not seem to be making connections, understanding cause and effect, using any typical social skills? Then I picked up a book on FAS. AHAA! THIS was IT! Fetal Alcohol Syndrome. My husband was distraught and grief stricken. I continued to read everything I could get my hands on about FAS and interventions as I continued in individual therapy safely processing my anger, grief, sadness, feeling so ill-equipped to deal with Dominic's many, many challenges. Dominic was a happy child. His affection was limited as was his fear of strangers. Dominic was completely indiscriminate with touching and talking with people wherever we went. He appeared to have limited or no social boundaries. He would wander off without any fear if given the opportunity. Although he would frequently attempt to kiss anyone he met, he failed to attach to my husband and me as a typical child would. He did not appear to understand cause and effect and any learning or redirection required near constant repetition. I thought I would go crazy (still do) with finding that almost everything I said or taught Dominic did not stick.

I often compare my parenting of my child with FAS to the movie "Groundhog's Day" where every day is a repeat of the previous day although I find my job far from humorous. His inability to handle change and his inability to control his impulses became more and more problematic. Meltdowns became a regular part of Dominic's day. He had many repetitive behaviors like flapping his hands, turning his head side to side, rocking his body from side to side while laying on his back, pushing on his groin, rubbing his forehead of the floor until he'd give himself rug burns. His balance, coordination and body awareness were all seriously impaired and he suffered many challenges with sensory integration dysfunction. Our once happy son had become trapped in his increasing frustrated little world. Our expectations in some ways echoed that which a parent raising a typical child's would, but our son was incapable of doing so many tasks and regulating his very own feelings and relationship with the world around him.

When Dominic was three and one-half, we sought the professional expertise of a psychologist and had a comprehensive psychological evaluation completed on Dominic. This gave us a roadmap to know more specifically how to continue to address Dominic's many challenges. Many people (professional's included) were completely clueless about what FAS was and how to treat or address it. So I spent time creating a document (Coping strategy number TWO) to give to everyone who worked with Dominic (Sunday school leaders, teachers, sitters, coaches, etc.). This document included an introduction to Dominic, the specific names for his many challenges (FAS, Sensory Integration Dysfunction, ADHD, etc.) as well as a very detailed clear outline of Dominic's many limitations. It had specific instruction/details on how to help him in each area and ended with a list of Dominic's many strengths as well as an invitation for the reader to borrow any resources I owned to use in their work with Dominic. The frustration was still nearly unbearable at the lack of treatments, intervention or anything to address my son's primary disability, FAS. I know I pushed Dominic to meet his various milestones and that everything my child did was WORK – from sitting in a chair (extremely weak core muscle, low tone, tires easily) to holding a pencil to throwing or catching a ball. Very few things felt fun as Dominic's limitations and challenges affect every area of his little life.

Dominic continued to participate in weekly OT, PT, and SLP therapy sessions while attending a developmental preschool from age three to age five. By the time Dominic reached four years of age, he was seen by a psychiatrist to begin medication in hopes of improving his precious quality of life. It was so painful to make this decision since my son was so small. It was at age 4 that Dominic was also diagnosed with High Functioning Autism. It blew me away to see how much was known about this disorder, how many treatments and even "cures" were available for a child with this diagnosis. Doors were opened for our son to begin to participate in a variety of additional and/or alternative treatments at that time. We started Dominic on a special diet, a variety of vitamins, probiotics, Omega 3s, etc. in addition to therapy and psychological medication. The greatest blessing came when Dominic began participating in an intensive one-on-one therapy called Applied Behavioral Analysis or ABA.

As a result of Dominic's work with his ABA therapist, he has been able to remain in a typical classroom. He completed one year of kindergarten in the public school with a lot of support. He was young and small for his age and had significant social and developmental delays. Thus we had him repeat kindergarten in a small local private school in a full day kindergarten classroom. His ABA therapist spends several hours in the classroom with Dominic to help keep Dominic on task as well as serve as a tutor, encourager, teacher and, best of all, surrogate frontal lobe for my son. Dominic requires a great deal of attention and energy to teach, parent and raise. He has no ability to hate. His love knows no bounds and he will never meet a stranger. He brings a lot of joy to people he meets and has a thirst for information and a curiosity and naivety that add to his charm. He has gone through so many challenges. He is not self-motivated, but is the hardest working child I have ever met. He is constantly being pushed and rises again and again to meet expectations and be successful. He will begin third grade in this same small private school this fall with his OT, PT and individual ABA therapist by his side.

In response to Dominic's many special needs, my home is filled with lots of structure, therapeutic play toys and a ton of visually posted schedules, lists, charts, rules, privileges, consequences and so on. Anything from remembering HOW to wash his hands to table manners to social boundaries when interacting with others is made available and clear for Dominic to use each day. Because anything my son learns one moment may be forgotten the next moment, day or week the above tools enable my husband and me to decrease our near constant verbal instruction or redirection. Although we use time-outs and removal of privileges to discipline Dominic whenever he displays negative or inappropriate behaviors after many warnings, the effect on his learning does not often create lasting change. Thus we view it as one more teaching tool and reminder of the appropriate versus inappropriate choices he must learn to be successful and kept safe.

Some of the coping strategies that we have taught or provided for Dominic include, but are not limited to, deep breathing, yoga, progressive muscle relaxation, a safe place (his bedroom) to relax and carry on some of the inappropriate, yet adaptive behaviors he does every day to regulate himself, an environment (including language) where he may freely express his feelings, ask questions and learn, a loving, conscientious team of professionals all working with him toward the common goal of helping him to be the best he can be.

It is unfortunate that where we live there are no true specialists in interventions that work for children who are alcohol affected. With no treatment or cure, we recognize that parenting, teaching, raising our son is a life long journey. We count among our many blessings that Dominic has been able to remain in a classroom with no more than eleven other children who have been with him in school for going on four years this fall. Dominic has never had a friend and still does not. No one calls to play with him. His friendship skills, unless completely prompted by an adult, remain very limited and his play is very narrowly focused on his main inertest – trains. I would say that his peers at school or in Sunday school tolerate him and, at times, help him by reminding him of rules, remaining patient despite his many irritating behaviors and, on very rare occasions, will teach him how to do something so that he can participate in an activity.

As a licensed social worker in the state of Indiana, I must obtain twenty hours of continuing education per year. So, I regularly attend conferences about attachment, autism, international adoption and fetal alcohol syndrome. This enables me to gain personal insight into the latest research available about my son's various challenges. More importantly, it enables me to connect personally with other parents and professionals whose lives have been deeply affected or touched by prenatal alcohol exposure. Coping strategy number THREE: knowing I am not alone in this unpredictable maze of fetal alcohol syndrome, has been so very helpful to me. I had failed to connect, or at least feel understood, in all the MOPS groups, Mom's Clubs, play groups, even in a group of moms I had met who adopted internationally as well. I even started a support group for parents of special needs children at my church, but still felt I needed the support of someone (others) who could relate to our specific journey.

At present and for the past eight years of my son's life, he has participated in weekly occupational, physical and speech therapies. He has had a lot of therapy to address his severe sensory issues, but nothing has been hugely helpful for him. Just this week my son is participating in an intensive sensory integration therapy program for fourteen days straight. After meeting with the director of the agency and consulting with our son's psychiatrist, all agreed Dominic could definitely benefit. No decision that I make about or for my son is taken lightly. I am at times faced with those who question or disagree with our decisions regarding my son. How far will I go to help my son be successful? How much will I pursue alternative and/or the most current interventions that work with alcohol-affected individuals? Will I ever stop looking for things that will help him be more independent? I suppose I will do whatever it takes. There is still so much we do not know about our son's disability. What will puberty be like for him? Will he hold a job some day? Will he ever live on his own? Get married? Be a father? I do think about the future but my energy and attention is required right here, right now to be the best mama my son (and other two children) needs. My husband, son and I celebrate each of Dominic's even smallest successes with great joy and pride. He has come so far and only God knows how far he will go. I feel exhausted yet privileged to be a part of his journey.

-Rachel Marie DeWald

A Story of FAS and Forgiveness

I'll never forget the first time I spoke my most shameful secret aloud to a stranger. It was March of 2003. I stood alone in my kitchen on the phone. Palms sweating, heart pounding, voice cracking, I said, "My son has Fetal Alcohol Syndrome." Imagine my surprise when she calmly answered, "So does mine" and asked about my family. I thought there would be blame and judgments! She made it clear that blame is not useful to anyone.

The question about my family was not easy to answer. I'd had three alcohol-exposed pregnancies. Stephen was born in 1988 after a planned pregnancy. I was a heavy drinker who still had some control. I could remember a few drinking episodes over the course of the pregnancy. Michael was born in 1991 when I was an unidentified alcoholic. Christina was born in 1994; I had a year of sober time, but had relapsed and experienced DTs. My children have a spectrum of prenatal alcohol exposure and effects. My husband, Paul, has had an amazing journey of his own throughout our eventful marriage.

I had plenty of experience with alcoholism, depression, and sexual trauma during childhood and adolescence. I became familiar with alcohol's effects as a preteen. I associated with people who drank like I did, so I didn't question my drinking. I was outwardly successful through school and into adulthood. I cut down my drinking as needed and continued to feel like a fraud in everything I accomplished.

Paul's and my family journey started with a planned pregnancy with Stephen. I stopped drinking with an effort some refer to as "white-knuckling"- a description of tremendous effort and attention with no support and variable success. I can remember a few drinking episodes through the course of the pregnancy, but Stephen had no obvious problems. I was depressed and felt utterly unable to care for him; I returned to work and occasional drinking which quickly escalated. I was into my first trimester with Michael by the time I realized I was pregnant. I thought I could stop as easily as I had with my first pregnancy, but alcohol had taken hold of my brain. I had severe depression, suicidal thinking, refractory vomiting, unstable appetite and weight fluctuation during Michael's pregnancy. I stopped for the 2nd trimester, but resumed episodic drinking later in the pregnancy. Michael and I both had withdrawal and he had feeding problems and failure to thrive from the start. I had a family intervention and got professional help with a psychiatrist and a few 12 step meetings. I relapsed and when Mike was almost two years old, I had medical catastrophe, my first inpatient addiction treatment, and a diagnosis of inflammatory cirrhosis. I was able to stay sober for almost a year and start dealing with the wreckage and shame caused by my drinking. Stephen was developing normally and attending regular preschool. Michael was evaluated and started Early Intervention. I progressed in my medical career with professional monitoring.

Multiple factors led to my final relapse; I binged over the period of a week and experienced DTs when I tried to stop on my own. I went from detox to long term halfway house treatment. Here I found out that I was well into my first trimester of a high risk pregnancy with Christina. In women's community, I finally dealt with undiagnosed and untreated physical, emotional and sexual trauma. I learned that I wasn't psychotic as I'd feared; the flashbacks that heralded each pregnancy and consequent relapse were triggered by hormonal sweeps. I talked about the depth of my shame at drinking during pregnancy and parenting, and the damage that had caused. I disclosed my shame and fear at having cirrhosis, and how it interferes with daily activities. I learned how to live day by day without drinking. I was discharged 71/2 months pregnant with a solid recovery and medical program, including a psychiatrist/ psychotherapist, addiction medicine doctor, 12 step meetings and sponsor, hepatologist, internist, an educated husband and obstetrition. After Christina was delivered, I had a bleeding crisis. When the children were 6, 3, and 4 months old, I was diagnosed with kidney cancer and had surgery. I had intermittent depressive symptoms, but not the suicidal thinking I had while I was drinking. Alcohol is certainly a factor in the biology, psychopathology, and management of suicide.

We weathered my health crises. After three years of trying, I was finally able to settle into permanent and useful sobriety.

There were three busy children in our home - Michael was the only one who seemed affected during the early years, but there was a very high level of activity overall. We have gradually figured out what intensive, daily supports Michael needs over the years. He was continually evaluated, monitored, and supported through Early Intervention, Preschool Handicapped, Multiply-handicapped kindergarten, and self-enclosed special education classes (after a failed mainstreaming attempt). He was classified eligible for special education and related services in the category Multiply Handicapped; he has mental retardation, and impaired vision, hearing, speech and communication. He was very speech delayed and had frequent ear, respiratory, and GI infections. He had multiple ENT and ophthalmologic procedures. He was consistently sociable, engaging, lovable, curious and inattentive as a boy. Any meds made him hyperactive and even aggressive. He was formally diagnosed with FAS at age 11 with information from multiple sources - developmental pediatrician, neuropsychologist, neurologist, occupational and speech therapists, learning consultant and social worker. He was also seen regularly for treatment by ENT, dentists, and an allergist. He was supported in Boy Scouts, soccer, Special Seals at the YMCA and religious education. He is highly successful at the Special Services School in our county; they accommodate him academically and provide support at his part- time job. He just turned 18 and has a relationship with a young woman he met at school; naturally our most immediate concerns are about safe sex and contraception. At home and in the community, we continue to test what he can learn and what experiences he can tolerate on a daily basis. Any change in routine is a stress that must be prepared for; he seems even less flexible as an adolescent.

Prenatal alcohol exposure has affected Stephen very differently. Stephen grew up intelligent, athletic, sociable, very verbal and capable. He hated homework and his teachers reported that he was talking too much, not paying attention, not working to his potential. He struggled with organizing homework and projects. At age 11, he had his first suicidal thoughts, safety plan and psychotherapy. He began an enduring habit of cooking and skateboarding to help balance his mood. He had his parents and a strong-willed girlfriend to help organize his time, activities, and peer interactions; he was an honor student in his vocational high school. The unmanageability set in aggressively when he moved out to go to college. He was quickly in poor health, academically unsuccessful, depressed, and experimenting with drugs. Many of his jobs have been overwhelming and short-term. It became obvious that he struggled to organize major tasks, in school and out. His time and money skills are suboptimal. His decisions regarding activities and peers were inflexible. We finally had him evaluated at the FASD Diagnostic Center in our state. His testing was affected by major mood disorders and wasn't conclusive for alcohol effects, but demonstrated a number of challenges common to affected individuals. I struggled with new shame and the realization that we were way behind in establishing what supports Stephen would need to be successful. He had spoken at conferences about being a sibling to a person with FAS. Now he struggles to incorporate his own effects into his approach to life.

Christina had a brief, intense alcohol exposure in the first trimester. She has had some reading difficulty that has improved with age, attention, and some support. She is 14 years old and has outstanding academic, social, and athletic success. She has only been partially evaluated at the FASD Diagnostic Center, by her choice.

Now you have an idea why I hesitated at a question about the family. Stephen, Mike, Christy and I have had multidimensional evaluations and interventions of varying intensity over many years. Mike and Christina take no meds; Stephen politely refuses antidepressants. I'm not always aware of the daily time, energy, and planning that is needed in our family until an objective observer points it out. Parenting our children is undoubtedly a much different journey for Paul than he could have expected. He is a successful Occupational Medicine physician with his own story. We both had medical education and clinical practice; knowledge isn't enough to prevent prenatal alcohol exposure. Alcohol use has to be assessed and treated as indicated. That sounds so straightforward, yet denial, shame and stigma, and depression kept me from seeking treatment for many years. Women with alcoholism have a long, fascinating history of struggle with the issues of enabling [7] and stigma [8-10]; stigma has often been tied to the presumption of promiscuity [11]. These women were compared to their Temperance Society counterparts in the 1820s and 1830s [12]. This prejudice was also expressed by some of the psychiatrists who treated them [13]. Women with mental illness and alcoholism were removed from families or poorhouses and placed in asylums in the 1800's. There, they were treated with water cures, minerals, and profound narcosis induced by barbiturates. Personal accounts have included "a living death, shackles, handcuffs, straightjackets, balls and chain, iron rings, and...other such relics of barbarism' [14]. Such deeply rooted prejudice is extremely difficult to eradicate, but historically showed the social and economic determinants of women's health. It continues to impact the field of addiction treatment today and it certainly affected me.

It took Michael a few years of discussion to realize that I'd used alcohol during my pregnancy with him. I asked his forgiveness and he asked me first if I was really sorry. Then I told him I hoped he could forgive me someday and he said" I don't mind. I love you mommy". Michael's question and declaration of love were precious gifts that led me to a significant, life-changing question of my own: "If he can forgive you this, who are you to not forgive yourself?" After all the years of self recrimination and blame, I finally understood what self-forgiveness feels like. The rest of the family has been just as generous with forgiving me. Forgiveness is the gift that motivates my involvement in FASD education and prevention. Shame kept me secretive and drinking; self forgiveness in recovery has put that shame on a leash. Self-forgiveness may seem like a sudden thing, but it is a product of years of work in a recovery program that emphasizes forgiving and asking for forgiveness with others. Forgiveness is a healing process that has to be acknowledged and maintained. It requires that harm be admitted and ongoing responsibility for damage be accepted. It has nothing to do with forgetting. Forgiveness has freed my children and me of the pervasive shame so destructive to birth families. It has freed us to recover, be creative, have fun, and help others.

Stephen and Christina have their own stories in this chapter. I asked Michael if he had anything to say about having FAS. He just shrugged and repeated his classic line "Tell them I don't mind". Michael doesn't spend time and energy wishing to be someone he's not. He has a straightforward approach to his routine, his day, his work and school duties, where Christina should go to high school, where I should work. He repeatedly reminds us all to go where we are loved.

-Mary DeJoseph - NJ / Northeast FASD Education and Research Center

Having a Brother with Fetal Alcohol Syndrome

How often do you see a six year old help a nine year old cross the street? How often do you see a fourth grader help a seventh grader with math homework? How often does an older brother solve the problem of what high school his younger sister should attend in one sentence? These are a few questions that go through my mind when asked what it is like to have a brother with Fetal Alcohol Syndrome (FAS). Michael is my brother before he is my brother with Fetal Alcohol Syndrome.

There are definitely challenges to having a brother with FAS. There are small things I had to adapt to, such as homework help and basic safety. When I was six and he was nine, I would assist him in crossing the street. Or when I was in fourth grade and he was in seventh grade, I would help him with his math homework. These were things that just became what I did, not something I questioned or analyzed. As I got older, I figured out why these little things were regular to me, but not to my friends. It was still okay with me.

The issues that affect me more are his emotional fluctuations and his inability to adapt to change. Because his mind only works about two-thirds his age, it is a constant struggle to remember his emotions and reactions are a bit behind what they "should" be. Michael's biggest issue (as well as mine) to deal with is his need for routine. Any change in his routine becomes a catastrophic event to his comfort level. It doesn't seem like it would be that serious of a problem, but it affects everything; from traveling to who drives him to work. When we ventured off to Alaska, he became so nervous and anxious that he got sick and threw up the first two days we were there.

The issues are as challenging as the positives are glorious. There are most definitely upsides to having Michael as my brother. Michael having FAS means that he sees things much differently then I or anyone else sees things. Some people may view that as a difficulty, but it has changed who I am completely. Being able to learn from him has given me the ability to voice my opinion (natural to me) yet understand how or what other people feel (natural to him). Compromising, calmly responding, being loyal to people, always being there, and loving people even though you know them completely, these are only a few things I have acquired from Michael.

A wonderful thing about Michael is his ability to understand one important thing and believe in it wholeheartedly. I was having trouble making a decision on which high school I should attend. I asked him and he answered, "I think you should stay in your school." My response, "Why is that?" And he said, "Because they love you there." That was it. The conversation was over. He didn't care that the average SAT scores were higher or the other schools had college credited courses or the graduation rates were higher. None of that mattered. They love me there and that was more than enough for him to see that was the only choice. Eventually I looked further into my school and found that they do have college accredited courses and maybe some scores were lower, but that's because there is a diverse student body. I decided to stay and, so far, I am having zero thoughts that I made a wrong choice and that is because Michael reminds me of the love.

-Christina DeJoseph

Impact of Prenatal Exposure to Alcohol on a Young Adult and His Family

When I was young I found out that my mom was very sick and that she could die. I only remember bits and pieces of those early years. My mom would go away for awhile or she would be in the hospital but I didn't know what to think then. I was too young. The sickness that plagued my mom was alcoholism and she had been sick for a long time. By the time I was born she was a successful doctor. I went through elementary school while my mom was in recovery and it had appeared that I was not affected by alcohol while in the womb. I went through school with the usual struggles of kids, but the support I had from my family allowed me to carry on without any noticeable problems. In fact, I excelled in certain classes, was repeatedly recommended for honors courses, and got along quite well with my classmates and teachers all the way through school. In high school, I was in National Honor Society, a gifted and talented program, and graduated in the top twenty percent of my class. Outwardly it had appeared that all this time I was a successful student and growing boy. However, it had been a long time and I had known something was wrong with me since kindergarten. Looking at the other kids around me, I knew there was something different about me but I could talk my way out of any suspicion that I needed help. I had trouble staying focused, completing certain tasks, and staying organized. However, I just figured it was me behaving incorrectly and I would keep it under the radar for nearly twenty years. No one even thought to question me about FAE or FAS.

My little brother, who was diagnosed with full-blown FAS when he was eleven, was a more obvious case. We knew Michael was multiply handicapped since he was very little and so his diagnosis came as no surprise. However, it had never occurred to me that Michael was handicapped. He was just my little brother. We shared a room from an early age and I looked after him as all older brothers do. I knew he had some odd behaviors but I understood him. My first thought when he was born was surprise; I had never met a baby before, being that I was only three years old myself. He was so little and looking back on it, his birth changed everything. My mom's sickness had become obvious and so she was going to begin recovery. My family carried on for the next few years with my mom coming and going from the hospital and in-patient recovery. I remember missing her terribly when she would be gone but knowing I had to keep looking after Michael and she would return to us soon. She had to travel out of state for some of her recovery and I remember the care packages and phone calls we would get from her. I could say those years were hard but I was just a kid and I knew how much love there was in our family and that we would get through this. I started to feel disconnected though. I was about six years old and it began to feel like I was drifting from family and then I started first grade. It occurred to me even at that early age that I wouldn't talk about how I felt because I didn't understand. I became worried that I was sick – plagued with an illness I could see none of the kids around me had. Then my little sister, Christina, was born. She, too, was beautiful and surprising when I first saw her in the hospital. Her entrance into the family was a loud one. It was determined after her birth that my mom had cancer and the doctors gave her a fifty-fifty chance of surviving the surgery that was needed to remove it. My mom survived but now she was going to have to learn how to be a mom and we were all going to have to learn how to be a family. My little sister would take the front seat, needing most of my parents' attention so Mike and I went on through school and our early years.

Now the whole period of my childhood is rather cloudy in my memory, mostly because I think I have tried to shut a lot of it out and so only feelings and sorted memories still come through. The trouble I have organizing my feelings and thoughts is probably also involved, making my memory like a scrapbook with large chunks basically let go. I remember my bedroom with my little brother and I remember some school and several family events but it's all very foggy up until around the end of grade school. This is when my life changed dramatically because I had become seriously depressed.

I had become overwhelmed all of a sudden in an entirely new way. I began to slip in school and become significantly disconnected again, but this time I knew something was wrong with me and I would have to come out about it. Still my ability to talk and reason my way out of things kept me from being honest and open with my family and the people in my school and so the true scope of my situation was still unknown to everyone in my life. I had become suicidal and my emotions began to run all over, but the theme was the same: I was getting worse and worse. No one could get though to me because I wouldn't let them and would never ask for help. It would take others telling me I needed help. I didn't really feel so young anymore and I started confronting the idea of death as a release from the chaos I felt in my heart and in my mind. I was smart and yet I couldn't get organized and I was full of emotion but I couldn't feel any connection with the people around me. My little sister at this point still demanded a lot of attention and we battled often. I was also battling with my dad frequently about all kinds of things, but mainly I think I knew I didn't want to be involved in the things he wanted for me. We clashed on so many things. My mom could see right through my chaos to the core and I think she recognized some of her own struggles in me so she became the one person I could open up to and I learned a lot about myself. In those years I felt challenged by everything around me and I started to shut down. Soon however my mom started to pull me out and she introduced me to an amazing woman psychiatrist who also could see through me ability to misdirect and so began to guide me back to world of the living. Life would not go right to smooth sailing though and this would not be my last encounter with depression and suicide.

In fact my adolescent life would be consistently rocked by the waves of my emotions. For months I would be fine and then for months I would go into a spell of internal chaos and pain often leading me to the desire to take my own life. I cried a lot and searched for someone or something to fill the hole in my heart. I tried a serious relationship in high school, seeking some feeling of connection, but that situation just further added to the insanity of that period. I became even more disconnected. All the while, my family was trying to get through to me and I was just drifting further from them. It was in high school though that it truly occurred to me that my little brother was handicapped and that he would always be a little different just like me. Our family was in Washington D.C. participating in an FAS and family documentary project. It was on the way home when we were stuck in traffic that my little brother started acting up. I was sitting in the front seat and I yelled back at him to calm down. After that I thought to myself, why can't he just be normal and act normal? I was washed over then by a wave of feeling. I had just realized that my little brother would never be "normal" and that our family would never be like other families. The next thought I had was that I loved him and I loved being a part of this special family.

It would not be long after this that I would start working with my mom doing FAS and family talks and my perspectives on my past and family would change. I started to learn about alcoholism and FAS and began telling my little story. I'll admit I'm nervous every time I stand up on a stage to tell people about myself. There are so many good stories to tell though and many memories that stand out with me and Mike. He has taught me so much about what's important and about myself, but he did so in such a graceful way that, if you didn't stop to think about it, you wouldn't even realize. All that I have learned in the last few years has helped me gain some perspective so I have conquered my suicidal tendencies knowing now that life is way too important to ever take it for granted that way again. I still battle a lot of emotional ups and downs, but I take life one day at a time now and carry on. My family still has challenges from time to time, but everyone carries on well and we are closer now for all that we have overcome.

About two years ago, I underwent testing for the first time to determine if I was at all affected by alcohol in the womb. The testing would determine that I was very intelligent but that the troubles I have always had with organizing and emotional instability could be linked to occasional drinking during my mom's pregnancy. We had thought all these years that I had been skipped over and that my little brother was the only one who was affected. It wasn't that my parents didn't see it but rather that I was again able to convince everyone that I was fine and that they needn't worry about me. Again I traveled under the radar and would later learn a truth about myself. Since kindergarten I was walking a different way than other kids around me, having come from a different place than the kids around me. I still was able to drift in with my peers but always felt distant from them and it is only now that a lot of the chaos and confusion I felt then is all starting to make sense. I wouldn't want anyone reading this to think that I feel slighted by the way my life has carried out so far; in fact, I feel quite the opposite. I have always felt my life has been many things but it has never been boring and for that I am very thankful. I would never wish to be anywhere else and now I can share my story and, hopefully, if there are any older brothers or sisters out there struggling, they can at least know they are not alone and even when thinking about death, there is still hope to be found everywhere. We just have to keep our eyes open for it.

Stephen DeJoseph

Suggested Reading/Viewing By and For Families Dealing with FASD

AL-ANON Family Groups. *From Survival to Recovery: Growing Up in an Alcoholic Home.* New York, NY: AL-ANON Family Groups.1994.

Alcoholics Anonymous World Services. *Living Sober.* New York, NY: Alcoholics Anonymous World Services.1975.

Barth, RP, Brodinsky D., & Freundlich M. *Adoption and Prenatal Alcohol and Drug Exposure.* Washington, DC: Child Welfare League of America, Inc. (2000).

Bobula J., & Bobula K. *Forgetful Frankie: The World's Greatest Rock Skipper.* Canada: Wildberry Productions. 2009.

Centers for Disease Control. *Fetal Alcohol Syndrome: Guidelines for Referral and Diagnosis.* Washington, DC: U.S. Department of Health and Human Services. 2004.

Chavez J., & Chavez, E. The ABC's of Fetal Alcohol Syndrome/Effect: A Handbook for Middle - Junior - Senior High School Teachers. Lewiston, ID: Chavez. 1993.

Children's Research Triangle. FASD Across the Span of Childhood: A Handbook for Parents and Providers. Chicago, IL: NTI Upstream. 2008.

Cole CK, Coles CD, Kanne Poulsen, M, Smith GH. *Children, Families, and Substance Abuse: Challenges for Changing Educational and Social Outcomes.* Baltimore, MD: Paul H. Brookes Publishing Company. 1995.

Conry J, Fast D. *Fetal Alcohol Syndrome and the Criminal Justice System.* Vancouver, Canada: British Columbia Fetal Alcohol Syndrome Resource Society. 2000.

Crowe J. *The Fatal Link.* Denver, CO: Outskirts Press, Inc. 2009.

Davis D. *Reaching Out to Children with FAS/FAE.* West Nyack, NY: The Center for Applied Research in Education. 1994.

Dorris M. *The Broken Cord.* New York, NY: Harper Perennial. 1989.

Double ARC. Triumph: Through the Challenges of Fetal Alcohol Syndrome. Findlay, OH: Kennedy Printing. 2004.

Falkner L. *I Would Be Loved*. College Station, TX: Virtualbookworm.com Publishing, Inc. 2002.

Hays Kids. Pathways to Success: A Fetal Alcohol Workbook. Cook, MN: Hays. 2009.

Hays Kids, Payne W. (Producer). (2005). *Pathways to Understanding: Raising Kids with Fetal Alcohol Spectrum Disorder*. [Seminar] New York, NY: Follow Productions.

Irene M. *Fetal Alcohol*. Bloomington, IN: AuthorHouse. 2004.

Kleinfeld J. *Fantastic Antone Grows Up*. Fairbanks, AK: University of Alaska Press. 2003.

Kleinfeld J, Wescott S. *Fantastic Antone Succeeds*. Fairbanks, AK: University of Alaska Press. 1993.

Kulp J. *The Whitest Wall*. Brooklyn Park, MN: Better Endings New Beginnings. 2008.

Kulp J. *Our FAScinating Journey*. Brooklyn Park, MN: Better Endings New Beginnings. 2002.

Kulp,L. *The Best I Can Be: Living with Fetal Alcohol Syndrome or Effects*. Brooklyn Park, MN: Better Endings New Beginnings. 2000.

Lesley C *Storm Riders*. New York, NY: Picador USA.2000.

Malbin D. *Trying Differently Rather Than Harder*. Portland, OR: Tectrice, Inc.2002.

McCreight B Recognizing and Managing Children with Fetal Alcohol Syndrome/Fetal Alcohol Effects: A Guidebook. Washington, DC: CWLA Press.1997.

Minnesota Department of Health. Guidelines of Care for Children with Special Health Care Needs: Fetal Alcohol Syndrome and Fetal Alcohol Effects. St. Paul, MN: Minnesota Department of Health. 1999.

Mitchell K. *Fetal Alcohol Syndrome: Practical Suggestions and Support for Families and Caregivers*. Washington, DC: National Organization on Fetal Alcohol Syndrome. 2002.

Morse BA, Weiner, L. *FAS: Parent and Child*. Boston, MA: Fetal Alcohol Education Program. 1993.

National Institute on Alcohol Abuse and Alcoholism. *Identification and Care of Fetal Alcohol-Exposed Children*. Bethesda, MD: National Institutes of Health. 1999.

National Institute on Alcohol Abuse and Alcoholism. *Identification of At-Risk Drinking and Intervention with Women of Childbearing Age*. Bethesda, MD: National Institutes of Health. 1999.

National Organization on Fetal Alcohol Syndrome*Making a Difference: Fetal Alcohol Spectrum Disorders Public Awareness Guide*. Washington, DC: National Organization on Fetal Alcohol Syndrome. 2007.

National Organization on Fetal Alcohol Syndrome*Karli and the Star of the Week*. Washington, DC: National Organization on Fetal Alcohol Syndrome. 2006.

National Organization on Fetal Alcohol Syndrome*Fetal Alcohol Spectrum Disorders: An Overview*. Washington, DC: National Organization on Fetal Alcohol Syndrome (DVD). 2004.

National Organization on Fetal Alcohol Syndrome-United Kingdom *A Child for Life*. London, England: National Organization on Fetal Alcohol Syndrome-United Kingdom (DVD). 2006.

Neafcy S. J*The Long Way to Simple: Fetal Alcohol Spectrum Disorders*. Brooklyn Park, MN: Better Endings New Beginnings. 2008.

Norgard K. *Hard to Place: A Crime of Alcohol*. Tucson, AZ: Recovery Resources Press. 2006.

Streissguth A. *Fetal Alcohol Syndrome: A Guide for Families and Communities*. Baltimore, MD: Paul H. Brookes Publishing Company. 1997.

Streissguth A, Kanter J. *The Challenge of Fetal Alcohol Syndrome: Overcoming Secondary Disabilities*. Seattle, WA: University of Washington Press. 1997.

U.S. Department of Health and Human Services. Reducing Alcohol-Exposed Pregnancies: A Report on the National Task Force on Fetal Alcohol Syndrome and Fetal Alcohol Effect. Washington, DC: U.S. Department of Health and Human Services. 2009.

U.S. Department of Health and Human Services A Call to Action: Advancing Essential Services and Research on Fetal Alcohol Spectrum Disorders, A Report of the National Task Force on Fetal Alcohol Syndrome and Fetal Alcohol Effect. Washington, DC: U.S. Department of Health and Human Services. 2009.

Substance Abuse and Mental Health Services Administration. *Recovering Hope: Mothers Speak Out about Fetal Alcohol Spectrum Disorders*. Washington, DC: U.S. Department of Health and Human Services. 2006.

University of New Mexico Department of Pediatrics, Fetal Alcohol Syndrome Growth Survey. *Fetal Alcohol Syndrome: A Handbook for Parents and Caregivers*. Albuquerque, NM: The University of New Mexico. 1999.

University of Washington Fetal Alcohol and Drug Unit. *Educating Children Prenatally Exposed to Alcohol and Other Drugs*. Seattle, WA: University of Washington Press. 1992.

Winokur MK. My Invisible World: Life with My Brother, His Disability, and His Service Dog. Brooklyn Park, MN: Better Endings New Beginnings. 2009.

Yurcek A. *Tiny Titan*. Brooklyn Park, MN: Better Endings New Beginnings. 2006.

REFERENCES

[1]   Greenfield S. Sex differences in substance use disorders. In Lewis-Hall, Freda MD, ed. Psychiatric Illness in Women: Emerging Treatments and Research. Washington DC: American Psychiatric Association Publishing, Inc. 2002.

[2]   U.S. Department of Health and Human Services. Reducing Alcohol-Exposed Pregnancies: A Report on the National Task Force on Fetal Alcohol Syndrome and Fetal Alcohol Effect. Washington, DC: U.S. Department of Health and Human Services. 2009.

[3]   Streissguth A. Fetal Alcohol Syndrome: A Guide for families and communities. Baltimore, MD: Paul H. Brookes Publishing Company. 1997.

[4]   U.S. Department of Health and Human Services. A Call to Action: Advancing Essential Services and Research on Fetal Alcohol Spectrum Disorders, A Report of the National Task Force on Fetal Alcohol Syndrome and Fetal Alcohol Effect. Washington, DC: U.S. Department of Health and Human Services. 2009.

[5]   Olson HC, Oti R, Gelo J. "Family Matters:" Fetal alcohol spectrum disorders and the family. Devel Disabil Res Rev 2009; 15: 235-249.

[6]   Jones KL, Smith DW, Ulleland CN, Streissguth AP. Pattern of malformation in offspring of chronic alcoholic mothers. Lancet 1973; 1: 1267-71.

[7]   Robe L. Co-starring famous women and alcohol: the dramatic truth behind the tragedies and triumphs of 200 celebrities. Minneapolis, Minnesota: Comp Care Publications. 1986.

[8]   Shorter E. A History of Psychiatry. New York, Chichester, Brisbane, Toronto: John Wiley & Sons, Inc. 1997.

[9]   Prestwich P. Female Alcoholism in Paris 1870-1920: The Response of psychiatrists and of families. Hist Psychiatry 2003; 14(3): 321-336.

[10]   Rothman DJ. Discovery of the Asylum: Social Order and Disorder in the New Republic. Boston, Toronto: Little, Brown, & Co. 1971.

[11]   Jamison K. Night Falls Fast: Understanding Suicide. New York: Alfred A Knopf. 1999.

[12]   Lunardini C. What every american should know about women's history: 200 events that shaped our destiny. Hollbrook, Mass: Bob Adams, Inc. 1994.

[13]   Sayers J. Mothers of Psychoanalysis. New York, London: WW Norton & Co. 1991.

[14]   Chesler P. Women and Madness, Revised and Updated. US, UK: Palgrave Macmillan. 2005.

CHAPTER 9

Translating Research into Action: Federal and State Initiatives

Deborah E. Cohen[1] and Susan A. Adubato[2],*

[1]*New Jersey Department of Human Services, Division of Developmental Disabilities, Hamilton, NJ and* [2]*University of Medicine and Dentistry – New Jersey Medical School, New Jersey FASD Education and Research Center, Newark, New Jersey, USA*

"For persons with developmental disabilities and their families, diagnosis is never an endpoint "

National Task Force on FAS/FAE, 2002

Abstract: Basic research into Fetal Alcohol Spectrum Disorders (FASD) is contributing much important information to our understanding of the dynamics of how alcohol affects developing neurological and physiological systems in unborn children. Clinical research is beginning to offer guidelines for intervention, treatment and services for women who may abuse alcohol and to children who are affected by prenatal exposures. It is equally important that, when the findings of research reach the point of utility, they be put into practice as standards of care. While the types and availability of services vary among states, most jurisdictions do support systems that can provide services and treatment to these populations. The purpose of this chapter is fourfold: 1. Provide an overview of the work that has been undertaken by federal agencies and associated task forces to develop innovative interventions and to encourage and reinforce the implementation of services on the state level; 2. Describe the service components that are generally available in each state; 3. Provide a description of service models that have been established or are evolving on the state level; and 4. Describe the role of voluntary agencies in the non-profit sector in establishing service systems for persons with FASD.

LEADERSHIP BY NATIONAL AGENCIES

Recognition that national governmental agencies needed to have open communication among them and to play a leadership role in research and prevention of FAS was acknowledged in the early 1990s. One of the earliest documents to address FAS, *Fetal Alcohol Syndrome and Pregnant Women Who Abuse Alcohol: An Overview of the Issue and the Federal Response,* was produced through interagency collaboration and published by the U.S. Department of Health and Human Services (USDHHS), Office of the Assistant Secretary for Planning and Evaluation, Office of Human Services Policy, Division of Children and Youth Policy in February 1992 [1]. Experts from the National Institute on Alcohol Abuse and Alcoholism (NIAAA), the Indian Health Service (IHS), the Centers for Disease Control (now "and Prevention") (CDC), and the Administration for Children, Youth and Family (ACYF) participated in writing this document. It is noteworthy for bringing together representatives from several federal agencies that are responsible for addressing alcohol abuse in women and its impact upon fetal development as well as for the broad range of issues it raised. One chapter in particular, "Gaps in Knowledge and Services", identified some components of a comprehensive service system and began the task of identifying the appropriate services needed by persons with FASD [1].

As described in previous chapters, the Institute of Medicine (IOM) published a report on FAS in 1996 that underscored the importance of a coordinated effort among federal agencies in addressing the myriad of issues associated with preventing and treating FASD [2]. One of the primary outcomes of the IOM report was the establishment of the Interagency Coordinating Committee on Fetal Alcohol Syndrome (ICCFAS) in October 1996 [3]. The IOM report noted that the responsibility for addressing the many issues relevant to FASD transcended the mission and resources of any single agency or program. It recommended that the NIAAA chair an effort to coordinate Federal activities on FAS and other disorders associated with prenatal alcohol exposure. As posited in its mission statement, "The challenge facing the ICCFAS is to improve communication, cooperation, and collaboration among disciplines that address health, education, developmental disability, research, justice, and social service issues relevant to FAS and related disorders caused by prenatal alcohol exposure" [3].

*Address correspondence to Susan A. Adubato: UMDNJ-NJMS New Jersey FASD Education and Research Center 30 Bergen Street ADMN 1608 Newark, NJ 07101, USA; E-mail: adubatsu@umdnj.edu

Meeting semi-annually, the membership of the ICCFAS is broad-based and includes representatives from the following agencies:

The Department of Health and Human Services (DHHS):

- Agency for Healthcare Research and Quality (AHRQ);
- Centers for Disease Control and Prevention (CDC);
- Health Resources and Services Administration (HRSA)'s Maternal and Child Health Bureau (MCHB);
- Indian Health Service (IHS);
- National Institutes of Health (NIH):
  - National Institute on Alcohol Abuse and Alcoholism (NIAAA) and
  - National Institute of Child Health and Human Development (NICHD);
- Substance Abuse and Mental Health Services Administration (SAMHSA);

The Department of Education (ED):

- Office of Special Education and Rehabilitative Services (OSERS); and

The Department of Justice (DOJ):

- Office of Juvenile Justice and Delinquency Prevention (OJJDP).

Early in their deliberations, members of the ICCFAS recognized that issues related to the behavior, social and health impacts of prenatal alcohol exposure were largely unknown and little research had been conducted in these areas. To learn more about these topics, the ICCFAS held a special focus session in September 1998 and published its proceedings, **Intervening with Children Affected by Prenatal Alcohol Exposure** [4]. These proceedings are one of the first documents to look more closely at specific state systems, e.g., mental health, developmental disabilities, special education, that are crucial to addressing the needs of persons with FASD.

The work of the ICCFAS continues. Its mission and accomplishments is summarized in its Progress Report and Five-Year Strategic Plan found at: (**http://www.niaaa.nih.gov/AboutNIAAA/Interagency/Pages/default.aspx**

In the late 1990s, advocacy agencies began to work with the U.S. Congress on two important pieces of legislation. These efforts resulted in: 1) the establishment of the National Task Force on Fetal Alcohol Syndrome and Fetal Alcohol Effects (FAE) (the Task Force) and 2) the founding of SAMHSA's Center for Excellence in FASD (the Center).

NATIONAL TASK FORCE ON FAS/FAE

In 1998, the U. S. Congress was made aware of the significant problems and costs associated with prenatal consumption of alcohol. In response, the Public Health Service Act, Section 299G (42 U.S.C. Section 280f, as added by Public Law 105-392) directed the Secretary of the U.S. Department of Health and Human Services (DHHS) to establish the Task Force [5]. The mission of the Task Force was to 1) foster coordination among all governmental agencies, academic bodies, and community groups that conduct or support FAS or FAE research, programs, and surveillance; and 2) otherwise meet the needs of populations impacted by FAS and FAE [5 – MMWR – Task Force]. CDC's National Center on Birth Defects and Developmental Disabilities (NCBDDD) was charged with the responsibility of administering the Task Force. As described in its charter, the functions of the Task Force were to:

- Advise persons involved in federal, state, and local programs and research activities of FAS and FAE regarding such topics as FAS awareness and education for relevant service providers and the general public (including school-aged children and women at risk), medical diagnosis for affected persons and their families;
- Coordinate its efforts with the DHHS ICCFAS; and
- Report, on a biennial basis, to the DHHS Secretary and relevant committees of Congress on the current and planned activities of the participating agencies [5].

Early in its operation, the Task Force formed two working groups: the Research Working Group and the Services and Public Awareness Working Group. The purpose of the Work Group was to evaluate existing FAS and ARND research and services and to make recommendations concerning actions needed to remedy deficiencies. Several of the recommendations posited by the Public Awareness Work Group spoke to the need to establish or improve services for persons with FASD at the state level. Recommendation 12, in particular, articulated this need by stating, "Develop a checklist of essential state services needed to prevent FAS and ARND, to treat persons with FAS and ARND and their families, and to better identify women at risk of having an alcohol-exposed pregnancy" [5]. (The complete list of all recommendations can be viewed at **http://www.cdc.gov/mmwr/preview/mmwrhtml/rr5114a2.htm**)

While the adverse effects of prenatal exposure are known, children who have been subjected to alcohol are often not referred for diagnostic evaluation or do not receive a correct diagnosis because of the absence of guidelines for referral and uniformly accepted diagnostic criteria. In 2002, Congress directed CDC to 1) develop guidelines for diagnosing FAS and other negative birth outcomes resulting from prenatal exposure to alcohol, 2) incorporate these guidelines into curricula for medical and allied health students and practitioners, and 3) disseminate curricula concerning these guidelines to facilitate training of medical and allied health students and practitioners.

In response to the Congressional mandate, CDC established a scientific working group (SWG) that consisted of persons with expertise in research and clinical practice regarding prenatal exposure to alcohol to develop diagnostic guidelines for FAS. The SWG worked closely with the Task Force to develop the guidelines. Both the SWG and the Task Force recognized that reaching consensus on the diagnostic criteria could not be the only outcome of their work. As a result, the ***Guidelines for Identifying and Referring Persons with Fetal Alcohol Syndrome*** goes beyond the primary Congressional mandate to include sections that address the implementation of:

- effective programs to educate women about the risks of consuming alcohol during pregnancy.

- efficacious screening tools to identify pregnant women who are consuming alcohol during pregnancy and use of brief interventions.

- effective programs to encourage the use of contraceptives by women who abuse alcohol [6].

The Guidelines also contributed to the growing body of knowledge regarding the educational and service needs of persons affected by prenatal exposure to alcohol and their families. The Guidelines can be accessed at: **http://cdc.gov/ncbdd/fasd/documents/RedAlcohPreg.pdf**

[§]Following the issuing of the Guidelines, the Task Force and CDC concentrated on identifying and supporting scientifically proven programs that reduced the consumption of alcohol among women, establishing the efficacy of screening and implementation of brief interventions for pregnant women. In its deliberations, the Task Force noted the importance of several societal variables:

Accessibility of Alcohol

Alcohol is a highly accessible and commonly consumed product that is integrated into many aspects of American culture, from special events to everyday life. However, it is one of the few socially acceptable products that is a major known contributor to disease, disability, and premature mortality [7]. Alcohol is a leading cause of morbidity and mortality in the United States [8,9]. Also, according to *Healthy People 2010* [10], substance abuse, which includes alcohol and illicit drug use, has been identified as 1 of the 10 leading health concerns that should be addressed and monitored to measure the health of the U.S general population. Moreover, among all substances of abuse, alcohol is the one most commonly consumed by women of childbearing age [11].

Reducing Alcohol-Exposed Pregnancies

The consumption of alcohol is pervasive in American society. SAMHSA's 2007 National Survey on Drug Use and Health documents that over 50% of all Americans report that they consume alcohol. While one 10-year national trend study of alcohol consumption during the period 1984–1995 [12] noted an overall decline in drinking rates during the study period, virtually no changes were found during the period 1990–1995, prompting the author to question whether or not the period of declining drinking rates might be over.

[§]*This section was written by R. Louise Floyd, RN, DSN and Mary Kate Weber, MPH, Centers for Disease Control and Prevention, National Center on Birth Defects and Developmental Disabilities, Prevention Research Branch, Fetal Alcohol Syndrome Prevention Team, Atlanta, GA and Mary J. O'Connor, PhD, ABPP, University of California at Los Angeles, Department of Psychiatry and Biobehavioral Sciences, David Geffen School of Medicine, Los Angeles, CA*

Similarly, another study looking at national binge drinking rates among adults during the period 1993–2001 [13] found that drinking rates had not declined and that the number of binge drinking episodes per capita actually had been increasing since 1995. Most recently, a national trend study of women of childbearing age (18–44 years) during the period 1991–2005 [14] found that there were no substantial changes in alcohol use and binge drinking rates among pregnant and non-pregnant women over the 15-year study period. These findings are especially troubling because drinking alcohol during pregnancy increases a woman's risk of having a baby with birth defects and developmental disabilities, including FASD.

The Task Force concluded that the implication of these findings might be daunting from a public health perspective and posed the question: Can it be that declines in alcohol use rates are relics of the past, and that the current rates will hold steady—if not increase in severity—over time (i.e., increasing per capita binge drinking rates)? As a response to these serious public health challenges, the Task Force gathered the facts of what interventions are currently known to be effective in the prevention of alcohol-exposed pregnancies (AEPs) and recommended the immediate implementation of these strategies in order to reduce adverse pregnancy outcomes for women and infants.

The Task Force produced a compilation report in March 2009. That report, *Reducing Alcohol-Exposed Pregnancies: A Report of the National Task Force on Fetal Alcohol Syndrome and Fetal Alcohol Effect* [15], reviewed existing evidence on prevention strategies to reduce alcohol use and AEPs, provided recommendations for promoting and improving these strategies, and offered future research directions in the field of FASD prevention. To read this important report, please go to: **http://www.cdc.gov/ncbddd/fasd/documents/FAS_guidelines_accessible.pdf**

While efforts to prevent prenatal alcohol exposure are ongoing at the local, state, and federal levels, the Task Force noted that chronic and binge drinking among women of childbearing age continue to persist, calling for a comprehensive approach to address alcohol use during pregnancy that should include both clinical and population-based alcohol use prevention strategies. It also reinforced the concept that it is also important to develop and maintain a continuum of evidence-based services and treatments for women of childbearing age to reduce the risk of AEPs and other adverse pregnancy outcomes. Table **1** summarizes the recommendations of the Task Force.

Table 1: Recommendations from the National Task Force on Fetal Alcohol Syndrome and Fetal Alcohol Effect

Universal Prevention[1]	
Recommendation 1:	Expand and test methodological approaches for assessing the effects of universal prevention strategies on alcohol use patterns and reproductive health outcomes of childbearing-aged women.
Recommendation 2:	Promote the implementation of effective population-based interventions for reducing alcohol-related harms in the general population, including women of childbearing age, as they are validated.
Selective and Indicated Prevention[2]	
Recommendation 3:	Ensure that funded intervention studies on alcohol use, abuse, and dependence include analyses of gender and age effects and examine pregnancy outcomes where possible.
Recommendation 4:	Promote the use of evidence-based intervention strategies tested in primary care, emergency rooms, and college settings for use in populations of childbearing-aged women at risk for an alcohol-exposed pregnancy.
Recommendation 5:	Establish formal alcohol screening, using validated instruments, and brief intervention programs that are culturally and linguistically appropriate for women of childbearing age.
Recommendation 6:	Expand the education and training of health and social service professionals in the areas of screening and intervening with women at risk for alcohol-exposed pregnancies.
Recommendation 7:	Ensure access to appropriate alcohol treatment services for women of childbearing age, especially those with treatment barriers, such as pregnant women and adolescents.
Recommendation 8:	Ensure that alcohol treatment options for all childbearing-aged women take into consideration their unique needs, such as pregnancy, co-occurring disorders, and other special treatment needs.
Recommendation 9:	Conduct further research aimed at implementing and evaluating treatment and intensive case-management approaches for women at highest risk of having a child with a fetal alcohol spectrum disorder.
Recommendation 10:	Promote research investigating interventions focused on the potential intergenerational effects of prenatal alcohol use on offspring.

[1]Universal prevention interventions attempt to promote the health of the general public or a particular group, regardless of risk.

[2]Selective and indicated prevention strategies are targeted and intensive falling along a continuum of care depending on the severity of the alcohol-related problem.

The CDC has continued to invest in state and university-based programs that address a broad range of training and service issues as recommended by the Task Force. Descriptions of these initiatives are available at: **http://www.cdc.gov/ncbddd/fasd/index.html**

SAMHSA'S CENTER FOR EXCELLENCE IN FASD

In 2000, Congress authorized the establishment of a FASD Center for Excellence in Section 519D of the Children's Health Act of 2000, (Section b of 42 USC 290bb-25d or Public Law 106-310) and appropriated funds to SAMHSA for this purpose. The FASD Center for Excellence (the Center) was launched in 2001 with six explicit mandates:

(1) study adaptations of innovative clinical interventions and service delivery improvement strategies for children and adults with fetal alcohol syndrome or alcohol-related birth defects and their families;

(2) identify communities which have an exemplary comprehensive system of care for such individuals so that they can provide technical assistance to other communities attempting to set up such a system of care;

(3) provide technical assistance to communities who do not have a comprehensive system of care for such individuals and their families;

(4) train community leaders, mental health and substance abuse professionals, families, law enforcement personnel, judges, health professionals, persons working in financial assistance programs, social service personnel, child welfare professionals, and other service providers on the implications of fetal alcohol syndrome and alcohol-related birth defects, the early identification of and referral for such conditions;

(5) develop innovative techniques for preventing alcohol use by women in child bearing years;

(6) perform other functions, to the extent authorized by the Secretary after consideration of recommendations made by the National Task Force on Fetal Alcohol Syndrome [16].

One of the first tasks undertaken by the Center was to organize a Steering Committee to help refine the mandates and provide guidance. At its inaugural meeting in February 2002, the Steering Committee formed workgroups to address the Center's six mandates and to identify best practices. Following a review of the existing clinical and community service interventions and treatment, the work groups concluded that there were a few pockets of services that might serve as models on which to build best practice systems. However, little science-based information existed on the efficacy of treatment programs for individuals with FASD, particularly with respect to age-specific interventions.

The Center, with guidance from the Steering Committee, has provided the leadership in delineating the components needed for an exemplary system of services for the prevention and treatment of FASD on the state level. These components are delineated in Table **2**:

Table 2: Matrix of State and Community Services for Prevention and Treatment of FASD

Prevention Education	
Universal	
	Public Education Campaigns
	Broadcast Media – PSAs and Paid Ads
	Alcohol Beverage Labeling
	Point of Sale Signs
	International FASD Prevention Day Campaigns
Specific	
	Physician Training and Continuing Education
	Medical Specialty Training, e.g., psychiatry
	Allied Health Professional Training
	Special Education Teacher Training
	School-Based FASD Health Education

Table 2: cont….

Prevention Education	
	Certified Alcohol and Drug Counselor Training
Indicated	
	Education of all Women of Child-Bearing Age
	Education of Women at High Risk
Women's Services	
Health Care	Universal Screening of all Women of Child-Bearing Age
	Universal Screening of all Pregnant Women
	Brief Intervention and Referral
	Postpartum Follow-Up Services
Addiction Treatment	Inpatient and Outpatient Services with Capacity to Include Children
	On-going Support Services, e.g., AA
	Employment Training Programs, e.g., PCAP
Children & Adolescents	
	Post partum Follow-up
	Child Evaluation Centers
	FASD Diagnostic Centers
	Early Intervention Services
	Therapeutic Services, e.g., PT, OT, Speech Language
	Preschool Handicapped Services
	Special Education
	Behavioral & Psychological Therapeutic Services
	Socialization & Recreational Programs
	Afterschool Programs
	Skills of Daily Living Education
	Vocational Education
	Family Life Education & Sexuality
Adult Services	
	Vocational Training
	Supported Employment
	Residential Services
	Money Management Training & Services
	Socialization & Recreational Programs
	Alcohol & Drug Prevention/Treatment Services
	Faith-Based Inclusion and Support
Family Services	
	Respite Care
	Financial Support, e.g., Medicaid, SSDI
	Parenting Education
	Family Support Groups
	Faith-Based Inclusion & Support Groups
	Guardianship Training
Juvenile & Criminal Justice	
	Family Court Judge Training
	Juvenile Justice System Training
	Institutional Training

(Adapted from the SAMHSA's Center for Excellence in FASD Steering Committee Minutes, February 2002).

States serve as the primary locus of activity for the development and implementation of programs and services for prevention of FASD as well as for clinical diagnosis and services for affected persons and their families. SAMHSA's FASD Center for Excellence provides the leadership to encourage and provide technical assistance to states:

- to have a designated State FASD Coordinator,

- to organize state-wide FASD Task Forces to enhance communication and service coordination,

- to educate communities about the affects of drinking during pregnancy,

- to develop and implement systems of intervention and care, and

- to provide leadership while undertaking other important actions.

The map below which is taken from SAMHSA's FASD Center for Excellence's State Page (http://www.fascenter.samhsa.gov/statesystemsofcare/statesystemsofcare.cfm) provides a snapshot of programs and initiatives that are underway in some states. A quick reference list of States by categories can be accessed here.

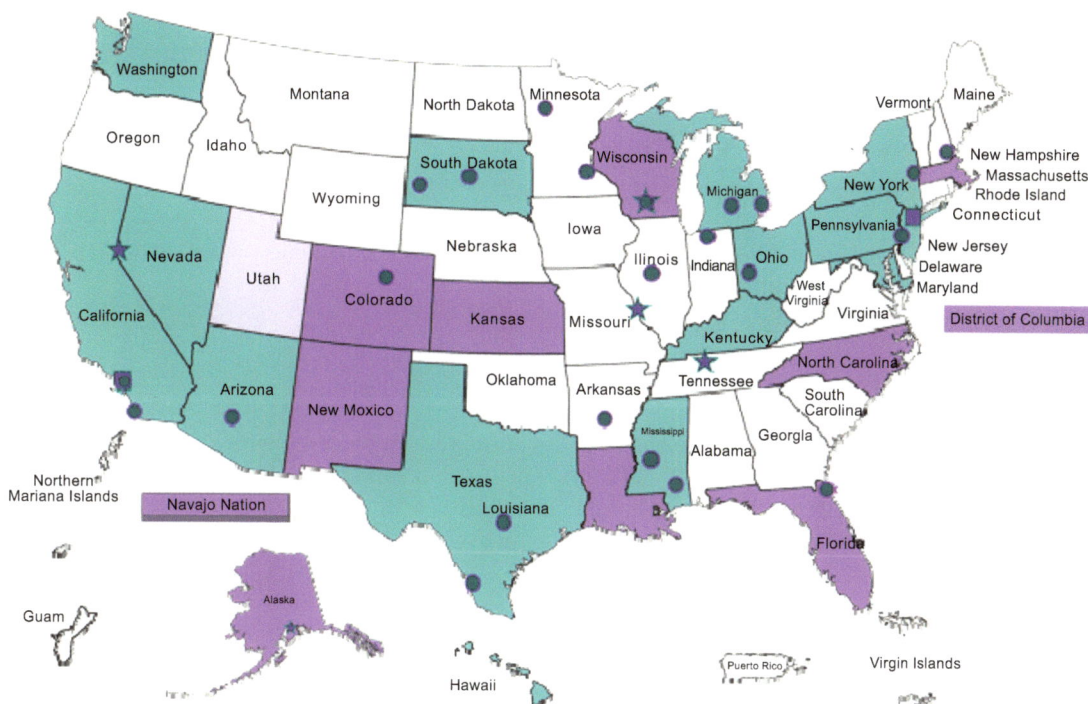

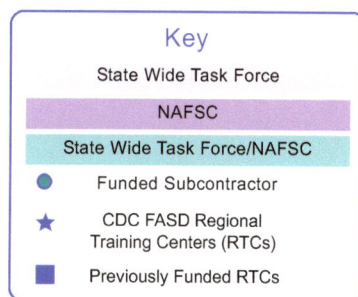

Key

State Wide Task Force	
NAFSC	
State Wide Task Force/NAFSC	
●	Funded Subcontractor
★	CDC FASD Regional Training Centers (RTCs)
■	Previously Funded RTCs

More information about the FASD Center for Excellence's subcontracts is available at: http://www.fascenter.samhsa.gov/

More information about CDC initiatives is available at: http://www.cdc.gov/ncbddd/fasd/index.html

The University of Washington maintains a database of the FAS Diagnostic and Prevention Network which can be accessed at: http://depts.washington.edu/fasdpn/htmls/nationwide.htm

A major initiative of the FASD Center for Excellence has been to provide the leadership for assisting states in addressing FASD. The Center has accomplished this by organizing the "Building FASD State Systems" (BFSS) and sponsoring annual meetings. A summary of the meetings is available at: http://www.fascenter.samhsa.gov/initiatives/bfssMeeting.cfm

One of the outcomes of the BFSS has been the establishment of the National Association of FASD State Coordinators (NAFSC). NAFSC's most important activities revolve around capacity-building and dissemination of science-based information on best practices and lessons learned from other States. NAFSC also seeks to:

- Provide information and resources.

- Provide mentorship and support to individuals involved in FASD efforts on a state level.

- Identify and share models for FASD prevention and treatment and involvement of service systems in addressing FASD.

- Establish and maintain a national identity for FASD.

- Advocate for all states to have a designated FASD Coordinator.

- Educate consumers, providers, researchers, and policymakers on FASD.

- Establish partnerships on a national and grassroots level.

There are currently 23 states in addition to the District of Columbia and Navajo Nation that have officially designated a FASD Coordinator. Additional information about NAFSC is available at http://www.fascenter.samhsa.gov/statesystemsofcare/nafsc.cfm

STATE AND TERRITORIAL SYSTEMS

As noted in the previous section, the FASD Center for Excellence has provided ongoing technical assistance to states to develop systems for preventing FASD and to provide services to individuals who have been affected by prenatal exposure to alcohol. However, several states initiated efforts to address prenatal consumption of alcohol and FASD prior to the advent of the Center. This section provides an overview of the evolution of FASD prevention and services in three states and the Common`wealth of Puerto Rico.

NEW JERSEY

New Jersey was one of the first states to begin to address FASD. In 1982, the first statewide conference on Fetal Alcohol Syndrome (FAS) was held for professionals working in the field of perinatal medicine. The first New Jersey Task Force was established a year later by the Governor's Advisory Council on Alcoholism within the NJ Department of Health (now the Department of Health and Senior Services (DHSS)). Over the next five years, the Task Force designed and conducted several programs and activities to increase public and professional awareness about the effects of alcohol on the developing fetus. Enough interest was raised through the media, the public education network and community organizations, such as the March of Dimes that, in 1993, the NJ State Legislature passed Public Law 1993, Chapter 43. This bill requires that warnings regarding the dangers of drinking alcohol during pregnancy be posted in all establishments that sell or serve alcoholic beverages.

During the 1980's, however, few direct services were available to address the specific issues of pregnant women who used or were addicted to alcohol. Systems to identify, manage and provide follow-up of these women and their infants were needed. In 1985, the Governor's Council on the Prevention of Mental Retardation published its report, ***Programs for Preventing the Causes of Mental Retardation*** [17]. This report summarized the status of prevention efforts in New Jersey at that time and presented recommendations on what actions the State needed to undertake to improve prevention efforts. One of the recommendations was the development of a more substantial systematic statewide approach to address FAS.

In 1988, the DHSS elected to implement this recommendation through the establishment of the FAS Prevention Project. The primary mission of the initiative was to provide a coordinated, statewide network of regionalized services to prevent the adverse effects of alcohol and substance use on the developing fetus and to promote healthy pregnancy outcomes. Hospitals and other agencies referred at risk women to Risk Reduction Specialists who provided direct drug and alcohol interventions and referrals to addiction treatment programs.

In its first twelve years of operation, the FAS Prevention Project staff identified thousands of women who were drinking during pregnancy and referred them to treatment services. However, despite its effectiveness, the FAS Prevention Program focused primarily on women who were already pregnant and who used clinic-based services. In addition, an evaluation conducted by the Center for Alcohol Studies at Rutgers University in 1996, was able to show the correlation between the Risk Reduction System and women's access to intervention and treatment services. However, it was unable to document a strong link between risk reduction services and infant health, both at birth and during development.

The DHSS also recognized that many persons who were suspected of having FAS were appearing with regularity in the judicial system. Partnering with other state departments, the DHSS sponsored a workshop on FAS for New Jersey Family Court Judges in 1993. The program included topics on recognizing FAS in teen defendants; sentencing issues for teens identified with FAS; and techniques for communicating with persons affected by FAS. This initiative has continued in New Jersey with periodic training programs being provided by the New Jersey FASD Education and Research Center (originally the Northeastern Regional FASD Training Center), The Arc of New Jersey and other organizations.

In 1998, the Office for Prevention of Developmental Disabilities (OPDD) in the New Jersey Department of Human Services (DHS), in partnership with the DHSS and several community organizations, sponsored a statewide conference regarding FAS. Ann Streissguth, Ph.D., was the keynote speaker. Following the conference, Dr. Streissguth provided information to representatives from OPDD, DHSS and community agencies on the legislation and program initiatives that were underway in Washington State and provided technical assistance for New Jersey to replicate some of these initiatives. This meeting resulted in the transfer of the FAS (now the FASD and other Perinatal Addictions) Task Force from the DHSS to the Governor's Council on the Prevention of Developmental Disabilities. The Governor's Council on Prevention, a legislatively established board, incorporated the FAS Task Force into its structure by making it a standing committee and appointed a member of the Governor's Council to serve as Chair. The Planning Committee for the conference as well as the FAS Risk Reduction Specialists and representatives of community service agencies became the initial members of the re-organized Task Force.

FETAL ALCOHOL SEPCTRUM DISORDERS AND OTHER PERINATAL ADDICTIONS TASK FORCE

As its first initiative, the Task Force investigated the status of FASD prevention and treatment programs in New Jersey. In 2001, the Governor's Council on Prevention and the Task Force submitted a report, ***Truth and Consequences of Fetal Alcohol Syndrome: Why New Jersey Should Be Concerned***, to Acting Governor Donald T. DiFrancesco [18]. The report included a recommendation for the establishment of FAS Diagnostic Centers. Acting Governor DiFrancesco included funds for the diagnostic centers in his Kids Needs Initiative, resulting in a state appropriation to DHSS to implement the recommendation. The report is available at http://www.state.nj.us/humanservices/opmrdd/fasd/FASbooklet.pdf

The Task Force continued its work. In 2003, in partnership with CDC, the NJ Task Force sponsored the 30th anniversary FAS Conference. Over 350 persons from the United States, Canada and Europe attended the event. Building on one of the workshops that was offered at the conference, the NJ FASD Task Force designed a public education campaign to inform all residents of the dangers of perinatal addictions. All ads included the phone number of the DHSS Family Health line as well as the address for the Task Force's newly designed and launched website, www.beintheknownj.org. Ads that have been developed for the campaign may be viewed at: http://beintheknownj.org/your-unborn-child-takes-part-in-everything-you-do/

Spanish Version

http://beintheknownj.org/your-unborn-child-takes-part-in-everything-you-dospanish-version/

http://beintheknownj.org/yes-you-can-protect-your-child-be-in-the-know/

Spanish Version

http://beintheknownj.org/yes-you-can-protect-your-child-spanish-version/

http://beintheknownj.org/every-baby-deserves-a-healthy-start-in-life/

Spanish Version

http://beintheknownj.org/every-baby-deserves-a-healthy-startspanish/

In 2007, the FASD Task Force submitted its five-year strategic plan, **Be in the Know**, to former Governor Jon Corzine. This plan is providing a roadmap for the work of the Task Force and providing methodology for tracking achievements   and   impact.   The   report   can   be   viewed   at: http://www.state.nj.us/humanservices/opmrdd/news/FAS07strategicplan.pdf

The Task Force also worked with the Department of Education to incorporate FASD education as part of the core curriculum standards for physical and health education. All NJ school children in middle and high schools are now required to be educated about the dangers of alcohol upon fetal development within their health curriculum.

FAS DIAGNOSTIC CENTERS

As noted above, New Jersey is now home to six FASD Diagnostic Centers which are based in established Child Evaluation Centers and are dispersed throughout the State. All staff were initially trained at the University of Washington to use the 4-Digit Diagnostic Code. Since opening their doors in 2002, the FASD Diagnostic Centers have screened over 12,000 for FAS. Of these children, 530 have been diagnosed with FAS and 375 with an FASD. Many of the children have been referred from the Child Welfare Agency (known as the Division of Youth and Family Services or DYFS) and Foster Care System. In addition to providing diagnostic services, staff of the Centers also assist in organizing family support groups, providing information about and referrals to appropriate services, and educating allied health and other service providers about FASD. Representatives from each of the FASD Diagnostic Centers are members of the FASD Task Force. In addition, the FASD Diagnostic Centers work closely with the Perinatal Addictions Specialists in the Risk Reduction System.

RISK REDUCTION SYSTEM

In 2002, the DHSS re-designed its FAS Risk Reduction Program. While the original program had primarily been hospital-based, the new Perinatal Addictions Prevention Project (PAPP) was based in each of the six regional Maternal and Child Health Consortia (MCHC). The PAPP provides professional education, professional training, and consumer education about the effects of alcohol and drug use during pregnancy. To ensure pregnant women receive appropriate assistance, the program also helps health professionals implement a prenatal screening tool (4P's Plus) for the early identification and treatment of high-risk behaviors.

The PAPP Risk Reduction Specialists have been successful recruiting, training and increasing the number of physicians who screen pregnant women. Fig. **1** shows all the pregnant women (N = 108,684) who were screened for high risk behaviors in the first four years of the program. The majority of these screenings were performed in hospital clinics. Similar to what has been documented by CDC and SAMHSA in their surveillance systems, 14 percent of the women reported that they consumed alcohol in the 30 days before they knew they were pregnant. Similarly, when women were asked if they had smoked cigarettes in the month before they knew they were pregnant, over 17% responded that they had smoked. If a screening reveals risk behavior, the women receive prevention education, are referred for a substance abuse assessment or enter treatment when appropriate.

Education is another important goal of the PAPP. In 2009, 355 programs were implemented that were designed to educate the general public about the risks of substance use during pregnancy. These educational programs reached 15,900 women and men. There were over 200 programs offered to raise awareness of the treating professionals and encourage their participation in the universal screening project.

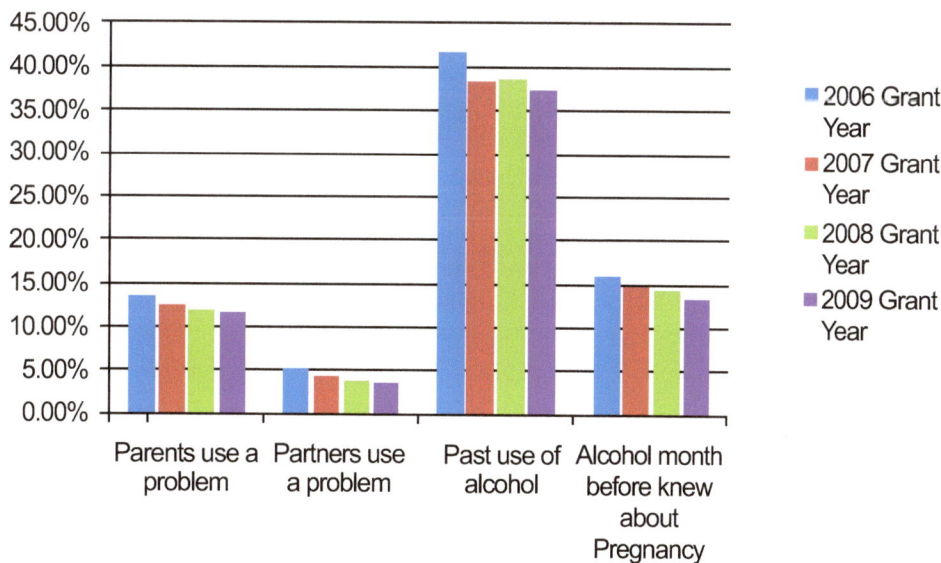

Figure 1: This figure shows results for all of the pregnant women screened for high risk behaviors, using the 4 P's Plus in the years 2006-2009.

Working with the PAPP and DHSS, the five Managed Care Companies that provide health care coverage for pregnant women enrolled in New Jersey Medicaid completed the development of a universal screening form, the Perinatal Risk Assessment, in 2009. The form is now used to screen all pregnant women who are insured by one of these companies. The form covers the medical history, psychosocial issues and also includes all of the 4P's Plus questions. Obstetric providers have to complete this form for all women with Medicaid upon entry into prenatal care. This ensures that these women are screened for alcohol, tobacco or other drug problems during their pregnancy. The Regional Risk Reduction Coordinators are available to assist obstetric providers to locate appropriate resources for women who need help. As is shown in the table above, the number of women who reported that they consumed alcohol in the month before they knew they were pregnant has been slowly decreasing over the four year period.

In addition to the Perinatal addiction specialists, the New Jersey Certification Board, which works with the Department of Human Services, Division of Mental Health and Addictions to Certify Alcohol and Drug Counselors (CACDs), implemented 6 hrs of mandatory training in prenatal alcohol exposure and FASD for all new and renewing CADCs, beginning in 2006. Two specialty certifications also are available for NJ CADCs: 36 hours for a Certified Perinatal Addictions Specialist, which includes training on prenatal alcohol use, and a 30 hr Women's Treatment certification, which includes a full day of training on prenatal substance use, including 3 hrs of prenatal alcohol use. This Women's Cert is mandatory for any CADC working in a woman's Treatment Center.

CHILD PROTECTION TRAINING

The Department of Children and Families, Division of Youth and family Services, the child protection agency of NJ, offers on-line training for various developmental disabilities. All new foster parents are mandated to take these courses. FASD has been included in the training manual for over 6 years. Basic information is provided on FASD, as well as state and national resources. This on-line course is up-dated bi-annually by a member of the FASD Task Force.

NEW JERSEY/NORTHEAST FASD EDUCATION AND RESEARCH CENTER

The New Jersey/Northeast FASD Education and Research Center is located on the campus of the University of Medicine and Dentistry of New Jersey – New Jersey Medical School (UMDNJ-NJMS) in Newark, NJ. The Center specializes in training about the effects of prenatal alcohol exposure and Fetal Alcohol Spectrum Disorders. Originally funded by the CDC, the center now receives funding through the NJ Office for Prevention of Developmental Disabilities. A curriculum for medical and allied health students and professionals was developed in conjunction with the original CDC grant. The New Jersey Center has since adapted that curriculum to suit various audiences. The amount of time needed for trainings can be personalized, depending on the needs of the individual organizations- from 1 hour to 2 days. The curriculum has been adapted for use with various professions, such as education, justice and legal, mental health, child protection, foster care, substance treatment, and state organizations. The modules available for training may be viewed at: http://beintheknownj.org/be-in-the-know-resources/be-in-the-know-about-the-new-jerseynortheast-fasd-education-and-research-center/. The CDC developed curriculum can be found at: http://www.cdc.gov/ncbddd/fasd/curriculum/

Since its inception in 2002, the New Jersey Center has trained over 8,200 professionals and families through conferences and designated workshops, covering 12 states and Washington, DC. While a major effort of the Center has been to bring the training to states throughout the Northeast and Central Atlantic States, staff continue to present at national conferences and at training programs in individual states throughout the country.

In addition, the Center provides technical assistance to other states and Puerto Rico in developing educational and state service programs. One of the most rewarding relationships has been New Jersey's work with the Institute for Developmental Disabilities at the Medical School in San Juan, Puerto Rico.

PUERTO RICO**

The New Jersey FASD Training Center began collaborating with and providing technical assistance to the Institute on Developmental Disabilities (IDD) in the Graduate School of Public Health of the University of Puerto Rico in 2006. This collaboration has been very successful and has resulted in training and technical assistant activities with

**This section was prepared, in part, by Annie Alonso, Ph.D. Director and Maria Reyes, MSW, Assistant Director, Institute of Developmental Disabilities, University of Puerto Rico, School of Public Health.*

different groups, including clinicians as well as public policy leaders. A total of 789 participants have been trained in FASD by the New Jersey Center staff. Forty percent of the trainees were physicians. A total of 1,531 individuals have been trained through the IDD.

In 2007, IDD offered a two–day training on FAS which was attended by an aide to a Puerto Rico legislator. This attendance resulted in the drafting of Legislative Bill No. 2014, a Point of Sale Signage Law that has been enacted in 16 states. After extensive education of legislatures and the Governor of Puerto Rico and with the consideration by the relevant Legislative Commissions, the bill was enacted. PR Act No. 79 of 2008 mandates that all places that sell alcoholic beverages display a wall chart warning about the negative effects on the fetus of alcohol consumption during pregnancy as well as putting a warning statement at the end of all wine and liquor lists on all restaurant and bar menus.

IDD included an objective to continue the trainings on FAS and to increase the awareness of risk of Developmental Disabilities in its strategic plan for 2008-2009. This objective includes the rights to services through the provision of preventive and health promotion education to at least 50 individuals from high risk populations. Approval from the Administration on Development Disabilities of this objective has resulted in the IDD continuing extensive trainings activities on the effects of the use of drugs, alcohol and tobacco during pregnancy. The program has expanded to provide training to community base organizations located at High Risk Communities. In addition, with the collaboration with the New Jersey FASD Education and Research Center, the Institute translated to Spanish, culturally adapted, revised and implemented the CDC curriculum on FAS. It has also provided the leadership to organize a FAS Committee that meets monthly and is working on a FAS prevention plan for Puerto Rico.

The IDD is continuing its collaboration with the New Jersey FASD Center and is focusing on training of physicians and other allied health professionals who work with high risk populations. It is promoting the development of an FASD Diagnostic Clinic that will screen, identify, evaluate and establish a service plan for individuals with an FASD. The IDD is working with the Department of Health to develop additional educational materials and a public education media campaign.

ALASKA'S FAS INITIATIVE PROJECT[***]

In 1997, Alaska's Department of Health and Social Services (DHSS) collaborated with two state representatives who recognized prenatal exposure to alcohol was a serious concern for the health of citizens in their region of the state and their constituents. This collaboration resulted in the first Fetal Alcohol Summit (FAS) being held in November 1997. The Summit participants put forth 103 recommendations that were grouped into four categories:

- Data, Surveillance and Diagnostics
- Public Policy
- Prevention
- Access to Services for Individuals Experiencing FAS

One of the most important outcomes of the Summit was the establishment of a centralized place in state government to provide leadership in addressing FAS. The mission of the Office of FAS is *"To prevent all alcohol-related birth defects and to improve the delivery of services to those individuals already affected by fetal alcohol spectrum disorders (FASD)."* The Office has assimilated the four categories of recommendations into the Alaska FAS Initiative Project and has elucidated four statewide goals:

- Prevent FASD;
- Screen and diagnose children as early as possible;
- Improve lifelong outcomes for individuals with FASD through improved services; and
- Document progress and evaluate program outcomes.

[***]*This section was prepared by L. Diane Castro, Prevention and Early Intervention Manager, State of Alaska Department of Health and Social Services Division of Behavioral Health.*

Three overarching principles guide the initiative: it is multidisciplinary, culturally responsive, and community-based. The approach aims directly at systems development, integration and change in an effort to coordinate existing systems and processes that have operated separately; to integrate service delivery and information management systems to the greatest possible extent; and to establish structures that will be self-sustaining into the future.

Initial funding of this project was through a one-time "start-up" grant from the Alaska Mental Health Trust Authority and contributions from each of the division of the DHSS; the total statewide budget in 1998 was approximately $300,000. In October 2000, Alaska was the recipient of a congressional earmark of $29 million ($5.8 million per year for 5 years). This earmark provided a great opportunity for Alaska in its efforts to reduce and prevent prenatal exposure to alcohol. Highlights of the 5-year grant award/earmark include:

- **Development of a sustainable network of Community-Based FASD Diagnostic Teams**. Over the 12 years since the Office of FAS was established, a total of 14 teams were established and are in some stage of development and implementation of services. During the five-years of federal funding, *Diagnostic Team Development Grants* were provided, with reduced amounts of funding available each year, to allow teams to become established in their existing service delivery system and not become dependent upon federal dollars for their ongoing operation. Currently, ten (10) community based teams are operating in Fairbanks, Tok, Bethel, Wasilla, Kenai, Kodiak and 2 teams in Anchorage, Juneau and Sitka. In addition, three communities that previously had teams are working to re-staff and rebuild their diagnostic capacity. Currently, teams that meet established criteria are funded for diagnostic services through a Provider Agreement process, where they are reimbursed for services rendered at a rate of $3,000 per completed diagnosis. The Alaska Legislature provided state general fund dollars for this purpose. In addition, through the state's only psychiatric hospital, Alaska Psychiatric Institute (API), a specialized team is in operation to address the needs of those youth who enter the system through API. All Alaska teams use the University of Washington 4-Digit Diagnostic Code process.

- **Development of two FASD Curricula and statewide training program.** In an effort to improve the education of the Alaska provider system about the effects and impact of prenatal exposure to alcohol, two curricula were developed: *FASD 101: Disabilities of Discovery: Insights into Brain-based Disabilities* and *FASD 201: Individualized Interventions and Supports.* (Visit http://www.hss.state.ak.us/fas/Resources/trainers/default.htm)

In addition, the Office of FAS worked in partnership with the Department of Education and Early Development to develop a web-based version of FASD 101 and a specialized FASD 101 directly focused on the educators and their role in understanding the impact of FASD on students. Since the early 1990's, Alaska has required all K-12 teachers to receive training on FAS and its impact on students. Due to the size and vastness of Alaska, it was decided that the only way to utilize these curricula to their capacity and to get the training available across Alaska was to develop a certified Training of Trainers model. In partnership with the University of Alaska, Family and Youth Services Training Center, the curricula were developed and a TOT process was established. Currently over 50 trainers have been certified to provide this training. A revision of FASD 101 was completed in state fiscal year 2009 and a revision of FASD 201 will be completed in state fiscal year 2010. Keeping the curricula updated with new information, research and evidence-based strategies that can assist our statewide multidisciplinary providers (from educators to clinicians to correctional officers to health care providers) is of great importance.

- **Development and presentation of a statewide multi-media public awareness campaign.** A three-phase public awareness campaign was developed in partnership with the Anchorage-based Nerland Agency. The campaign included TV, radio, and print ads, in addition to informational brochures, message pens, magnets and posters for follow-up to the on-air information. The ads were aimed at women who are social drinkers who are able to stop drinking, but are unaware of the damage alcohol could do to their growing fetus; to the family, friends and community members of high-risk women who may not be able to stop drinking on their own—the message was "Thankfully there are people who can help…" The final message was aimed at the Alaska medical community, utilizing doctors, speaking to their colleagues with the message "As a medical provider it is my responsibility to tell women not to drink during pregnancy." The campaign continued for approximately 5 years before funding ended. It was very successful and generated a great deal of conversation, questions, follow-up referrals and a general changing of the social norm about alcohol and pregnancy. Visit http://www.hss.state.ak.us/fas/Resources/media.htm

- **FAS Surveillance Project.** In partnership with the Division of Public Health and the Alaska Birth Defects Registry (ABDR), a clear and consistent process for reporting prenatal exposure to alcohol was developed. Alaska law allows reports to the ABDR for prenatal exposure to occur up to the age of 6. All reports to the registry are reviewed through direct medical record abstractions, with determinations of FAS using the CDC FAS case definition developed through a 5-state FASSNET partnership (Alaska was one of the 5 states). New FAS prevalence trend data for birth years 1996 through 2002 were released in February 2010, showing a marginally significant decrease in the overall prevalence rate, with a significant decline of 49% among our Alaska Native infants. The increased FAS risk for Alaska Natives fell from 17 times that of non-Natives in 1996-1998 to five times higher in 2000-2002. Prevention activities of the Alaska FAS Initiative project likely contributed to this substantial reduction in FAS risk for the Alaska Native population during 1996-2002; unfortunately there was no measurable effect on reducing the prevalence of FAS among non-Native infants.

- **Medicaid Waiver Demonstration Project.** In December 2006, Alaska received a five-year federal award to improve services to young Alaskans with co-occurring diagnoses of Serious Emotional Disturbance (SED) and a Fetal Alcohol Spectrum Disorder (FASD). This demonstration project is allowing Alaska to begin developing "practice to research" service delivery approaches that will improve the long-term outcomes for youth with these diagnoses and to help them remain in home and community-based services instead of receiving services in out-of-state in residential psychiatric treatment centers. A rigorous evaluation is being conducted to establish what waiver services are showing the greatest overall improvement of quality of life for these young people.

Alaska's FAS Initiative project has made significant and lasting systems change in the way the State addresses all aspects of prenatal exposure to alcohol, from promotion to prevention to early intervention to life-long services for individuals and their families. Service systems have improved, services have increased, and the overall impact of FASD on multiple service delivery systems has decreased. There is still much work to be done; there is new information, research and data to be incorporated into ongoing prevention and service delivery work; and the acceptance of alcohol in the state often impedes good decision-making and policy determinations. The Alaska legislature supports the FASD efforts with funding and legislative action and remains committed to continue the efforts that were started in 1998. Alaska has made great strides in reducing the impact of prenatal exposure to alcohol and the associated disabilities. The commitment, effort and passion of those involved with this initiative continue.

http://www.adn.com/2010/02/19/1148098/fas-rate-among-natives-declining.html

COLORADO FASD STATE SERVICES[****]

Colorado began services related to Fetal Alcohol Spectrum Disorders (FASD) Prevention in 1989. Some of these services were initiated due to new grant funding in the state but other services took hold at this time due to providers recognizing a need for services that currently were not in place. Some of the efforts described here were developed specifically for Fetal Alcohol Syndrome (FAS) or Fetal Alcohol Spectrum Disorders but others had a broader focus and included exposure to all prenatal drugs.

In 1989, *Colorado Responds to Children with Special Needs (CRCSN)*. The Birth Defects Monitoring and Prevention Program at the Colorado Department of Public Health and Environment (CDPHE) began conducting surveillance and prevention activities for FAS. The multidisciplinary advisory board that developed the policies and criteria for the Birth Defects Registry included FAS and emphasized linking affected children and their families with services and resources in their communities.

In addition to CRCSN's basic mandate to monitor and prevent FAS, the CDC have funded five successive projects, all of which have included FAS:

- Disabilities Prevention Program (1989-1995)
- Fetal Alcohol Syndrome Prevention and Surveillance (1992-1997)

[****]*This section was written by Pamela Gillen, ND, RN, CACIII, Director, COFAS Prevention Program, University of Colorado Denver, Anschultz Medical Campus, Colorado AHEC System*

- Population Based Surveillance of Fetal Alcohol Syndrome (FASSNET) (1997-2003)

- FAS Prevention Project (FASSLink) (2003-2009)

- FAS Surveillance (2009-2014)

Colorado is the only state that has been funded by the CDC for all four consecutive FAS surveillance projects.

Fetal Alcohol Syndrome Prevention and Surveillance (1992-1997)

This was a cooperative agreement with CDC and six other states. In Colorado, CRCSN partnered with the Colorado Alcohol and Drug Abuse Division (ADAD) to integrate the prevention of FAS with the monitoring of affected births. In 1996, an RFP process established for a statewide FAS and other prenatal drug prevention coordinator out of ADAD to ensure ongoing FAS prevention in Colorado once the funding was gone. CRCSN developed a surveillance system. CRCSN and ADAD along with support from the Colorado Fetal Alcohol and Substance Abuse Coalition developed six packets of information for health care providers, human service professionals, families, educators and the justice system that became national models. The project developed a curriculum for traditional substance abuse treatment programs that integrated information about FAS and curriculum for juvenile justice workers. The project actively supported the Colorado Fetal Alcohol and Substance Abuse Coalition.

Population Based Surveillance of Fetal Alcohol Syndrome (FASSnet) (1997-2003)

CRCSN was also one of five states awarded cooperative agreements by CDC to develop a population-based surveillance system for fetal alcohol syndrome. The system, FASSNet, created a case definition, an electronic data collection tool, provider education, and produced prevalence estimates of FAS in four of the participating states.

FAS Prevention Project (FASSLink) (2003-2009)

CDPHE, in partnership with the University of Colorado Health Sciences Center, **C**olorado **F**etal **A**lcohol **S**yndrome **P**revention **O**utreach **P**roject (COFAS-POP), was awarded a third cooperative agreement from CDC for FAS prevention and surveillance. CRCSN worked primarily to revise FASSNet based on the data and experience gained during the years of its development. The result was FASSlink conducting FAS surveillance in the seven-county Denver metropolitan area. The project actively supported NOFAS Colorado, the non-profit that evolved from the Colorado Fetal Alcohol and Substance Abuse Coalition.

COFAS-POP focused on the prevention of alcohol-exposed pregnancies and developed two components, a **Community Intervention** and an **Individual Level Intervention**.

Community Intervention

> **Personal Decisions** is the name of the Community Intervention program. It consists of a Self-Guided Intervention promoted through a media campaign and is directed at all women of childbearing age between 18 to 44 years. When a woman calls, she talks with a health professional who screens her for the project by asking questions related to her drinking and to her use of contraceptives. An Information Packet modeled after the Personal CHOICES materials were mailed to women who met the eligibility criteria.

Individual Level Intervention

> The Individual Level component involved contracts with the four county public health departments utilizing nurses, social workers and substance abuse counselors to provide intervention for women. The intervention is based on a stepped care model using motivational interventions, moderate to intensive case management, or group interventions.

- **Personal Choices** is the first level of intervention and is brief.

- **Personal Skills** is the moderate level of case management.

- **Personal Support** is the most intense level of case management.

FAS Surveillance (2009-2014)

CRCSN is currently funded by a multi-site cooperative agreement to refine the FASSnet/FASSlink system to conduct population-based surveillance for FAS. CRCSN received a national State Leadership Award for its work in FAS surveillance and prevention.

In 1990, NOFAS Colorado began as the Colorado Fetal Alcohol and Substance Abuse Coalition out of growing concern around the medical, educational and social problems that professionals and families were facing regarding prenatal alcohol and drug exposure. The mission of this organization is to be a forum for agencies and families to collaborate on prevention, identification, and intervention of prenatal alcohol and drug exposure, and to be a unified voice in the community. The Colorado Fetal Alcohol and Substance Abuse Coalition became an affiliate member to the National Organization of Fetal Alcohol Syndrome (NOFAS) in 2006. Over the years the coalition and more recently NOFAS Colorado has provided a multitude of services across Colorado.

In 1993 The Special Connections program began. This program, jointly managed by the Department of Health Care Policy and Financing and the Division of Behavioral Health within the Colorado Department of Human Services, is designed as a case management and treatment program for pregnant women in Colorado. The goals of the programs are to help reduce or stop substance use among pregnant women during and after their pregnancy. In addition the focus is to help women have a healthy infant, continue to maintain the family as a unit and improve parenting practices of the family. Over the past few years, there has been a significant increase in expenditures for this program, which reflects two things: 1) an increase in the utilization of residential treatment services; and 2) the waiver which allows Special Connections participants to continue their treatment up to 1 year post-partum, assuming continued eligibility for Medicaid.

In 1996, the University of Colorado developed the statewide Colorado FASD/ATOD Substances prevention outreach project, now known as COFAS. The COFAS program was funded due to the increasing rates of women drinking during childbearing age in Colorado. The lack of providers' skills around identification and screening of risky drinking behaviors, lack of skills in addressing women's substance use behaviors and lack of information on how and where to refer women for treatment or intervention services makes this project necessary with medical care that is state-of-the-art, comprehensive and effective.

COFAS is a statewide FASD and prenatal substance abuse prevention outreach program housed within the Colorado Area Health Education Center (AHEC) System within the University of Colorado Denver. The Colorado AHEC System is a partnership between the University of Colorado Denver (UCD) and five community based AHECs. By linking UCD's academic resources with local educational, health care and human service agencies, the AHEC System establishes a statewide network of agencies and groups who provide educational and related services to communities throughout the state.

COFAS's mission is inclusive of the AHEC mission as well as working to reduce the incidence of prenatal alcohol and drug exposure across the state of Colorado.

COFAS received funding from "March of Dimes Colorado State Chapter Community Grant Program Increase Availability of Prevention Services" category for a one-year "Rethink Your Drink" public service announcement educational campaign, an informational health clinic video, and informational Internet video podcasts. This podcast "Between Girls" can be viewed on the COFAS website at:
http://www.ucdenver.edu/life/services/AHEC/ProgramAreas/cofas/AlcoholUseinPregnancy/Pages/Prevention.aspx#betweengirls

"Rethink Your Drink" was designed to educate women about the health risks of drinking alcohol while pregnant, and the permanent affects alcohol can have on the developing fetus. The program is also for women who are not yet pregnant, but are drinking and engaging in unprotected intercourse, and for those who are drinking and do not realize they are pregnant. These posters can be viewed at:
http://www.ucdenver.edu/life/services/AHEC/ProgramAreas/cofas/AlcoholUseinPregnancy/Pages/AlcoholUseinPregnancy.aspx

The Colorado Fetal Alcohol Spectrum Disorders Commission was established by legislation in 2009. This legislation also mandated that every vendor licensed in the state to sell alcohol beverages was encouraged to post a health warning sign to inform patrons that the consumption of alcohol during pregnancy may cause birth defects, including FAS. The Colorado FASD Commission is implementing the following recommendations:

1. Expand efforts to promote universal prevention;

2. Expand selective prevention efforts for targeted audiences;

3. Modify classification systems to include FASD as approved conditions so that persons with FASDs are eligible for federal and state disabilities benefits;

4. Insure access to diagnostic services;

5. Intensify research initiatives and coordination among Colorado agencies.

Colorado has also instituted various FASD prevention programs. In 2005, Peer Assistance Services Inc. was awarded a grant from the Substance Abuse and Mental Health Services Administration, Center for Substance Abuse Prevention. The goal of this initiative was to implement a comprehensive approach to reducing alcohol consumption during pregnancy among at-risk women of childbearing age in the Colorado community. Peer Assistance assisted staff at organizations working with at-risk families and individuals to implement evidence-based strategies such as screening and brief interventions to reduce alcohol use during pregnancy. The at-risk families included families with a parent in recovery from addiction, teen parents, families in homeless shelters or transitional housing, families with a parent or youth currently in prison or juvenile corrections, and families with a parolee member who has a substance abuse history.

The Juvenile Court of Colorado's 17th Judicial District is integrating FASD screening, diagnosis, and intervention within the Juvenile Delinquency and Child Welfare courts of Adams and Broomfield Counties. The goal of the FASD Project is to improve the functioning of children and youth with an FASD who come before the court. The Project objectives include preventing or limiting out-of-home placement, improving school attendance, improving academic performance and reducing recidivism. All children on Probation and children ages 3-4 who are removed from their parents because of substance abuse are screened to see if they were prenatally exposed to alcohol. Those who were prenatally exposed are evaluated to determine their functioning and then the FASD staff work with their treatment team to implement the recommendations of the evaluation team.

SBIRT Colorado (Screening, Brief Intervention, Referral to Treatment)

In September, 2006, the Colorado Office of the Governor was awarded a five-year grant from the Substance Abuse and Mental Health Services Administration to expand the continuum of healthcare to include Screening, Brief Intervention, Referral to Treatment practices in healthcare settings statewide. SBIRT, as a standard practice, is being implemented in healthcare settings including hospitals, primary care settings, HIV and other clinics in urban, rural and frontier communities across the state. Over the course of five years, 125,000 patients will be screened for substance use and provided the appropriate services including a brief intervention or referral to brief therapy or treatment. Clinical guidelines have been developed and will be disseminated to primary care providers statewide to assist in delivering SBIRT services. The mission is to integrate screening and brief intervention as a best practice to addressing substance misuse as a healthcare issue in settings statewide. The grant is administered by the Colorado Division of Behavioral Health and managed by Peer Assistance Services, Inc.

In 2009, the Colorado Department for Public Health and Environment (CDPHE) partnered with the Denver Metro Health Clinic (DMHC), an urban STD clinic that is part of the Denver Public Health (DPH) program, received funding from CDC to implement the Project CHOICES, a successful research project, into an urban STD clinic. The grant, Reducing Risks for an Alcohol-Exposed Pregnancy (AEP) in High Risk Women Attending Sexually Transmitted Diseases (STD) Clinics in Urban Settings, is in the initial set up phase of its project.

For more information about Colorado's initiatives to prevent FASD, visit: **http://www.fascenter.samhsa.gov/state systemsofcare/states/colorado.cfm#statewebsite**

ROLE OF VOLUNTARY AGENCIES

Voluntary, non-profit agencies have played an instrumental role in bringing much attention to the issues associated with the consumption of alcohol during pregnancy as well as to their effects on fetal and child development. These organizations advocated for the establishment of the National Task Force on FAS/FAE as well as for SAMHSA's FASD Center for Excellence.

The National Organization of Fetal Alcohol Syndrome (NOFAS) is the leading voice and resource of the Fetal Alcohol Spectrum Disorders (FASD) community. Founded in 1990, NOFAS is the only international non-profit organization committed solely to FASD primary prevention, advocacy and support.

NOFAS seeks to create a global community free of alcohol-exposed pregnancies and a society supportive of individuals already living with FASD. NOFAS effectively increases public awareness and mobilizes grassroots action in diverse communities and represents the interests of persons with FASD and their caregivers as the liaison to researchers and policymakers. By ensuring that FASD is broadly recognized as a developmental disability, NOFAS strives to reduce the stigma and improve the quality of life for affected individuals and families. More information about NOFAS, its affiliates and its programs is available at **http://www.nofas.org/about/**

NOFAS has organized an affiliate network in states across the country and in the United Kingdom. Information about FASD efforts in individual affiliates can be obtained by visiting the sites below:

NOFAS Affiliate Network

NOFAS Alaska,

NOFASCA, (No Direct Link Available)

Beginnings of San Luis Obispo (California),

NOFAS Colorado,

NOFAS Connecticut,

NOFAS Georgia,

NOFAS Illinois (Trinity Services),

NOFAS Kentucky (Bluegrass Regional Prevention Center),

NOFAS Michigan (Macomb County Fetal Alcohol Resource Education and Support),

MOFAS,

NOFAS MISSOURI (St. Louis ARC - Missouri Fetal Alcohol Spectrum Disorder Action and Care Team)

NOFAS Missouri, St. Louis ARC-Missouri Fetal Alcohol Spectrum Disorder Action and Special Needs Advocates and Parents (Nebraska),

NOFAS New Hampshire,

NOFAS New Jersey (Beintheknownj.org),

NOFAS New Mexico (University of New Mexico Center on Substance Abuse, Alcoholism and Addictions-CASAA FAS Prevention Program,

The Fetal Alcohol Syndrome Support Network of NYC and Long Island, Inc-FASSN

National Council on Alcoholism and Drug Dependence-Rochester Area

NOFAS North Carolina

NOFAS Ohio (Double ARC)

NOFAS of Northeast Ohio

Fetal Alcohol Syndrome Consultation and Education and trainings Services. Inc (FASCETS)

NOFAS South Dakota (The University of South Dakota Center for Disabilities)

NOFAS Tennessee

NOFAS United Kingdom

Utah Fetal Alcohol Coalition (UFAC)

NOFAS Virginia

NOFAS Washington State

Family Empowerment Network (FEN-Wisconsin)

Orchids FASD Services, Inc

FUTURE DIRECTIONS

Over the course of the past 20 years, federal, state and voluntary agencies have become more committed to addressing issues associated with prenatal exposure to alcohol. As research moves into the realm of practical application, these organizations will continue to play key roles in translating findings into initiatives that enhance prevention of prenatal exposures to alcohol as well as into those that ameliorate the effects. Opportunities for education about these exposures are no longer solely in the province of medical services; state agencies and universities need to continue to work to insure that FASD issues are incorporated into High School Family Life Education curricula and College social and community services education.

Much of the action to address FASD is happening on the state level. Legislation, policies and programs will increase as awareness of the importance of not consuming alcohol grows among the general population. In addition, increasing the numbers of physicians and allied health professionals who are trained to recognize and diagnose FASD will likely result in adapting present special education and service systems programs to meet **lifelong** needs of persons with FASD.

REFERENCES

[1]   USDHHS, Office of the Assistant Secretary for Planning and Evaluation. Fetal Alcohol Syndrome and Pregnant Women Who Abuse Alcohol: an Overview of the Issue and the Federal Response. February 1992.

[2]   Stratton K, Howe C, Battaglia F (Ed.) Fetal Alcohol Syndrome: Diagnosis, Epidemiology, Prevention and Treatment. Institute of Medicine National Academy Press, Washington, D.C. 1996.

[3]   USDHHS, National Institute of Alcohol and Alcohol Abuse, http://www.niaaa.nih.gov/AboutNIAAA/Interagency/aboutICCFAS.htm

[4]   USDHHS, National Institute of Alcohol and Alcohol Abuse, Intervening with Children Affected by Prenatal Alcohol Exposure. Proceedings of a Special Focus Session of the Interagency Coordinating Committee on Fetal Alcohol Syndrome, September 10 – 11, 1998.

[5]   Weber MK, Floyd RL, Riley EP, Snider DE. National Task Force on Fetal Alcohol Syndrome and Fetal Alcohol Effect: Defining the National Agenda for Fetal Alcohol Syndrome and Other Prenatal Alcohol-Related Effects. Morbidity and Mortality Weekly Review, September 20, 2002/51(RR14); 9-12.

[6]   Bertrand J, Floyd RL, Weber MK, *et al.* National Task Force on FAS/FAE Fetal Alcohol Syndrome: Guidelines for Referral and Diagnosis: Atlanta GA: Centers for Disease Control And Prevention 2004 Contract No.: Document Number.

[7]   Babor T, Caetano R, Caswell S, *et al.* Alcohol: No ordinary commodity. New York: Oxford University Press Inc.; 2003.

[8]   McGinnis JM, Foege WH. Actual causes of death in the United States. JAMA 1993; 270: 2207–12.

[9]   Mokdad AH, Marks JS, Stroup DF, Gerberding JL. Actual causes of death in the United States [erratum appears in *JAMA* 2005, 293-4]. JAMA. 2004; 291: 1238–45.

[10] U.S. Department of Health and Human Services. Healthy people 2010: Understanding and improving health (2nd edition, Volume 1). Washington, DC: U.S. Government Printing Office; 2000.

[11] Floyd RL, Jack BW, Cefalo R, *et al.* The clinical content of preconception care: alcohol, tobacco, and illicit drug exposures. Am J Obstet Gynecol 2008; 199(6B): S333–9.

[12] Greenfield TK, Midanik LT, Rogers JD. A 10-year national trend study of alcohol consumption, 1984-1995: is the period of declining drinking over? Am J Public Health 2000; 90(1): 47–52.

[13] Naimi TS, Brewer RD, Mokdad A, Denny C, Serdula MK, Marks JS. Binge drinking among US adults. JAMA 2003; 289(1): 70–5.

[14] Denny CH, Tsai J, Floyd RF, Green PP. Alcohol use among pregnant and non-pregnant women of childbearing age- United States, 1991-2005. MMWR Morb Mortal Wkly Rep 2009; 58(19):529–32.

[15] Barry KL, Caetano R, Chang G, *et al.* Reducing alcohol-exposed pregnancies: A report of the National Task Force on Fetal Alcohol Syndrome and Fetal Alcohol Effect. Atlanta, GA: Centers for Disease Control and Prevention; 2009.

[16] Public Law 106-310

[17] New Jersey Governor's Council for the Prevention of Mental Retardation. Programs for Preventing the Causes of Mental Retardation. The Arc of New Jersey, 1985.

[18] New Jersey Governor's Council on the Prevention of Developmental Disabilities. Truth and Consequences of Fetal Alcohol Syndrome: Why New Jersey Should Be Concerned. 2002.

AFTERWORD

Some Thoughts from a Doting Aunt:

Never, Never Underestimate the Power of Neurological Development,

Love and, Perhaps, Good Nutrition

Matt arrived when he was six weeks old. As an only child, an only grandchild and an only nephew, this infant was a gift to my family. At his first post partum visit a few weeks later, Matt's pediatrician pronounced him to be a perfect and healthy little boy. This was 1980, however, and even though Matt's face was already showing some of the dysmorphic features that would become more prominent over the next few months, most pediatricians had never heard of Fetal Alcohol Syndrome (FAS) at the time.

Our small family was fortunate for several reasons. First, because it was a semi-private adoption, my sister (mom) and brother-in-law (dad) were better informed about Matt's birth parents' backgrounds than is typical and, later when we needed it, were able to get some information about Matt's birth mother's behaviors during pregnancy. Thus, we knew that Matt's birth parents had been high school sweethearts who had gone off to college. Matt's birth mother got pregnant during the summer between her freshman and sophomore years, but, as happens too often, did not know she was pregnant when she returned to college. Matt's birth father was on the football team and his birth mother, it seems, partied hearty after every game. Once she realized she was with child, Matt's birth mother left school for the rest of the year, lived with an aunt, stopped drinking alcohol and received good prenatal care. While Matt was small at birth, he was within the normal ranges and his Apgar score was good. Matt's birth parents wanted to complete college and decided that the best course of action would be to put him up for adoption. We learned later that, after graduation, they had gotten married and had additional children.

The second fortunate circumstance is that Matt's adopted mom was a teacher who was greatly attuned to child developmental issues. While she suspected problems early on, Matt's delayed speech and language resulted in mom insisting that Matt be screened for developmental disorders at age three by his pediatrician. When the screenings showed clear delays, he recommended that Matt be assessed by a pediatric neurologist which led to our third fortuitous event. We all lived in the Boston area where there were a few pediatric neurologists who were familiar with the effects of prenatal exposure to alcohol and the telltale facial abnormalities. As a result, Matt received a diagnosis of FAS when he was still young. The neurologist predicted that Matt would have severe intellectual disabilities and would not be able to read, write or understand mathematics.

Matt's diagnosis was re-confirmed by another pediatric neurologist when he was five and preparing for his first Individual Education Plan (IEP) for Special Education (SPED). This time, however, Matt's intelligence tests showed that he was far from having "mental retardation" as his scores showed then, and have consistently done so ever since, an above average IQ. Aptitude and behavioral tests, however, have drawn a different picture, reflecting difficulties in abstract reasoning, memory and recall, language usage and comprehension, and other problems. Both his fine and gross motor skills were good and his mechanical abilities excellent.

The fourth area in which our family was fortunate pertains to Matt's education. Throughout his elementary and middle school years, Matt's mom was greatly involved with his school systems, first by operating an after school tutoring program and later by working as a permanent substitute teacher. As a result, mom got to know everyone involved in Matt's education and worked with them to ensure that her son got the academic attention he needed. Matt was never in separate special education classrooms, but was mainstreamed with time spent in Resource Rooms for additional help. Despite the initial prediction and while he did struggle mightily, Matt learned to read, write and perform arithmetic functions. However, he also experienced serious attention deficits, was unable to sit still as long as required and was often disruptive in the classroom. By Thursday night, he had it! Matt had reached the limits of his self-control and would have a melt down from the pressures of trying to learn, keep up with his peers, and behave appropriately within the social norms. Ritalin did help to contain these educational and behavioral issues, but finding the proper dosage was challenging and the medication needed to be altered frequently.

When he was nine years old, Matt and his parents moved from the Boston area to the southern Catskills in New York. Even the arrival of a promised puppy did not resolve the difficulties this change brought. Matt struggled to keep up in the classroom with cohorts who did not know or accept his learning problems. He found it challenging to make new friends and often got into trouble by trying to please them and be accepted by them.

Being of normal intelligence was both a blessing and a curse. It was a joy to realize that Matt could learn and have a future that was largely self-sufficient. However, as Matt struggled to fit into his new environment, he also became aware that he was somehow different than his peers were. He was old enough to recognize that learning came easily to most of his classmates while he wrestled to remember the lessons of the day; that none of them had trouble sitting still and attending to instructions; that none of his peers took medication; that most of them were larger than he was. The latter issue was particularly striking as Matt's postnatal growth retardation manifested itself completely during adolescence. Although Matt has always had a good appetite and enjoyed nutritious foods, including fresh vegetables and fruit, he has remained of short stature, even though both of his birth parents were tall. Matt began to act out more frequently, often expressing his frustrations, fears, and feelings of rejection and depression by telling lies, seeming to be conscience-less, throwing tantrums, and putting holes in walls with his fists. Matt's parents responded appropriately by investing in large amounts of spackle, hiring a good contractor and finding a psychiatrist to treat their son. It was impossible to locate a psychiatrist who was familiar with the psychological aspects of FAS, but, over the years, we have found that those who were trained to treat children with Attention Deficit and Hyperactivity Disorder (ADHD) were of benefit to Matt.

Matt reached the high point of his adolescence when he was thirteen. He decided that he wanted to give a present to his grandfather by participating in a complete Bar Mitzvah. For over a year, Matt memorized his Torah (Five Books of Moses) and Haftorah (Old Testament Prophets) portions in Hebrew by listening to audio tapes. He also learned all the blessings and wrote and presented a speech. Coincidently and ironically, one of Matt's readings was from Judges 13:7 in which an angel tells Samson's future mother, "Behold, thou shall conceive and bear a son: And now, drink no wine or strong drink....". Many of Matt's friends from Boston came for the celebration and he has always said that "my Bar Mitzvah was the happiest day of my life." Unfortunately, after all the months of preparation for and excitement of the week-end, Matt crashed hard when it was over and severe depression set in. After experiencing several instances of rejection and anti-Semitism by peers, a school system that no longer met his educational needs and verbal abuse by an adult, his parents decided to send Matt to a private school that specialized in working with students with ADHD and other learning disabilities. The additional benefit was that the school was located in New Jersey near to where Matt's aunt lived. So, when Matt was fourteen, he started over again, or so his family believed.

As it turned out, Matt began to live the life described by Ann Streissguth in her 1996 study. He had shown signs of being attracted to cigarettes and alcohol at an early age. Unfortunately, the school Matt attended was not well-supervised and alcohol, tobacco and drugs were readily available. He was suspended several times for being in possession of these substances. Matt had a girlfriend two years his senior with whom he was engaged in an intense sexual relationship. He experienced clinical depression severe enough that his psychiatrist placed him on bed rest and medication for almost a month, during which he moved into his aunt's home. When he was well enough to return, Matt announced that he did not want to live at the school any longer and moved in with his aunt permanently. At the end of the year, Matt and the school administrators agreed that a parting of the ways would be best. However, Matt did not want to return to New York, so was enrolled in the public school where his aunt lived.

For the next year and half, Matt seemed to hold his own at the local school. He made friends, some of dubious distinction and influence. He found a nicer, new girlfriend and became involved in some after school activities. He did struggle with some of the class work, but the additional support from the Resource Room helped him to continue to learn and remain motivated. At the same time, Matt experienced periods of depression, confusion, belligerence, increased lying and secretiveness. Although Matt had known from an early age that he had been adopted, he seemed to blame his parents for his troubles and limited his interaction with them. This erratic behavior continued until the doorbell rang very early one morning in January, 1997. When his aunt answered the door, she found four police standing on her stoop with a warrant to arrest Matt for selling drugs.

One night in juvenile detention convinced Matt that this was not the future he sought. Matt's parents and aunt appeared in court the next day with the guarantee that this young man would be sent to a Substance Abuse

Treatment Center in New York. Matt completed his junior year in high school while at the center and returned to his original school system for his senior year. Thus, Matt lived the remaining characteristics described by Streissguth: involvement with the criminal justice system and interrupted schooling.

Matt performed well during his senior year in high school, particularly in his vocational education program, but remained depressed and an outsider. As the year was ending, it was clear that some plans were needed for post-graduation. Matt had always shown an interest in and a talent for cooking and now expressed a desire to pursue this as a career. He was accepted into a respected college and, the following September, began a new adventure. Unfortunately, Matt was unable to maintain the requirements of the program, missed one class too many and, three weeks before the end of his freshman year, was asked to leave. He then relocated to New Hampshire where he spent the summer working in a coastal tourist town. Matt decided to spend the winter in New Hampshire but seemed to spend most of his time unemployed and living out of his car. He spent one very cold week-end in lock-up for being with a companion who had been passing bad checks. The following August, Matt concluded that homelessness and poverty left a lot to be desired, so he headed south for New Jersey where his parents now lived.

During the next few years, Matt held many jobs, primarily in the food and catering industry. With help and support from his parents and aunt, he settled into his own apartment with a pet ferret. He made some new friends and re-acquainted himself with old ones, re-established relationships with his parents and aunt and, for the most part, grew up and achieved a great degree of independence. After several years of working in the food industry, Matt changed career paths and began working in customer services where new talents were discovered and cultivated. After his girlfriend moved to Boston, Matt decided it was time for him to return to his New England roots and moved there as well.

Matt's childhood and adolescence were stormy and unsettling. When he was about fifteen, Matt wanted to know what was "wrong" with him and why did he seem so different than his friends. His mom and aunt explained that his birth mom had drunk alcohol while she was pregnant and what the consequences had been for him. When Matt experiences an emotional low, he thinks about what greater heights he might have achieved and wonders, if he does have children, will they be like him?

Now, at age thirty, Matt has achieved a level of maturity that his parents and aunt had doubted he would ever be able to attain. From the three year old whose parents were told he would never learn, Matt has developed into a bright, articulate young man. His reading and comprehension abilities show evidence of great improvement, reinforcing recent proposals that our neurological systems continue to develop during young adulthood. Matt has learned to adapt and cope. He compensates for his tendency to be disorganized by making lists and checking them often. Matt's become the go-to guy when it's time to plan a trip or a camping week-end. He has hopes and aspirations. This young man has been in a steady and healthy relationship for over a year, has thoughts of getting married, having children and being a good father to them. He wants to be successful in a career and has recently returned to school to train to become an electrician. When Matt makes his mind up to do something, he can achieve his goal.

Matt has become much more than we ~ or his first neurologist ~ ever expected. While he certainly had a difficult adolescence, it is hard now to distinguish between what was extreme teen-age angst and what were severe consequences of prenatal exposure to alcohol. What is clear is that Streissguth's mitigating factors ~ a stable, loving home, early diagnosis, and access to appropriate services ~ were all present for Matt and greatly influenced his life. Today, Matt is in a "seriously committed" relationship, he is in the process of buying a house and he is completing the educational process to become a certified electrician. For a child and now adult who loves good food, we wonder what part nutrition may also have played in maximizing Matt's neurological development and thus his attainment of such a high degree of maturity and independence.

Debbie Cohen

INDEX

A

Addiction- 54, 72, 78, 134, 137, 139, 140, 157, 158, 162, 164, 186, 190
Adolescence – 37, 51, 75, 103, 127-143
Alaska - 194-196
Antioxidants – 31
ARBD – 10, 12, 18, 19, 21, 26, 129, 132, 137
ARND – 4, 5, 9, 12, 16, 17-21, 25, 26, 43, 44, 45, 48, 52, 55, 59, 183

B

Behavior regulation – 64, 66, 68, 69, 73, 74, 76, 81, 86, 94, 95, 103

C

β-carotene - 31
Canadian Guidelines – 17, 18, 19, 21, 48
CDC – 43, 140, 143, 152, 181-182, 182-185
CDC Guidelines – 6-10, 16, 17, 18, 19, 21, 24-25, 48
Cell adhesion molecules - 31
Cellular antioxidant properties - 31
Choline – 33, 36, 44, 131, 133
Colorado – 159, 196-199
Competence – 50, 78, 79, 84, 86, 87, 103, 155, 156
Co-occurring disorders – 43, 45-46, 48, 49, 51, 127, 131, 137, 140, 141, 142, 185
Corpus callosum – 6, 11, 54, 56, 109, 130
Criminal Justice – 45, 148, 151, 152, 153, 154, 187, 204
Cyanidin-3-glucoside - 31

D

Dental care – 58, 127, 128, 132, 135
Developmental disabilities – 44, 57, 65, 66, 67, 72, 77, 82, 84, 87, 101, 106, 108, 109, 118, 150, 182, 184, 193
Diagnosis – 4-26, 35, 44, 46, 47, 48-52, 54, 55, 56-57, 64, 71, 75, 80, 82, 94, 103, 137-141, 149, 156, 183, 188
Drug therapy – 58
DSM-IV – 48, 49, 51, 53, 138

E

Early Intervention – 22, 66-107, 127, 187
Educational interventions – 108-122
Environmental enrichment – 37, 88, 91
Executive functioning – 6, 8, 9, 46, 48, 51, 52, 56, 74, 86, 89, 90, 92, 103, 109, 111, 113, 120, 121, 129
Exercise – 37, 91, 131, 132

F

FAE – 11, 12, 14, 18, 19, 26, 44, 45, 46, 56, 130
False confessions - 155
Folic acid - 35
Four Digit Diagnostic Code – 10, 12, 13, 15, 16, 17, 191, 195